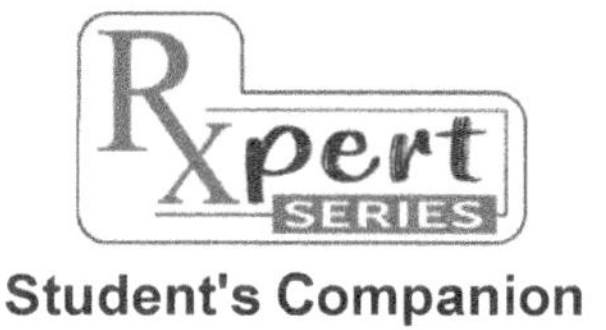

Student's Companion

Biochemistry

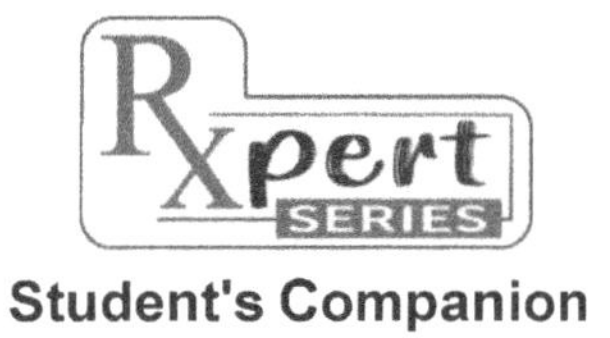

Student's Companion

Biochemistry

Dr. G. Saravanan
M. Pharm., Ph.D.
Professor
Department of Pharmaceutical Chemistry,
MNR College of Pharmacy,
Sangareddy, Hyderabad, TS, India.

Dr. V. Alagarsamy
M. Pharm, PhD, FIC, FRSC
Professor and Principal,
MNR College of Pharmacy,
Sangareddy - 502 294,
Hyderabad, TS, India.

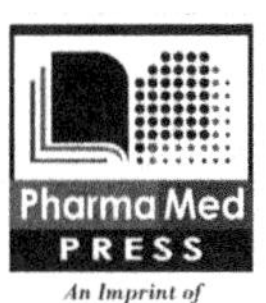

PharmaMed Press
An imprint of BSP Books Pvt. Ltd.,
4-4-309/316, Giriraj Lane,
Sultan Bazar, Hyderabad - 500 095.

Biochemistry

by *G. Saravanan and V. Alagarsamy*

Published by:

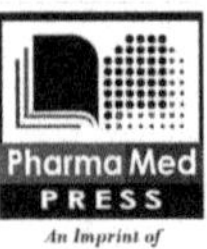

PharmaMed Press

An imprint of BSP Books Pvt. Ltd.,

4-4-309/316, Giriraj Lane, Sultan Bazar, Hyderabad - 500 095.

Phone: 040-23445688; Fax: 91+40-23445611

E-mail: info@pharmamedpress.com

www.pharmamedpress.com/pharmamedpress.net

ISBN: 978-93-95039-36-9 (Hardback)

Preface

The branch of science dealing with the study of all the life processes such as control and coordination within a living organism is called Biochemistry. A sub-discipline of both chemistry and biology, biochemistry may be divided into three fields: structural biology, enzymology and metabolism. Over the last decades of the 20th century, biochemistry has become successful at explaining living processes through these three disciplines. Much of biochemistry deals with the structures, functions, and interactions of biological macromolecules, such as proteins, nucleic acids, carbohydrates, and lipids. They provide the structure of cells and perform many of the functions associated with life. The findings of biochemistry are applied primarily in medicine, nutrition, and agriculture. Biochemistry covers a range of scientific disciplines, including genetics, microbiology, forensics and medicine.

Biochemistry is essential to understand the following concepts. a) The chemical processes which transform diet into compounds that are characteristics of the cells of a particular species; b) The catalytic functions of enzymes; c) Utilizing the potential energy obtained from the oxidation of foodstuff consumed for the various energy-requiring processes of the living cell; d) The properties and structure of substances that constitute the framework of tissues and cells; e) To solve fundamental problems in medicine and biology.

The vast academic experience helped us to realize the need of the B. Pharm., students for a book that can help them to easily understand the subject. Many of our students also insisted us publish a book after getting themselves inspired of learning biochemistry with at most ease and simplicity from our clear and illustrative lecture notes. The main object of this book is to attract the B. Pharm., students, so that they feel an urge to explore and understand the basics of biochemistry.

This book is an effect of our vision to discover the best book on biochemistry especially for B. pharmacy second semester students, which consists of five units as per revised PCI syllabus. Unit - 1 deal with the biomolecules and bioenergetic basics. In this part, each biomolecule is discussed in a simplified manner with clear definition, classification, properties, and significance. For easy understanding and revision, classifications of biomolecules were schematically represented, and properties and biological significance were given point by point. Unit - 2 to Unit - 4 deals with biomolecules metabolism. One of the major highlights of this book is the presentation of metabolism of biomolecules which clearly distinguish this book from the rest of the available books on the market. Metabolic pathways were represented both in structural form and theoretical form along with the type of reaction, name of the enzyme responsible, and energetic aspects. The changes that take place in each biochemical reactions are highlighted in the structure for an easy understanding of the reaction. Detailed explanation was given for every reaction of various metabolic pathways with the reasoning of enzyme name and energetic calculation. In the applicable places, regulation, inhibitors, and metabolic disorders of biochemical reactions were also discussed. Unit - 5 deals with enzyme including classification, mechanism of action, inhibition, kinetics, co-enzymes, isoenzymes and applications in a student-friendly manner. Probable questions including multiple-choice questions with key, short answers, and long answers are given at end of each chapter add colors to this book. Hence, this book facilitates the students to understand the subject more easily and interestingly. We welcome suggestions and constructive criticism from all corners of the academic community.

Dr. G. Saravanan & Dr. V. Alagarsamy

Acknowledgement

A warm response to Prof. V. Alagarsamy's earlier Books on the "Text Book of Medicinal Chemistry", "Pharmaceutical Chemistry of Natural Products" (Published by Elsevier), Pharmaceutical Inorganic Chemistry, Organic Chemistry – A Comprehensive Approach and Pharmaceutical Organic Chemistry (Published by Pharma Book Syndicate) prompted us to author Pharmaceutical Biochemistry – A Comprehensive Approach. The success of this book made us to write this book on "Biochemistry", covering entire syllabus prescribed by the Pharmacy Council of India (PCI) for B. Pharm., second semester students.

We wish to place on record our heartfelt thanks to everyone who has made this book possible, especially our beloved teachers from the first standard to the doctoral program. We dedicate this book to the many hundreds of budding graduates and pharmacy students, whom we have taught over the years, and our teachers who have encouraged us to convert our class notes into textbook to reach a wide range of academic community.

We are immensely grateful to Prof. K. Chinnaswamy and Dr. B. Suresh (Pro-Chancellor, JSS University; Ex-President, Pharmacy Council of India) for their constant support and inspiration extended to us to author this book.

We gratefully acknowledge the constant and continuous encouragement and moral support extended by Shri. M. N. Raju, Chairman, and Mr. M. Ravi Varma, Vice-Chairman, MNR Educational Trust, Hyderabad, for our entire academic and research pursuit, is a great motivation for us in taking up this new challenge.

We thank all the faculty members of the Faculty of Technology, Osmania University, Hyderabad for their constant support in all our academic activities.

We thank Mr. Anil Shah, Managing Director, PharmaMed Press for recognizing and inviting us to write this book. The friendly interaction experienced with the Pharma Book Syndicate, Mr. Naresh (Production Manager), and his team offered cordial support, which always made us furnish our input to make this Book one of the Best. Getting such a cooperative and energetic team encourages the authors to continue their writing always. We thank them wholeheartedly for accepting all views while designing the book and helping us reach this target.

Individually Dr. Saravanan expresses his sincere thanks to his grandfather (Mr. R. Narayanasamy), grandmother (Ms. N. Janaki), father (Mr. V. Govindaraj), mother (Ms. G. Nagathilagam), father-in-law (Mr. T. R. Raja), mother-in-law (Ms. R. Rajathi), uncle (Mr. N. Manikandan & Mr. N. Thirupathi Vasagan), brother (Mr. G. Veeraputhiran), and cousin (Mr. R. Ramanarayanan & Mr. R. Lakshmana Kumar) for their kind encouragement and moral support throughout his career. The stimulation he got from his wife (Ms. R. Murugalakshmi) to reach this target is more than enzymes, and the patience and cooperation extended by his children (S. Veeraeshwaran and S. Veerakanishka), made him think of the goal without any diversion. He also expresses his sincere thanks to his friends especially Dr. T. Panneer Selvam, Dr. P. Dinesh Kumar, Dr. C. R. Prakash, Dr. K. Selvaraj, Dr. P. Parasuraman, and Dr. N. Kiruthiga for their support in his career.

Most of all, we thank The Almighty God for his endless blessings, knowledge, and strength to make this book possible.

G. Saravanan
sarachem1981@gmail.com
WhatsApp: +91-9963023257
V. Alagarsamy
drvalagarsamy@gmail.com
WhatsApp: +91-7674893936

Contents

UNIT – 3 : LIPID METABOLISM AND AMINO ACID METABOLISM

UNIT - 4 : NUCLEIC ACID METABOLISM

UNIT - 5 : ENZYMES

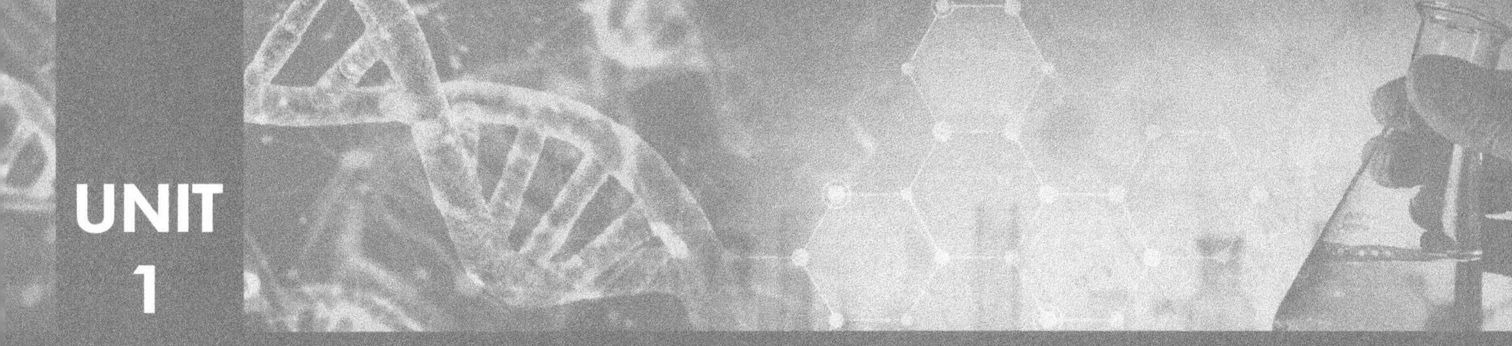

UNIT 1

Biomolecules and Bioenergetics

Biomolecules or Macromolecules

Life is composed of lifeless chemical molecules. About 6,000 and 1,00,00 different types of molecules are present in bacterium and man, respectively. Among these only few are characterized till now. Proteins, nucleic acid (such as DNA and RNA), polysaccharides and lipids are the important macromolecules or biomolecules composed of amino acids, nucleotides, monosaccharides and fatty acids, respectively. Strictly speaking lipids are not polymers but fatty acids are present in majority of lipids. The building blocks and functions of important biomolecules of cells are summarized in Table 1.1.

Table 1.1 Building blocks and functions of important biomolecules of cells.

S. No	Macromolecules or Biomolecules	Repeating Unit or Building Blocks	Important Functions
1	Protein	Amino acids	Static and dynamic functions of cell and fundamental basis of structure.
2	Deoxyribonucleic acid (DNA)	Deoxyribonucleotides	Storehouse of genetic information.
3	Ribonucleic acid (RNA)	Ribonucleotides	Essentially needed for biosynthesis of protein.
4	Glycogen or Polysaccharide	Glucose or monosaccharide	Storage form of energy to meet short term demands.
5	Lipid	Fatty acid, glycerol	Structural components of membrane and storage form of energy to meet long term demands.

Carbohydrates

In nature carbohydrates are the most abundant organic molecules and widely distributed in plants and animals. They are synthesized in plants by photosynthesis and serves as storage of energy (e.g. starch and glycogen) and source of energy (e.g. sugars). Earlier, carbohydrates were regarded as the **hydrates of carbon i.e., C(H_2O)** (carbo indicates "carbon"; hydrates indicates "water"), hence they are named as carbohydrates. The hydrogen and oxygen are present in the same ratio as in water, hence the term hydrates is added. They are primarily composed of carbon, hydrogen and oxygen. **$(CH_2O)_n$ or $C_nH_{2n}O_n$ (where n > 3)** is the empirical formula of most of the carbohydrates. **Example:** Glucose ($C_6H_{12}O_6$), ribose ($C_5H_{10}O_5$), etc. But some non-carbohydrates also appear as hydrates of carbon. **Example:** Formaldehyde (CH_2O; HCHO), acetic acid ($C_2H_4O_2$; CH_3COOH), lactic acid ($C_3H_6O_3$; $CH_3CH(OH)COOH$) and inositol ($C_6H_{12}O_6$). In addition, some genuine carbohydrates do not satisfy this empirical formula. **Example:** Rhamnose, ($C_6H_{12}O_5$), digitoxose ($C_6H_{12}O_4$), rhamnohexose ($C_7H_{14}O_6$). Therefore, carbohydrates are not always considered as hydrates of carbon. The general formula for polysaccharides is **$(C_6H_{10}O_5)_n$**.

Carbohydrates are defined as optically active polyhydroxy aldehydes or ketones or compounds which produce them on hydrolysis. Nitrogen, phosphorus, or sulfur is also present in some of the carbohydrates apart from the carbon, hydrogen and oxygen. Because of their sweet taste, the simpler members of carbohydrate family are also known as saccharides (In Latin, **saccharum means "sugar"**).

Classification of Carbohydrates

Based on solubility, crystal structure and taste, carbohydrates are broadly classified into two major types as,

1. Sugars
2. Non-sugars or polysaccharides or glycans

1. **Sugars:** Sugars are soluble in water, crystalline in structure and are sweet in taste. Further based on the number of sugar molecules present sugars are classified into two categories
   A. Monosaccharides
   B. Oligosaccharides

   A. **Monosaccharides:** In Greek, mono means "single" and in Latin, saccharum means "sugar", hence monosaccharides are composed of single sugar molecules. Monosaccharides are defined as polyhydroxy aldehydes or ketones which cannot be hydrolysed to simpler sugars. Monosaccharides having more than four carbon atoms possess cyclic structures. In nature the most commonly found monosaccharides are D-glucose (aldohexose) and D-fructose (ketohexose). In nucleic acids, nucleotides and nucleosides, aldopentoses such as D-ribose and 2-deoxy-D-ribose are present.

   Based on the nature of carbonyl group, present monosaccharides are further sub divided into two types.

   (i) **Aldoses or Aldose sugar:** Carbonyl group present is aldehyde, hence aldoses are monosaccharides composed of polyhydroxy aldehydes.

   (ii) **Ketoses or Ketose sugar:** Carbonyl group present is ketone, hence ketoses are monosaccharides composed of polyhydroxy ketones.

   These aldose and ketose sugars are further divided into several types based on the number of carbon atoms in the molecules as follows.

   (a) **Trioses:** Tri means "three", hence trioses are monosaccharides made up of three carbon atoms. **Example:** Glyceraldehyde (Aldotriose) and dihydroxy acetone (Ketotriose).

   (b) **Tetroses:** Tetra means "four", hence tetroses are monosaccharides made up of four carbon atoms. **Example:** Erythrose, threose (Aldotetrose) and erythrulose (Ketotetrose).

   (c) **Pentoses:** Penta means "five", hence pentoses are monosaccharides made up of five carbon atoms. **Example:** Ribose, arabinose, xylose, lyxose (Aldopentose) and ribulose, xylulose (Ketopentose).

   (d) **Hexoses:** Hexa means "six", hence hexoses are monosaccharides made up of six carbon atoms. **Example:** Allose, altrose, glucose, mannose, gulose, idose, galactose, talose (Aldohexose) and allulose, fructose, sorbose, tagatose (Ketohexose).

   (e) **Heptoses:** Hepta means "seven", hence heptoses are monosaccharides made up of seven carbon atoms. **Example:** Glycero mannoheptose (Aldoheptose) and sedoheptulose (Ketoheptose).

   (f) **Nanoses:** Nano means "nine", hence nanoses are monosaccharides made up of nine carbon atoms. **Example:** Neuraminic acid (Ketonanose).

   B. **Oligosaccharides:** In Greek, oligo means "few" and in Latin, saccharum means "sugar", hence oligosaccharides are composed of few (two to ten) sugar molecules. In oligosaccharides short chain of monosaccharide units or residues are present and are linked by characteristic linkages known as glycosidic linkage. On hydrolysis these carbohydrates yield two to ten monosaccharide molecules. Hence, further based on the number of monosaccharide units formed on hydrolysis they are divided into various classes as follows.

   (i) **Diasaccharides:** In Greek, di means "two" and in Latin, saccharum means "sugar", hence disaccharides are composed of two sugar molecules i.e, two monosaccharide residues. These two monosaccharide residues are attached covalently by an O-glycosidic bond, which is formed when a hydroxyl group of one monosaccharide reacts with the anomeric carbon of the other monosaccharide. These sugars on hydrolysis give two moles of the monosaccharides. **Example:** Maltose on hydrolysis yields two molecules of α-D-glucose (α-1,4-glycosidic linkage); Lactose on hydrolysis yields one molecules each of β-D-glucose and β-D-galactose (β-1,4-glycosidic linkage); Sucrose on hydrolysis yields one molecules each of α-D-glucose and β-D-fructose (1,2-glycosidic linkage); Isomaltose on hydrolysis yields two molecules of α-D-glucose (α-1,6-glycosidic linkage); Cellobiose on hydrolysis yields two molecules of β-D-glucose (β-1,4-glycosidic linkage).

(ii) Trisaccharides: In Greek, tri means "three" and in Latin, saccharum means "sugar", hence trisaccharides are composed of three sugar molecules i.e, three monosaccharide residues. These sugars on hydrolysis give three moles of the monosaccharides. Most oligosaccharides consisting of three or more units do not occur as free entities but are linked to non-sugar molecules (lipids or proteins) in glycoconjugates. **Example:** Raffinose on hydrolysis yields one molecule each of α-D-glucose, β-D-fructose and α-D-galactose or sucrose and α-D-galactose

(iii) Tetrasaccharides: In Greek, tetra means "four" and in Latin, saccharum means "sugar", hence tetrasaccharides are composed of four sugar molecules i.e, four monosaccharide residues. These sugars on hydrolysis give four moles of the monosaccharides. **Example:** Stachyose on hydrolysis yields one molecule each of α-D-glucose and β-D-fructose and two molecules of α-D-galactose.

(iv) Pentasaccharides: In Greek, penta means "five" and in Latin, saccharum means "sugar", hence pentasaccharides are composed of five sugar molecules i.e, five monosaccharide residues. These sugars on hydrolysis give five moles of the monosaccharides. **Example:** Verbascose on hydrolysis yields one molecule each of α-D-glucose and β-D-fructose and three molecules of α-D-galactose.

2. **Non-sugars or Polysaccharides or glycans:** (Non-sugars are insoluble in water and forms colloids, non-crystalline in structure and are tasteless (not sweet in taste). In Greek, poly "means" many and in Latin, saccharum means "sugar", hence polysaccharides are composed of many sugar molecules i.e, many monosaccharide residues. These sugars on hydrolysis give many moles of the monosaccharides. Chemically they are long chain or polymers of monosaccharides. Some polysaccharides, such as cellulose, are linear chains; others, such as starch, glycogen, are branched. Glycosidic linkage can be formed at any one of the hydroxyl group of monosaccharides that's why branches are occurring in polysaccharides. Further based on composition i.e., repeating units, polysaccharides are further classified into two categories as,

   A. Homopolysaccharides or homoglycans

   B. Heteropolysaccharides or heteroglycans

   A. Homopolysaccharides or homoglycans: (In Greek homo means "same", poly means "many" and in Latin, saccharum means "sugar", hence homopolysaccharides are composed of same sugar molecules i.e, same monosaccharide residues. Only a single type of monosaccharide is obtained on hydrolysis of homopolysaccharides. They are further classified into two types based on monosaccharide present as

   (i) Glucosan: They are polymers of glucose i.e., repeating unit is glucose. **Example:** Starch, glycogen, cellulose, dextrans, dextrins, chitin, etc.

   (ii) Fructosan: They are polymers of fructose i.e., repeating unit is fructose. **Example:** Inulin, etc.

   B. Heteropolysaccharides or heteroglycans: (In Greek hetero means "different", poly means "many" and in Latin, saccharum means "sugar", hence heteropolysaccharides are composed of different sugar molecules i.e, different monosaccharide residues. Mixture of few monosaccharide or its derivatives is obtained on hydrolysis of heteropolysaccharides. Mucopolysaccharides are heteroglycans made up of repeating units of sugar derivatives namely amino sugars and uronic acids. Mucopolysaccharides are commonly known as glycosaminoglycans (GAG). Some of mucopolysaccharides are found in combination with proteins to form proteoglycans or mucoids or mucoproteins. In proteoglycans 5 % protein and 95 % carbohydrates are present. Various examples of mucopolysaccharides are, keratan sulphate, heparin, dermatan sulphate, chondroitin sulphate, hyaluronic acid, etc.

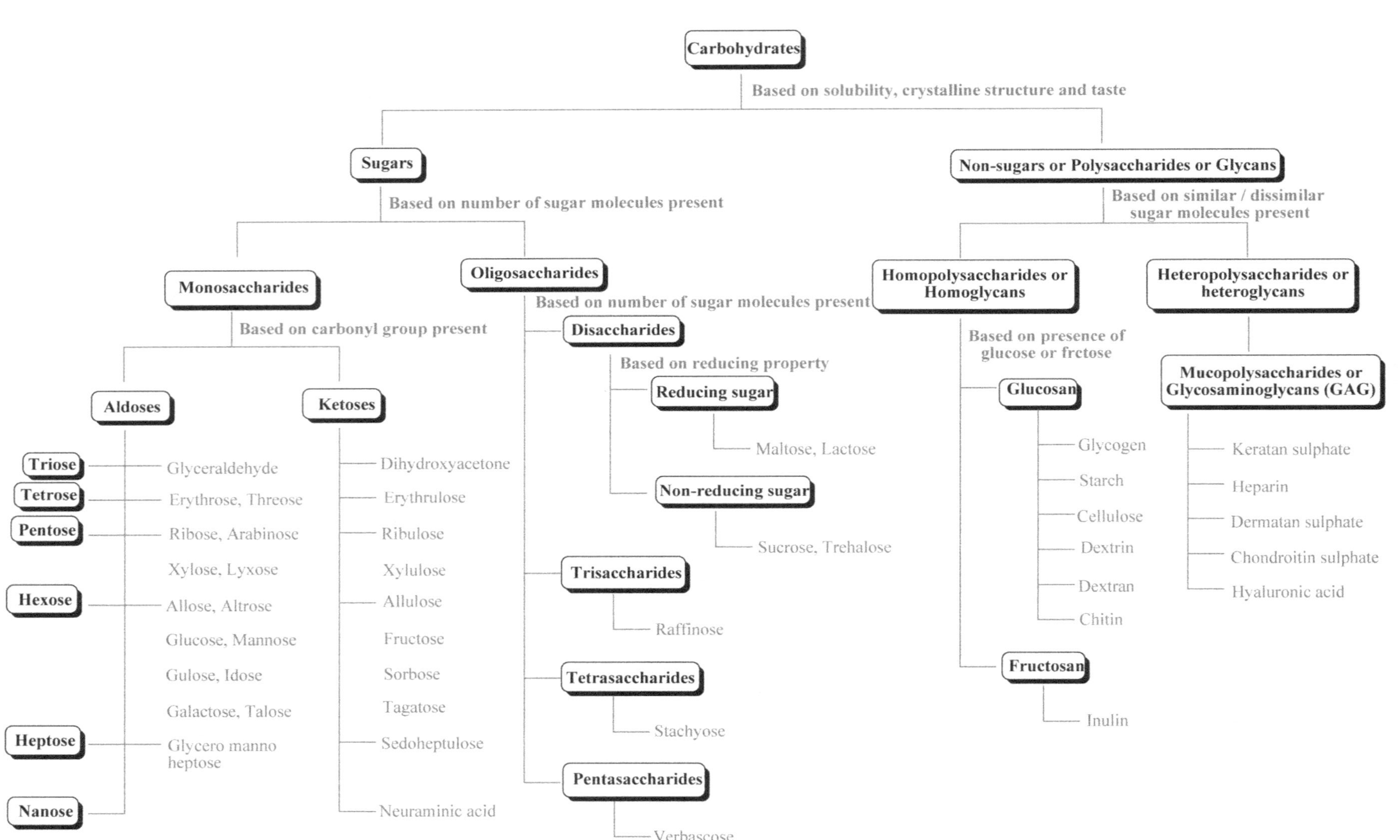
Carbohydrates
Based on solubility, crystalline structure and taste
Sugars
Non-sugars or Polysaccharides or Glycans
Based on number of sugar molecules present
Based on similar / dissimilar sugar molecules present
Monosaccharides
Oligosaccharides
Homopolysaccharides or Homoglycans
Heteropolysaccharides or heteroglycans
Based on carbonyl group present
Based on number of sugar molecules present
Aldoses
Ketoses
Disaccharides
Based on reducing property
Reducing sugar
Maltose, Lactose
Non-reducing sugar
Sucrose, Trehalose
Based on presence of glucose or frctose
Glucosan
Glycogen
Starch
Cellulose
Dextrin
Dextran
Chitin
Fructosan
Inulin
Mucopolysaccharides or Glycosaminoglycans (GAG)
Keratan sulphate
Heparin
Dermatan sulphate
Chondroitin sulphate
Hyaluronic acid
Triose
Tetrose
Pentose
Hexose
Heptose
Nanose
Glyceraldehyde
Erythrose, Threose
Ribose, Arabinose
Xylose, Lyxose
Allose, Altrose
Glucose, Mannose
Gulose, Idose
Galactose, Talose
Glycero manno heptose
Dihydroxyacetone
Erythrulose
Ribulose
Xylulose
Allulose
Fructose
Sorbose
Tagatose
Sedoheptulose
Neuraminic acid
Trisaccharides
Raffinose
Tetrasaccharides
Stachyose
Pentasaccharides
Verbascose

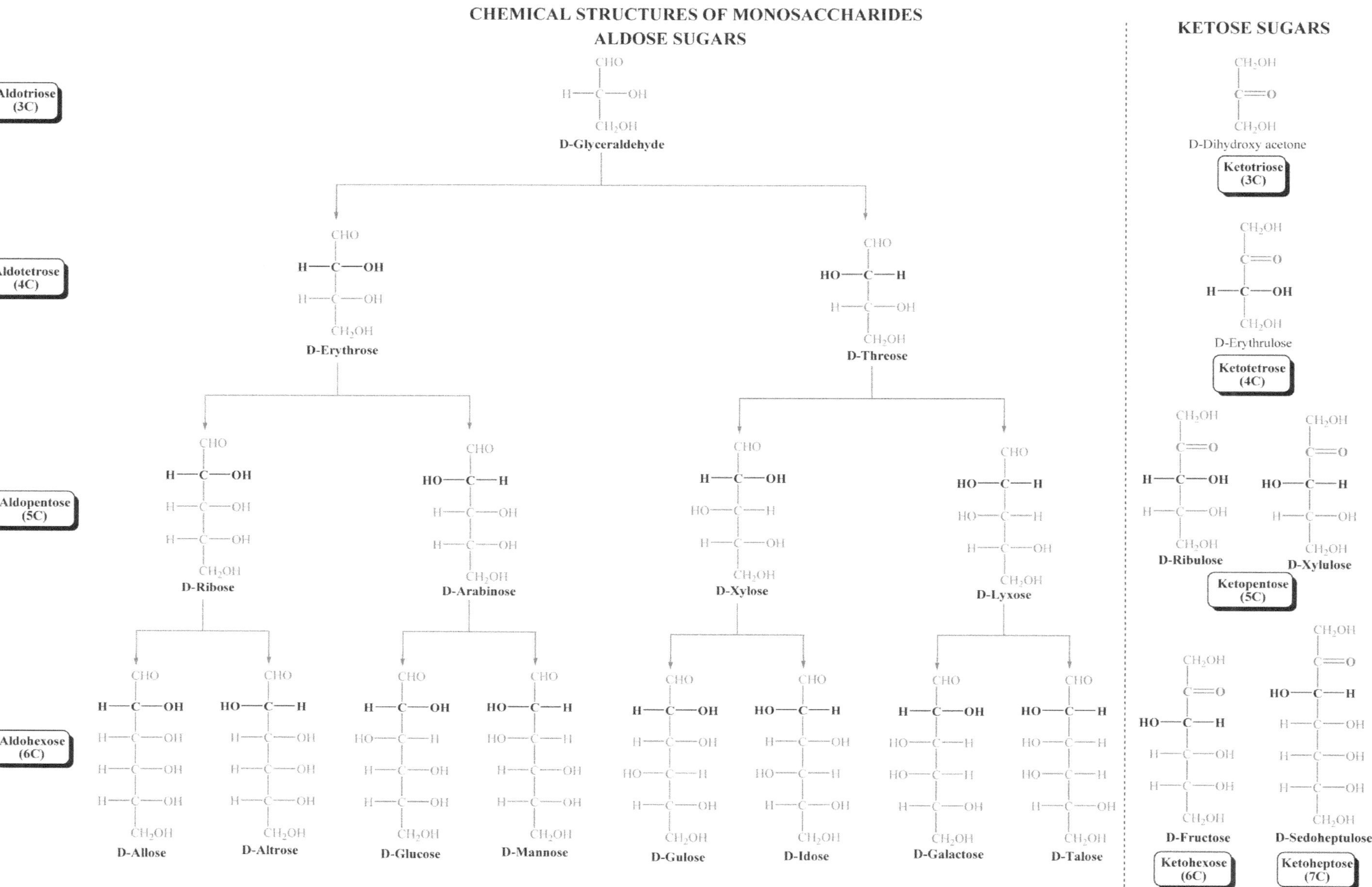
CHEMICAL STRUCTURES OF MONOSACCHARIDES
ALDOSE SUGARS
Aldotriose (3C)
D-Glyceraldehyde
Aldotetrose (4C)
D-Erythrose
D-Threose
Aldopentose (5C)
D-Ribose
D-Arabinose
D-Xylose
D-Lyxose
Aldohexose (6C)
D-Allose
D-Altrose
D-Glucose
D-Mannose
D-Gulose
D-Idose
D-Galactose
D-Talose
KETOSE SUGARS
D-Dihydroxy acetone
Ketotriose (3C)
D-Erythrulose
Ketotetrose (4C)
D-Ribulose
D-Xylulose
Ketopentose (5C)
D-Fructose
D-Sedoheptulose
Ketohexose (6C)
Ketoheptose (7C)

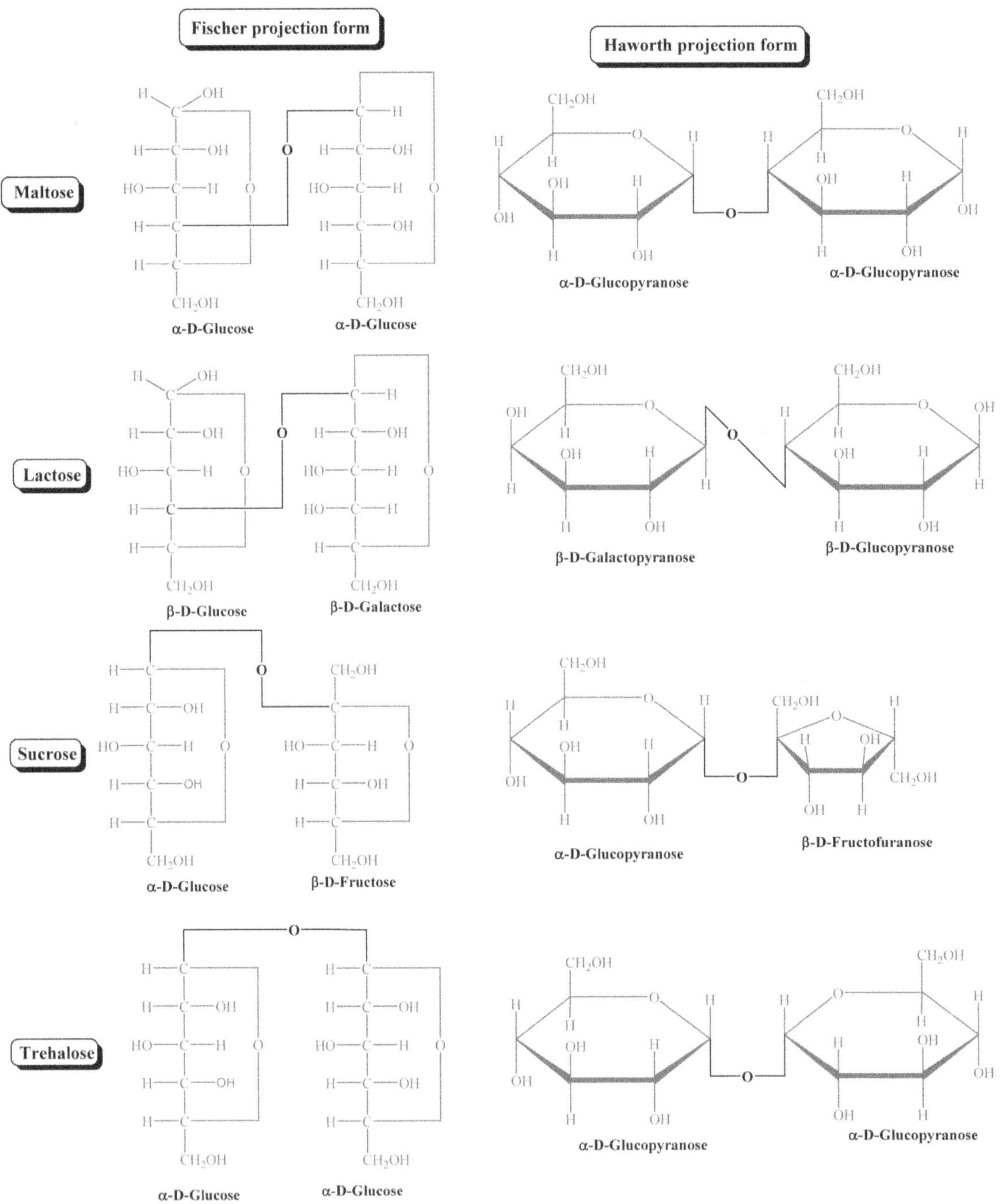

Chemical Nature of Carbohydrates

The followings are some important structural aspects of carbohydrates particularly monosaccharides. They are,

1. Stereoisomerism (D- & L-isomers)
2. Optical activity
3. Configuration of D-aldoses and D-Ketoses
4. Epimers
5. Enantiomers & Diastereomers
6. Anomers
7. Mutarotation

1. **Stereoisomerism:**

   The important characteristic of monosaccharides is stereoisomerism. Compounds possessing same molecular formula, but different structural formula are termed as stereoisomer. Asymmetric or chiral carbon is defined as carbon attached to four different atoms or groups. The number of possible isomers (2^n) of given compound is determined from the number of chiral carbon (n) present. Four asymmetric carbons are present in glucose, hence 16 isomers are possible.

   D- & L-isomers: The spatial arrangement of hydrogen (-H) and hydroxyl (-OH) group on the carbon atom that is adjacent to the terminal primary alcohol carbon (penultimate carbon or in glucose it is C-5 or in glyceraldehyde it is C-2) will determine whether the monosaccharide is D- or L-isomer. In D-isomer the hydroxyl (-OH) group is present in right side whereas in L-isomer the hydroxyl (-OH) group is present in left side. The simplest asymmetric carbon possessing monosaccharide is glyceraldehyde. Hence, it is chosen as reference monosaccharide to represent all other monosaccharides structure. The D- and L-isomers are mirror images of each other. In mammalian tissue, the naturally occurring monosaccharide are mostly D-isomers only. In addition, D-series of monosaccharide is specifically metabolized by the enzyme machinery of the cell.

D-Glyceraldehyde   L-Glyceraldehyde   D-Glucose   L-Glucose

2. **Optical activity:**

   The characteristic feature of the asymmetric carbon is optical activity. The optical isomers rotate the plane polarized light into either right side or left side. When normal light (disperse in all direction) is passed into nickel prism it will be converted in to plane polarized light (disperse in only one direction). If optical isomers rotate the plane polarized light into right side, it is known as dextrorotatory compound and is denoted by the symbol "d or +", whereas if optical isomers rotate the plane polarized light into left side, it is known as levorotatory compound and is denoted by the symbol "l or -". Generally, based on the structural relationship with glyceraldehyde optical isomers are denoted as D(+), D(-), L(+) and L(-). Racemic mixture contains equal amount of d- and l-isomers and does not exhibit any optical activity because dextrorotatory and levorotatory activities cancel each other. The term dextrose is used for glucose solution in medical practice because of dextrorotatory nature of glucose.

3. **Configuration of D-aldoses and D-ketoses:**

   The configurations of various D-aldoses are mentioned by increasing the chain length by one carbon atom at a time in Kiliani Fischer synthesis. Among various aldoses, the most predominant which occurs in nature is glucose.

   There are five D-ketoses which are physiologically important are D-erythrulose, D-ribulose, D-xylulose, D-fructose and D-sedoheptulose. The configuration of various D-aldoses and D-ketoses are mentioned under chemical structures of monosaccharides.

4. **Epimers:**

   Epimers are defined as two compounds differing from each other around a single specific carbon (other than anomeric carbon) in their configuration. The reaction involving interconversions of epimers is known as epimerization and the enzyme involved is *epimerase*. **Example:** Glucose and mannose (C-2 epimer because they differ in their configuration around C-2); Glucose and galactose (C-4 epimer because they differ in their configuration around C-4).

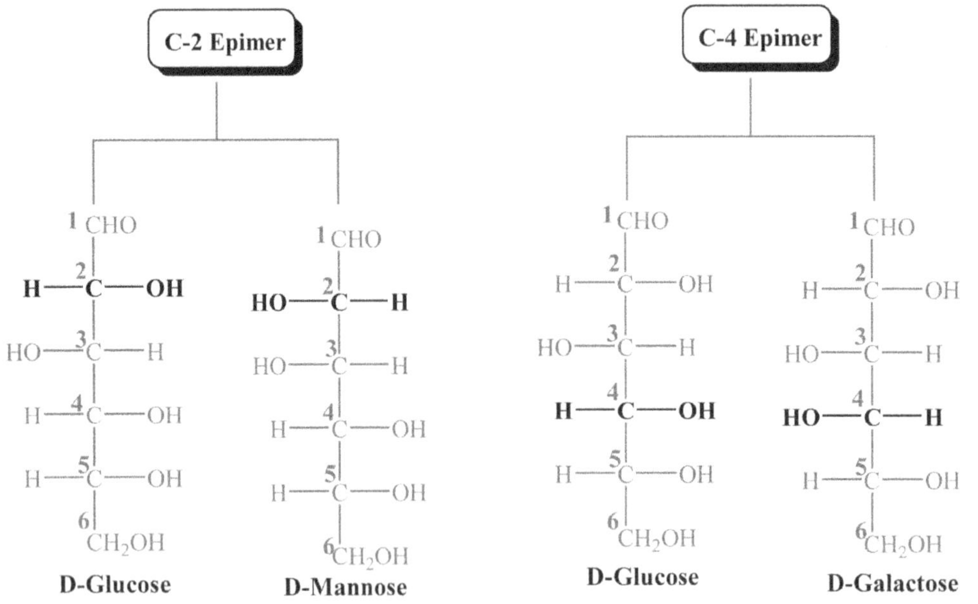

C-2 Epimer

D-Glucose D-Mannose

C-4 Epimer

D-Glucose D-Galactose

5. **Enantiomers & Diastereomers:**

Enantiomers: The stereoisomers which are mirror images of each other are known as enantiomers. The D- and L-isomers are mirror images of each other, hence they are enantiomers. **Example:** D-Glucose and L-glucose.

Diastereomers: The stereoisomers which are not mirror images of each other are known as diastereomers. **Example:** D-Glucose and D-mannose.

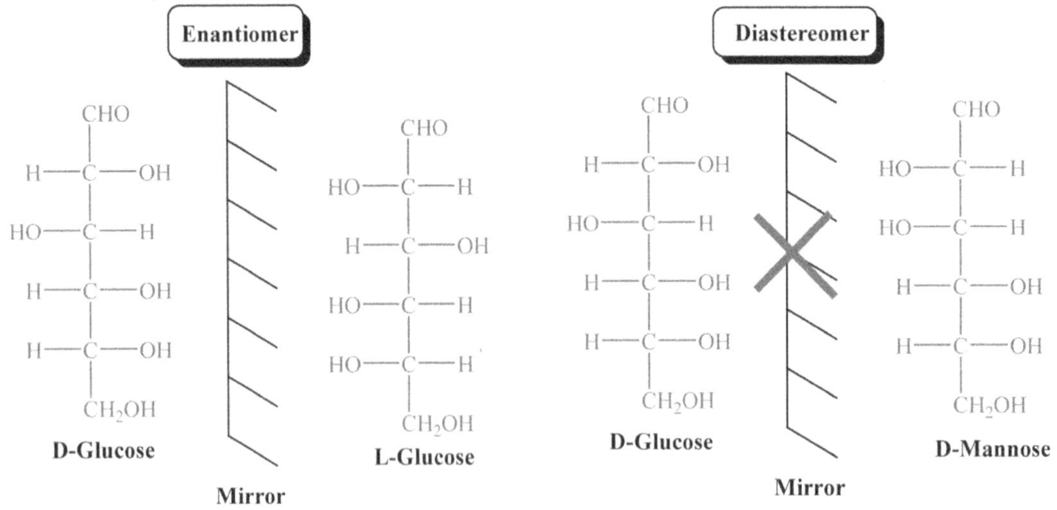

Enantiomer

D-Glucose Mirror L-Glucose

Diastereomer

D-Glucose Mirror D-Mannose

6. **Anomers:**

Two isomers differ from each other around a single specific carbon i.e., anomeric carbon in their configuration is known as anomers. Anomeric carbon is the functional group carbon atom which is involved in the formation of hemiacetal or hemiketal. Simply the two isomers differing only in the configuration of C-1 (in aldoses) or C-2 (in ketoses) are known as anomers, while such a carbon atom is known as anomeric carbon atom. **Example:** The α-and β-cyclic forms of D-glucose. In Haworth ring structure of D-glucose if the hydroxyl (-OH) group of anomeric carbon is present on the opposite side to the terminal primary alcoholic (-CH_2OH) group then it is known as α-D-glucose. Similarly, if the hydroxyl (-OH) group of anomeric carbon is present on the same side to the terminal primary alcoholic (-CH_2OH) group then it is known as β-D-glucose.

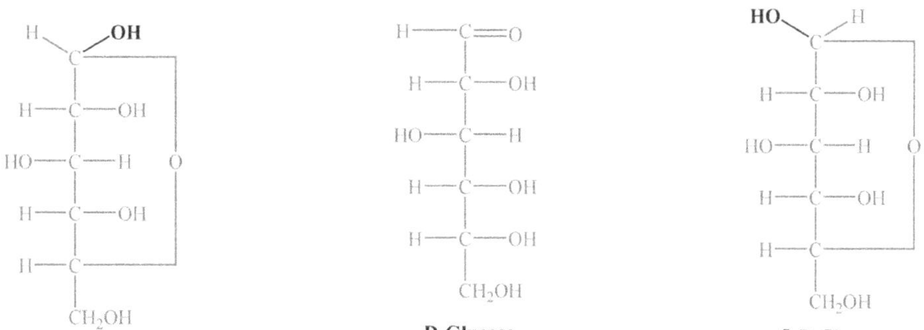

α-D-Glucose D-Glucose (Open chain form) β-D-Glucose

Fischer projection: Anomeric form of D-glucose

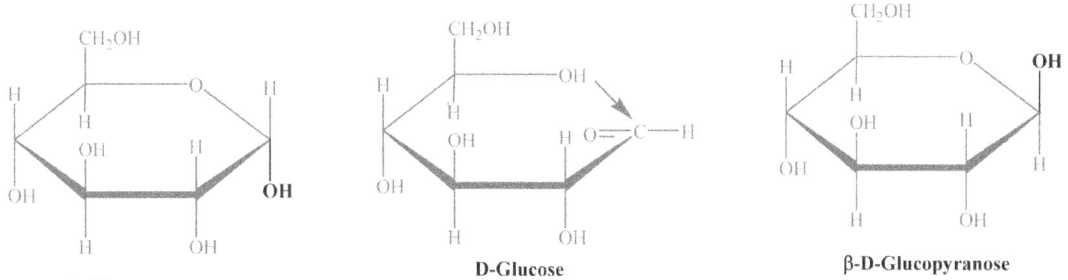

α-D-Glucopyranose D-Glucose (Acyclic form) β-D-Glucopyranose

Haworth projection: Anomeric forms of D-glucose

7. **Mutarotation:**

   Two distinct configurations (α and β) of the hemiacetals and hemiketals can occur when the cyclic structure open and re-closes due to the rotation of carbon atom bearing the reactive carbonyl group. The carbon atom which is involved in this rotation is known as anomeric carbon and the obtained two forms are termed as anomers. Mutarotation is defined as the change in specific optical rotation representing the interconversion of α- and β-forms to an equilibrium mixture.

   Example: The specific optical rotation of freshly prepared solution of α-D-glucose and β-D-glucose in water is + 112.2 ° and + 18.7 ° respectively. But the specific optical rotation of both α-D-glucose and β-D-glucose gradually changes and attains equilibrium with a constant value of + 52.7 ° due to mutarotation of glucose. The equilibrium mixture contains 36 % of α-D-glucose, 63 % of 7-D-glucose and 1 % of open chain form.

	α-D-Glucose ⇌	Equilibrium mixture ⇌	β-D-Glucose
Specific optical rotation	+ 112.2 °	+ 52.7 °	+ 18.7 °

Biological Significance of Carbohydrates

1. For all organism carbohydrates are the principal dietary source of energy (4 Cal/g).
2. Carbohydrates are used as a precursor for the synthesis of many organic compounds like fats and amino acids. Degradation products of carbohydrates act as "promoters" or "catalysts".
3. In the form of glycoprotein and glycolipids carbohydrates participate in the cell membrane structure and important cellular functions like cell growth, adhesion and fertilization.
4. For many organism carbohydrates are the structural components including cellulose fiber of plants, exoskeleton of some insects and the cell wall of microorganisms.
5. The immediate energy demands of the biological systems are satisfied by carbohydrates as glycogen (storage form of energy).

6. To the mammals except ruminant, glucose is the most important energy source of carbohydrates.
7. In medicinal practice dextrose is frequently used.
8. Erythrocytes and brain cells utilize glucose solely for energy purposes.
9. Glucose can be converted to glycogen (storage form of energy), galactose (component of lactose) and ribose (nucleic acid component).
10. High concentration of fructose is present in the semen which produces energy for motility of sperms. Sperms utilize fructose for energy. Fructose is formed in the seminiferous tubular epithelial cells from glucose.
11. Large amount of maltose present in several food preparations particularly baby foods are produced by hydrolysis of grains. Disaccharides are easily digestible from the nutritional point of view.
12. The lactose is synthesized from glucose in lactating mammary gland by the duct epithelium. For the newborn baby good source of energy is lactose present in breast milk.
13. A non-pathogenic *Coliform bacillus (E. coli)* usually ferments lactose, whereas pathogenic *Typhoid bacillus* does not ferment lactose generally. This test is used to distinguish two microorganisms.
14. *E. coli* and *A. aerogenes* present in milk converts milk to lactic acid in many organisms.
15. Osmotic condition of the blood is changed when sucrose is administered parentrally which causes flow of water from the tissues into blood.
16. Inulin a homoglycans composed of fructose is used in estimation of GFR (Glomerular filtration rate) to assess the renal function. It is also used for the estimation of body water i.e., ECF (extra cellular fluid).
17. Heparin is a mucopolysaccharide used as anticoagulant.
18. Cellulose is non-digestible carbohydrates which decrease the intestinal absorption of glucose and cholesterol thereby increases bulk of faeces. Hence, cellulose is used to avoid constipation.
19. In joints the mucopolysaccharide hyaluronic acid act as shock absorbent and lubricant.
20. Hyaluronidase is an enzyme present in semen that degrades the gel (contains hyaluronic acid) present around ovum. Hence, it may lead to effective penetration of sperm into the ovum.
21. The solutions of dextrin are used as "mucilages".
22. The solution of dextran having molecular weight approximately 75,000 has been used as plasma expander.
23. In constipation, agar is used as laxative and agar is used in agar plate for culture medium preparation.
24. Certain derivatives of carbohydrates are used as drugs. **Example:** Cardiac glycosides like digoxin and digitoxin and antibiotics like aminoglycosides and streptomycin.
25. Antifreeze glycoprotein present in antarctic fish is responsible for their survival below -2 °C.
26. Derangement of glucose metabolism is seen in diabetes mellitus, glycogen storage diseases and galactosemia.
27. Certain pathological conditions such as cataract, nephropathy is due to the accumulation of sorbitol and dulcitol in the tissues.

Lipids

In Greek, lipos means "fat". **Lipids are defined as organic compounds which are relatively insoluble in water and soluble in organic solvents like alcohol, ether, etc, potentially related to fatty acids and utilized by the living cells**. Chemically, lipids are esters of fatty acids.

The polar groups present in lipids are much smaller than their non-polar portion, hence, they are insoluble in water. Although they have several uses in medicine and industries, the function of oils and fats is mainly the storage of energy. Lipids are the chief concentrated storage form of energy and they play a role in cellular structure and various other biochemical functions. It is a heterogeneous group of compounds and are mostly small molecules. Lipids differ from the rest of body compounds because of their hydrophobic and non-polar nature. Lipids are not polymers like polysaccharides, proteins and nucleic acid.

Throughout the plant and animal kingdom, lipids are distributed widely. In plants, they occur in the seeds, nuts and fruits. In animals, lipids are stored in adipose tissues, nervous-tissues, and bone marrow. Neutral lipids are uncharged lipids. **Example:** Monoacylglycerol, diacylglycerol, triacylglycerol, cholesterol and cholesteryl esters.

Classification of Lipids

Based on the composition, lipids are broadly classified into four major types as follows.

They are,

1. Simple lipids
2. Compound lipids (or) Complex lipids
3. Derived lipids
4. Miscellaneous lipids

1. Simple lipids:

These lipids, upon hydrolysis, yield one or more fatty acids and an alcohol. Generally, simple lipids are esters of fatty acids. The simple lipids are further classified based on nature of the alcohol present into two major types as,

(a) Fats & oils

(b) Waxes

(a) Fats and oils or triacylglycerols: These are esters of fatty acids with glycerol. Fats and oils are glyceryl esters of higher fatty acids like palmitic, stearic, oleic, linoleic, and linolenic acids. In fats and oils (triglyceride), one molecule of glycerol is linked with three molecules of higher fatty acids by ester linkage.

CH_2—OH, HO—CH, CH_2—OH (Glycerol) + HO—C(=O)—R_1, HO—C(=O)—R_2, HO—C(=O)—R_3 (Fatty acids) —Esterification, $-3\ H_2O$→ CH_2—O—C(=O)—R_1, R_2—C(=O)—O—CH, CH_2—O—C(=O)—R_3 (Triglycerides or Triacylglycerol)

Glycerol **Fatty acids** **Triglycerides or Triacylglycerol**

Triglycerides are of two types based on the nature of fatty acids. If all the three fatty acids attached to glycerol are identical or same, then the triglycerides are known as simple triglycerides. Incase if three fatty acids attached to glycerol are not identical or different, then the triglycerides are known as mixed triglycerides. Natural fats are mainly composed of mixed triglycerides. As these glycerides have no free acidic or basic groups, they are often termed as neutral fats.

The composition of fats and oils are the same but they differ in their physical appearance at room temperature (RT). They are distinguished on the basis of their melting ranges. The oils are liquids at ordinary temperature while the fats are solids or semisolids (This distinction is not quite sharp and depends upon the climate and seasonal variation. **Example:** Coconut oil, sesame oil, and ghee are liquids in summer and solids in winter in our country). Fats are solid at room temperature and contain mostly saturated fatty acids like stearic and palmitic acids. Hence, melts at higher temperature. (**Example:** Vegetable fats like cocoa butter and animal fats like bone tallow, mutton tallow and lard).

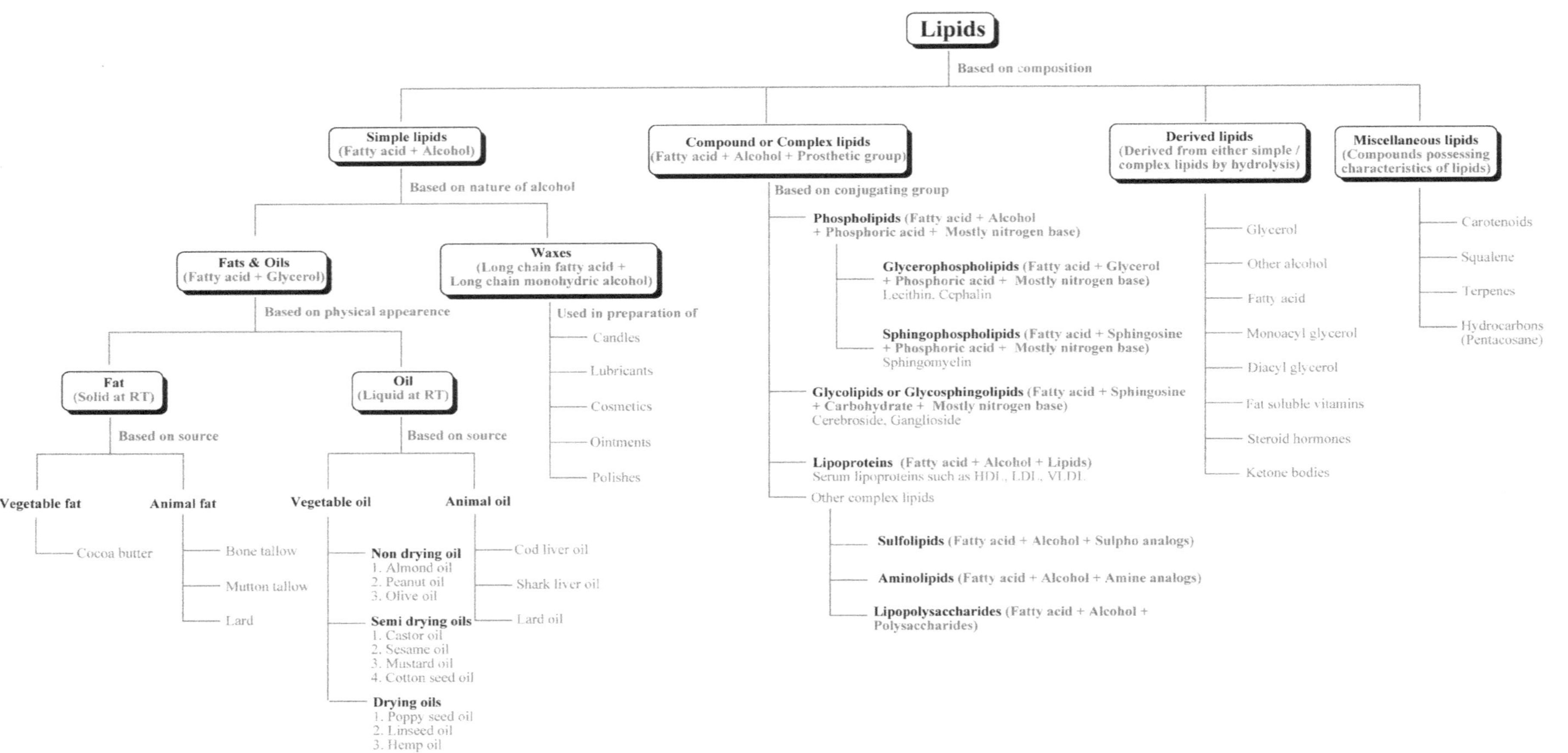
Lipids
Based on composition
Simple lipids (Fatty acid + Alcohol)
Based on nature of alcohol
Fats & Oils (Fatty acid + Glycerol)
Based on physical appearence
Fat (Solid at RT)
Based on source
Vegetable fat
Cocoa butter
Animal fat
Bone tallow
Mutton tallow
Lard
Oil (Liquid at RT)
Based on source
Vegetable oil
Non drying oil
1. Almond oil
2. Peanut oil
3. Olive oil
Semi drying oils
1. Castor oil
2. Sesame oil
3. Mustard oil
4. Cotton seed oil
Drying oils
1. Poppy seed oil
2. Linseed oil
3. Hemp oil
Animal oil
Cod liver oil
Shark liver oil
Lard oil
Waxes (Long chain fatty acid + Long chain monohydric alcohol)
Used in preparation of
Candles
Lubricants
Cosmetics
Ointments
Polishes
Compound or Complex lipids (Fatty acid + Alcohol + Prosthetic group)
Based on conjugating group
Phospholipids (Fatty acid + Alcohol + Phosphoric acid + Mostly nitrogen base)
Glycerophospholipids (Fatty acid + Glycerol + Phosphoric acid + Mostly nitrogen base)
Lecithin, Cephalin
Sphingophospholipids (Fatty acid + Sphingosine + Phosphoric acid + Mostly nitrogen base)
Sphingomyelin
Glycolipids or Glycosphingolipids (Fatty acid + Sphingosine + Carbohydrate + Mostly nitrogen base)
Cerebroside, Ganglioside
Lipoproteins (Fatty acid + Alcohol + Lipids)
Serum lipoproteins such as HDL, LDL, VLDL
Other complex lipids
Sulfolipids (Fatty acid + Alcohol + Sulpho analogs)
Aminolipids (Fatty acid + Alcohol + Amine analogs)
Lipopolysaccharides (Fatty acid + Alcohol + Polysaccharides)
Derived lipids (Derived from either simple / complex lipids by hydrolysis)
Glycerol
Other alcohol
Fatty acid
Monoacyl glycerol
Diacyl glycerol
Fat soluble vitamins
Steroid hormones
Ketone bodies
Miscellaneous lipids (Compounds possessing characteristics of lipids)
Carotenoids
Squalene
Terpenes
Hydrocarbons (Pentacosane)

Oils are liquid at room temperature and contain mostly unsaturated fatty acids like oleic acid. Hence, melts at lower temperature. (**Example:** Non-drying oils like almond oil, peanut oil, and olive oil, semi drying oils like castor oil, sesame oil, mustard oil and cotton seed oil, and drying oils like poppy seed oil, linseed oil and hemp oil).

(b) **Waxes:** These are esters of long chain fatty acids and long chain monohydric alcohols or sterols. The alcohols present in the waxes are other than glycerol. This alcohol may be aliphatic or alicyclic in nature. In general, the waxes are used in many industries for the production of candles, lubricants, cosmetics, ointments, polishes, etc.

2. **Complex lipids (or) compound lipids:**

These lipids contain additional or prosthetic groups such as phosphoric acid, proteins, carbohydrates, sulphate, nitrogen base, etc. along with fatty acids and alcohol. Based on the nature of additional groups present, the complex lipids are further subdivided into many types as follows.

(a) **Phospholipids:** In this complex lipid, the prosthetic group present is phosphoric acid. Most of the phospholipids also contain nitrogen bases. Based on the alcohol present in the phospholipids, it was further subdivided into two categories as,

1. **Glycerophospholipids:** It is composed of fatty acids, glycerol, phosphoric acid, and nitrogen bases. **Example:** Lecithin and cephalin.
2. **Sphingophospholipids:** It is composed of fatty acids, sphingosine (alcohol), phosphoric acid and nitrogen bases. **Example:** Sphingomyelin.

(b) **Glycolipids:** It is otherwise known as glycosphingolipids because of the presence of alcohol sphingosine. It is composed of fatty acids, sphingosine (alcohol), carbohydrate and nitrogen bases. **Example:** Cerebroside and ganglioside.

(c) **Lipoproteins:** It is composed of fatty acids, alcohol and lipids. **Example:** Serum lipoproteins such as HDL, LDL and VLDL.

(d) **Other complex lipids:** Among various other complex lipids, sulpholipids, aminolipids, and lipopolysaccharides are important.

3. **Derived lipids:** These compounds possess characteristics of lipids and are obtained either from simple or complex lipids by hydrolysis. **Example:** Glycerol, fatty acid, other alcohol, monoacylglycerol, diacylglycerol, fat soluble vitamin, steroid hormones and ketone bodies.
4. **Miscellaneous lipids:** Large numbers of compounds possess the characteristics of lipids and these compounds come under miscellaneous lipids. **Example:** Carotenoids, squalene, hydrocarbons like pentacosane, terpenes, etc.

Biological Significance of Lipids

1. Lipids are the concentrated fuel reserve of the body which is the most important role of lipids.
2. Lipid also acts as an insulating material and protects the internal organs.
3. In addition, lipids also give shape and smooth appearance to the body.
4. Dietary fat is important for the sufficient absorption of the essential fatty acid and fat-soluble vitamins from the food.
5. Lipids, particularly phospholipids and cholesterol are the major constituents of biological membrane structure and regulates the membrane permeability.
6. Lipids serve as a source of fat-soluble vitamins such as vitamin A, D, E, and K.
7. Some biologically active materials which serve as important building blocks of compounds like acetic acid are derived from lipids.
8. Lipids, especially steroid hormones and prostaglandins are important cellular metabolic regulators.
9. The cellular respiration and the conformation of ETC is maintained by the phospholipids particularly lecithin, cephalin and cardiolipin.

10. From the intestine, fats are absorbed by the participation of phospholipids.
11. Lipoproteins are involved in the transport of lipids and the phospholipids are necessary for the synthesis of different lipoproteins.
12. Phospholipids are regarded as lipotropic factors because in the liver it prevents the accumulation of fat.
13. Unsaturated fatty acids and arachidonic acids are released from phospholipids only. Eicosanoids such as prostaglandins, thromboxane, prostacyclins, etc. are biosynthesized from archidonic acid and unsaturated fatty acids only.

Fatty Acids

The simplest forms of lipids are fatty acids. In natural fats and oils, fatty acids occur mainly as esters but do occur in the unesterified form as free fatty acids. Fatty acids are carboxylic acids with hydrocarbon side chains. Fatty acids of natural fats are usually straight chain derivatives, containing even numbers of carbon atoms, as they are synthesized from two carbon units. The chain may be saturated or unsaturated. Compared to plant origin fatty acids (contain epoxy, keto and hydroxyl group and cyclopentane ring in structure), animal origin fatty acids possess a simple structure.

Classification of Fatty Acids

Fatty acids are classified in many different ways as follows,

1. Classification based on total number of carbon atoms
2. Classification based on length of hydrocarbon chain
3. Classification based on nature of hydrocarbon chain

1. Classification based on total number of carbon atoms

Fatty acids are broadly classified into two major types based on the total number of carbon atoms present is even number or odd number.

(a) **Even number of carbon atom chain fatty acids:** The total number of carbons present in this fatty acid is an even number (2, 4, 6 and similar series). In general, even carbons (14 to 20 carbons) are present in most of the fatty acids that occur in natural lipids. The reason behind this concept is the occurrence of fatty acid biosynthesis with sequential addition of two carbon units. **Example:** Palmitic acid (contains 16 carbons in total), stearic acid (contains 18 carbons in total), etc.

(b) **Odd number of carbon atom chain fatty acids:** The total number of carbons present in this fatty acid is an odd number (1, 3, 5 and similar series). Odd numbered fatty acids are present in milk and are also found in microbial cell walls. **Example:** Propionic acid (contains 3 carbons in total), valeric acid (contains 5 carbons in total), etc.

2. Classification based on length of hydrocarbon chain

Based on the length of the hydrocarbon chain present in fatty acid, it was broadly classified into three major types. They are,

(a) **Short chain fatty acids:** This fatty acid consists of 2 to 7 carbon atoms.

(b) **Medium chain fatty acids:** This fatty acid consists of 8 to 15 carbon atoms.

(c) **Long chain fatty acids:** This fatty acid consists of 16 and above (usually up to 24) carbon atoms.

3. Classification based on nature of hydrocarbon chain

Fatty acids are subdivided into two major groups based on the nature of hydrocarbon chains, particularly saturation conditions. They are,

(a) **Saturated fatty acids:** Unsaturation (double or triple bonds) is absent in these fatty acids. CH_3-$(CH_2)_n$-COOH is the general structural formula of saturated fatty acids. They are named by adding the suffix "-anoic" after the hydrocarbon with the same number of carbon atoms.

Example: Propanoic acid, pentanoic acid or valeric acid, n-hexadecanoic acid or palmitic acid, n-octadecanoic acid or stearic acid, etc.

(b) **Unsaturated fatty acids:** Unsaturation (double or triple bonds) is present in these fatty acids. In systematic name, the suffix "-enoic" is added after the hydrocarbon with the same number of carbon atoms. Depending on the number of unsaturated bonds present or the degree of unsaturation, it is further classified into two different types as follows,

1. **Monounsaturated (Monoethenoid, monoenoic) fatty acids:** Contains one double bond. **Example:** Palmitoleic acid and oleic acid.
2. **Polyunsaturated (polyethenoid, polyenoic) fatty acids:** It is commonly known as PUFA and contains two or more double bonds. These fatty acids are not synthesized by the body due to the lack of double bond introducing enzymes beyond 9 to 10 carbons. It is necessary to take through dietary sources. Hence, PUFA is also called as **essential fatty acid.** **Example:** Linoleic acid, linolenic acid and arachidonic acid.

Nomenclature of Fatty Acids

1. Systematic nomenclature of fatty acids is based on the name of hydrocarbons with the same number of carbon atoms. In systematic nomenclature, the final 'e' in the name of the hydrocarbon is replaced by the suffix 'oic acid'. **Example:** Propanoic acid (the corresponding hydrocarbon is 'propane'. In this, final 'e' is replaced by the suffix 'oic acid' i.e., "propane – e + oic acid = propanoic acid")
2. In general, saturated fatty acids end with a suffix 'anoic acid'. **Example:** Octanoic acid and decanoic acid. Similarly, unsaturated fatty acids with double bonds end with a suffix 'enoic acid'. **Example:** Octadecenoic acid (oleic acid) and hexadecenoic acid (palmitoleic acid).
3. The C-1 would be carboxyl carbon of a fatty acid and the C-2 would be α-carbon, the C-3, C-4, C-5 and C-6 would be β, γ, δ and ε carbon, respectively. The end methyl carbon is known as the ω carbon or n-carbon atom.

$$\underset{\omega}{\overset{n+6}{CH_3}} - \overset{7\ to\ (7+n)}{(CH_2)_n} - \underset{\varepsilon}{\overset{6}{CH_2}} - \underset{\delta}{\overset{5}{CH_2}} - \underset{\gamma}{\overset{4}{CH_2}} - \underset{\beta}{\overset{3}{CH_2}} - \underset{\alpha}{\overset{2}{CH_2}} - \overset{1}{COOH}$$

Table 1.2 List of biochemically important fatty acids.

S.No.	Common name	IUPAC name	Structure	Codes
I. Saturated fatty acids				
1	Acetic acid	n-Ethanoic acid	CH_3COOH	2: 0
2	Propionic acid	n-Propanoic acid	CH_3-CH_2-COOH	3: 0
3	Butyric acid	n-Butanoic acid	CH_3-$(CH_2)_2$-COOH	4: 0
4	Valeric acid	n-Pentanoic acid	CH_3-$(CH_2)_3$-COOH	5: 0
5	Caproic acid	n-Hexanoic acid	CH_3-$(CH_2)_4$-COOH	6: 0
6	Caprylic acid	n-Octanoic acid	CH_3-$(CH_2)_6$-COOH	8: 0
7	Capric acid	n-Decanoic acid	CH_3-$(CH_2)_8$-COOH	10: 0
8	Lauric acid	n-Dodecanoic acid	CH_3-$(CH_2)_{10}$-COOH	12: 0
9	Myristic acid	n-Tetradecanoic acid	CH_3-$(CH_2)_{12}$-COOH	14: 0
10	Palmitic acid	n-Hexadecanoic acid	CH_3-$(CH_2)_{14}$-COOH	16: 0
11	Stearic acid	n-Octadecanoic acid	CH_3-$(CH_2)_{16}$-COOH	18: 0
12	Arachidic acid	n-Eicosanoic acid	CH_3-$(CH_2)_{18}$-COOH	20: 0
13	Behenic acid	n-Docosanoic acid	CH_3-$(CH_2)_{20}$-COOH	22: 0
14	Lignoceric acid	n-Tetracosanoic acid	CH_3-$(CH_2)_{22}$-COOH	24: 0

Table 1.2 contd...

II. Unsaturated fatty acids				
15	Palmitoleic acid	cis-9-Hexadecenoic acid	CH_3-$(CH_2)_5$-CH=CH-$(CH_2)_7$-COOH	16: 1: 9
16	Oleic acid	cis-9-Octadecenoic acid	CH_3-$(CH_2)_7$-CH=CH-$(CH_2)_7$-COOH	18: 1: 9
17	Linoleic acid	cis, cis-9,12-Octadecadienoic acid	CH_3-$(CH_2)_4$-CH=CH-CH_2-CH=CH-$(CH_2)_7$-COOH	18: 2: 9, 12
18	Linolenic acid	All cis-9,12,15-Octadecatrienoic acid	CH_3-CH_2-CH=CH-CH_2-CH=CH-CH_2-CH=CH-$(CH_2)_7$-COOH	18: 3: 9, 12, 15
19	Arachidonic acid	All cis-5,8,11,14-Eicosatetraenoic acid	CH_3-$(CH_2)_4$-CH=CH-CH_2-CH=CH-CH_2-CH=CH-CH_2-CH=CH-$(CH_2)_3$-COOH	20: 4: 5, 8, 11, 14

4. For indicating the number and position of the double bonds, various conventions are used. **Example:** In fatty acids, the presence of a double bond between carbon atoms 9 and 10 is indicated by Δ^9. The number of carbon atoms, the number of double bonds, and the positions of the double bonds are widely indicated by using this convention only.

$$\overset{18}{CH_3}-(CH_2)_4-\overset{13}{CH}=\overset{12}{CH}-\overset{11}{CH_2}-\overset{10}{CH}=\overset{9}{CH}-(CH_2)_7-\overset{1}{COOH}$$

Linoleic acid $[C_{18}, \Delta^{9,12}]$

$$\overset{18}{CH_3}-\overset{17}{CH_2}-\overset{16}{CH}=\overset{15}{CH}-\overset{14}{CH_2}-\overset{13}{CH}=\overset{12}{CH}-\overset{11}{CH_2}-\overset{10}{CH}=\overset{9}{CH}-(CH_2)_7-\overset{1}{COOH}$$

Linolenic acid $[C_{18}, \Delta^{9,12,15}]$

$$\overset{20}{CH_3}-(CH_2)_4-\overset{15}{CH}=\overset{14}{CH}-\overset{13}{CH_2}-\overset{12}{CH}=\overset{11}{CH}-\overset{10}{CH_2}-\overset{9}{CH}=\overset{8}{CH}-\overset{7}{CH_2}-\overset{6}{CH}=\overset{5}{CH}-(CH_2)_3-\overset{1}{COOH}$$

Arachidonic acid $[C_{20}, \Delta^{5,8,11,14}]$

5. In biochemistry, fatty acids are represented in shorthand notation using numbers instead of writing the full structures. The general rule followed is that the total number of carbon atoms are written first, followed by the number of double bonds present, and finally the first carbon position of the double bonds starting from the carbonyl end. **Example:** Palmitic acid is written as 16: 0, oleic acid is written as 18: 1: 9 and arachidonic acid is written as 20: 4: 5, 8, 11, 14.
6. Various saturated and unsaturated fatty acids which are biologically important are listed in the Table 1.2.

Biological Significance of Fatty Acids

1. Fatty acids are the cellular fuel sources of the body.
2. Fatty acids are the composition of hormones and lipids.
3. Fatty acids play a role in the modification of proteins.
4. Essential fatty acids are the major lipids present in the biological membrane and are required for the membrane structure and function.
5. Essential fatty acids are useful for the transportation of cholesterol.
6. Essential fatty acids prevent fatty liver.
7. Essential fatty acids are useful for the synthesis of eicosanoids such as prostaglandin, prostacycline, thromboxane, leukotriene, etc.

8. Fatty acids are involved in a wide range of biological signaling pathways.
9. Fatty acids play a role in signal-transduction pathways.
10. Some skin-care products contain fatty acids, which can helps to maintain healthy skin appearance and function.
11. Commercially fatty acids are used not only in the production of numerous food products but also in soaps, detergents, and cosmetics.
12. Fatty acids, particularly omega-3 fatty acids, are also commonly sold as dietary supplements.

Nucleic Acids

Nucleic acids are the polynucleotides and nucleotides are composed of nitrogen base, pentose sugar and phosphate group. Nucleic acids primarily serve as repositories and transmitters of genetic information. The pentose sugar present in RNA and DNA is ribose and 2-deoxyribose, respectively. Either directly or indirectly, nucleotides participate in almost all biochemical processes. Nucleotides are the structural components of nucleic acids such as DNA and RNA and co-enzymes. In addition, several metabolic reactions are also regulated by nucleotides.

Classification or Types of Nucleic Acids

Nucleic acids are broadly classified into two major types based on the sugar molecules present in them. They are,

1. Deoxyribonucleic acid or DNA
2. Ribonucleic acid or RNA

1. **Deoxyribonucleic acid or DNA:** It is a polymer of deoxyribonucleotides composed of deoxyribose sugar, nitrogen bases such as purines (adenine & guanine), pyrimidines (thymine and cytosine) and phosphate group.
2. **Ribonucleic acid or RNA:** It is a polymer of ribonucleotides composed of ribose sugar, nitrogen base such as purines (adenine & guanine), pyrimidines (uracil and cytosine), and phosphate group.

Chemical Nature of Nucleic Acids

Nucleic acids are chemically polynucleotides held by 3′- and 5′-phosphate bridges or nucleic acids are built up by the monomeric units known as nucleotides. Upon hydrolysis, nucleic acids produce nucleotides. Further, the hydrolysis of nucleotides produces nucleosides and phosphoric acid. Hence, **nucleotides are defined as phosphate esters of nucleosides**. Hydrolysis of nucleoside produces nitrogen base and sugar. Nucleosides are chemically composed of nitrogen base and sugars. In nucleic acids, there are two different types of nitrogen bases such as purines and pyrimidines are present. Adenine and guanine are two purine nitrogen bases and thymine, cytosine and uracil are three pyrimidine nitrogen bases present in nucleic acid. Out of three pyrimidine nitrogen bases, thymine and cytosine is present in DNA and cytosine and uracil is present in RNA. In nucleic acids, two different types of sugar molecules such as ribose and deoxyribose are present. In that, deoxyribose sugar is present in DNA and ribose sugar is present in RNA.

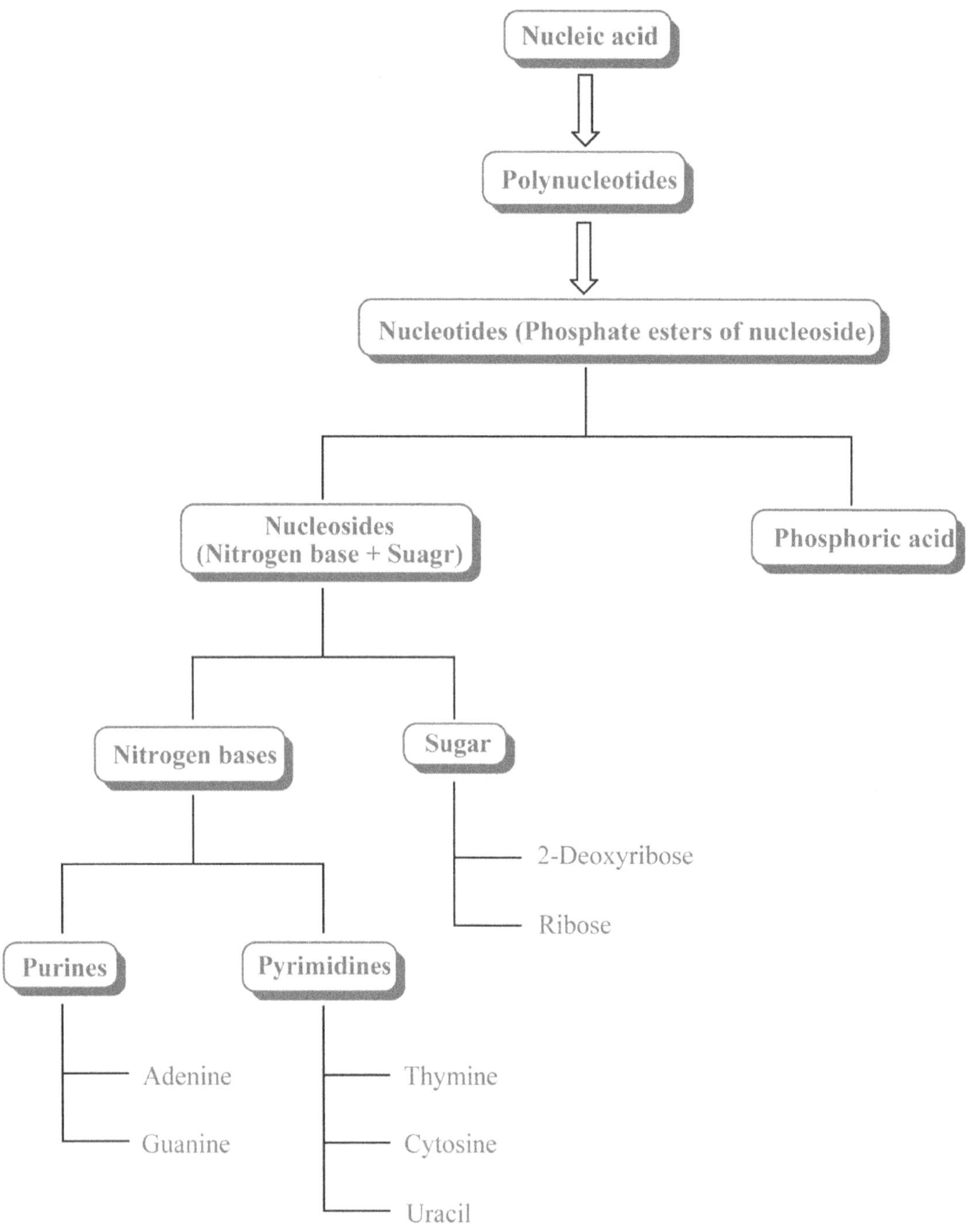

Nitrogen Bases

Nitrogen bases are chemically aromatic heterocyclic compounds. Two types of nitrogen bases present in nucleic acid are mentioned below.

1. Purines
2. Pyrimidines

In general, purines are numbered in anti-clockwise direction whereas pyrimidines are numbered in clockwise direction. The general structures of purines and pyrimidines are represented in the below structures.

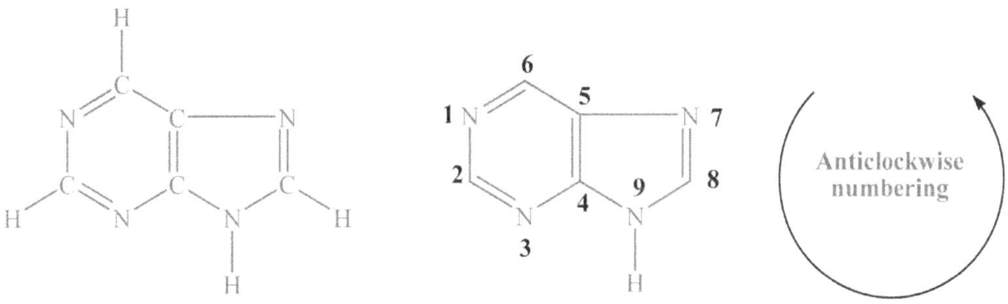

Anticlockwise numbering

General structure of purine nitrogen base

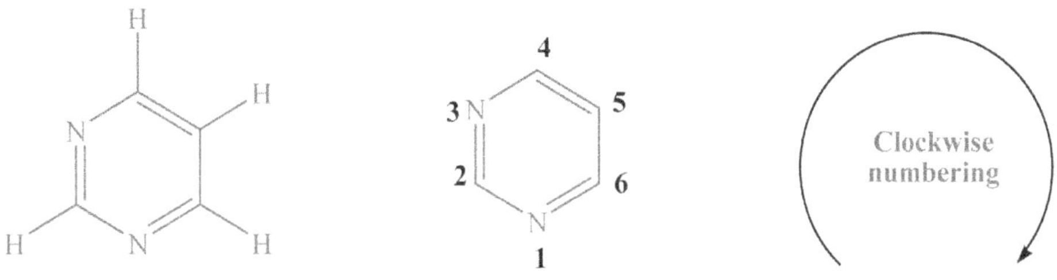

Clockwise numbering

General structure of pyrimidine nitrogen base

Purines: Adenine and guanine are the two purine bases present in the nucleic acids. Both adenine and guanine are present in DNA and RNA. Existence of molecules in a lactam (keto) form and lactim (enol) form is known as tautomerism. Purine with an oxo (C=O) functional group exhibits tautomeric forms as follows.

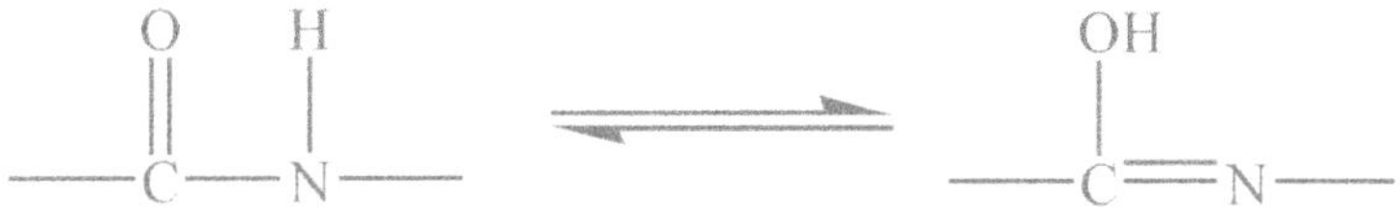

Lactam form or Keto form ⇌ **Lactim form or Enol form**

Table 1.3 Chemical structures of nitrogen bases.

S. No.	Name of base	Chemical name	Lactam form or Keto form	Lactim form or Enol form
A. Purine bases				
1	Adenine	6-Aminopurine (or) 9H-Purin-6-amine	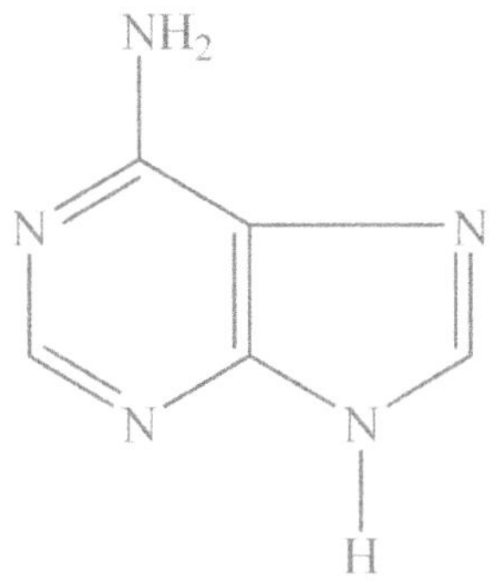	----
2	Guanine	2-Amino-6-oxopurine (or) 2-Amino-1H-purin-6(9H)-one	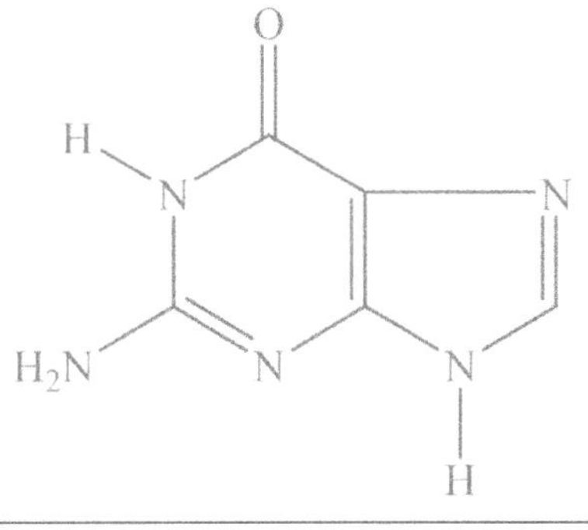	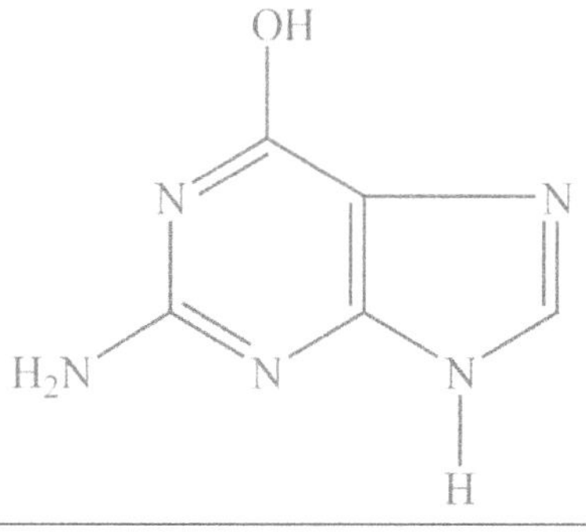

Table 1.3 contd...

S. No.	Name of base	Chemical name	Lactam form or Keto form	Lactim form or Enol form
B. Pyrimidine bases				
3	Thymine	2,4-Dioxy-5-methylpyrimidine or 5-Methyluracil	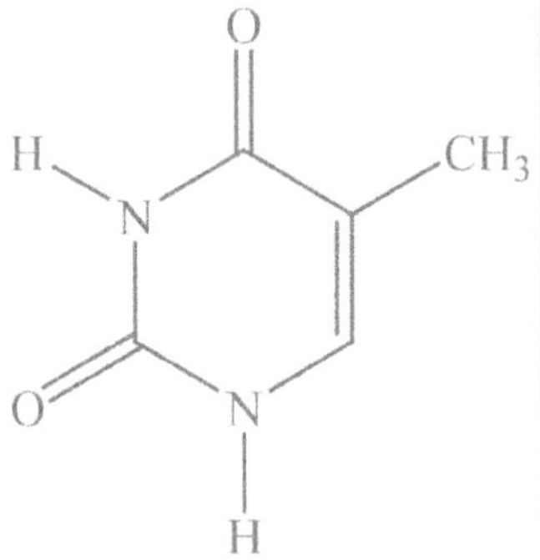	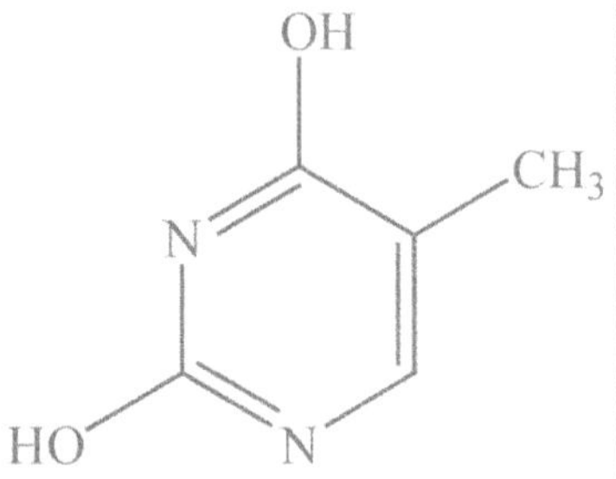
4	Cytosine	2-Oxo-4-aminopyrimidine	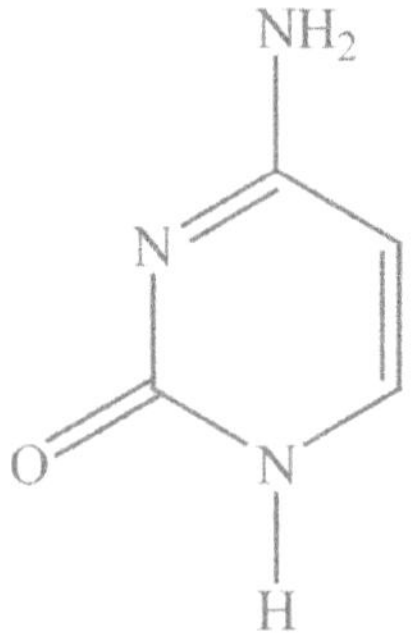	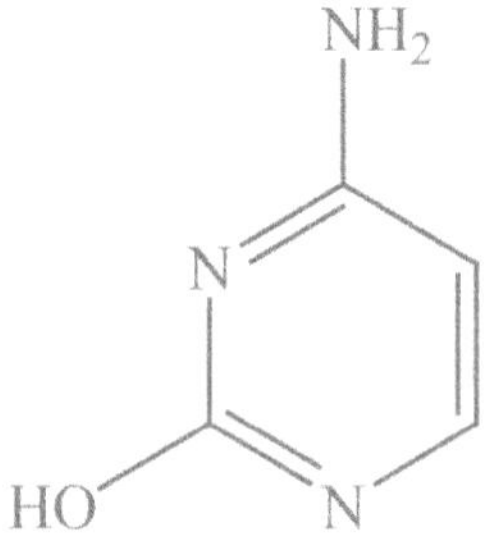
5	Uracil	2,4-Dioxypyrimidine (or) Pyrimidine – 2, 4 (1H, 3H) - dione	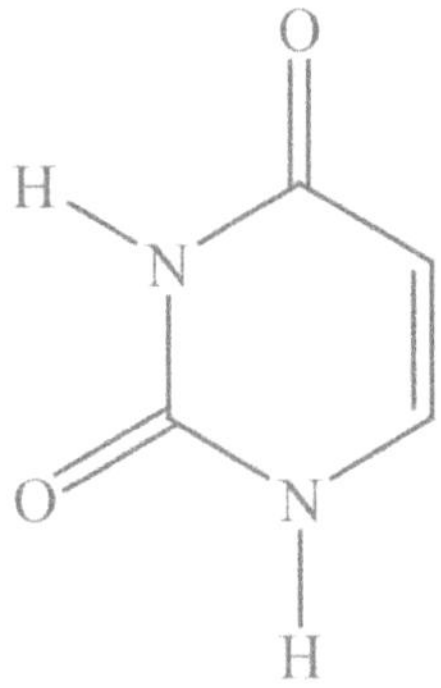	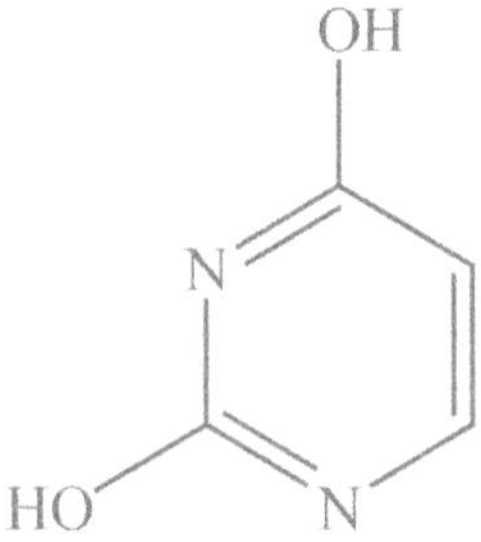

Pyrimidines: Thymine, cytosine and uracil are the three pyrimidine bases present in the nucleic acids. Thymine is present only in DNA and uracil is present only in RNA. Cytosine is present in both DNA and RNA. Like purines, pyrimidines with oxo (C=O) functional groups exhibit tautomeric forms. At physiological pH lactam forms are predominantly present. Chemical structures of various purine and pyrimidine nitrogen bases are listed in Table 1.3.

Sugars

Nucleic acid contains pentose sugars (five carbon monosaccharides) such as ribose and 2′-deoxyribose. For differentiation from nitrogen base numbering, sugar molecule numbers are represented with an associated prime (′). The two sugars mentioned above are differing in their structure at C-2′ only. Deoxyribose possess one less oxygen at C-2′ compared to ribose. DNA contains 2′-deoxyribose and RNA contains ribose sugar.

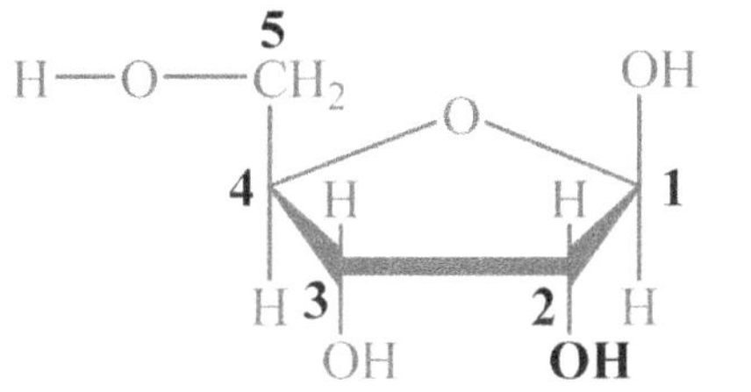

β-D-Ribose

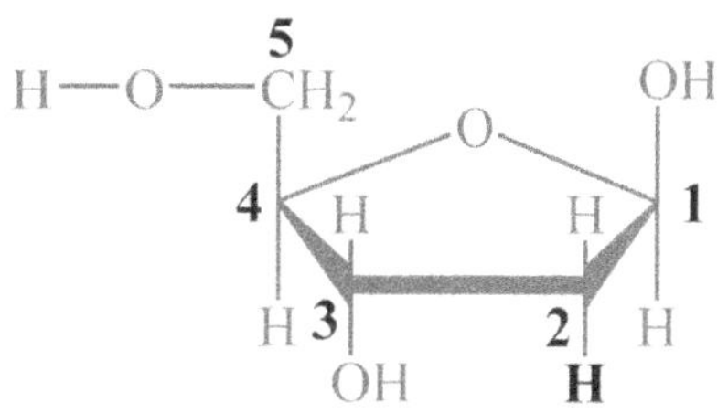

β-D-2-Deoxyribose

Nomenclature of Nucleotides

Nucleosides are formed when pentose sugars are added to the nitrogen bases. If the sugar attached is ribose it is called ribonucleoside. The ribonucleosides of bases adenine, guanine, cytosine and uracil are adenosine, guanosine, cytidine and uridine, respectively. If the sugar attached is 2-deoxyribose then it is called deoxyribonucleoside. The prefix deoxy is added to the corresponding ribonucleoside name to get the deoxyribonucleoside name. The deoxyribonucleosides of bases adenine, guanine, cytosine and thymine are deoxyadenosine, deoxyguanosine, deoxycytidine and deoxythymidine, respectively.

When a nucleoside is attached to a single phosphate moiety, the term mononucleotide is used. For example, adenosine attached to single phosphate moiety is named as adenosine monophosphate (AMP) which is composed of adenine, ribose and phosphate moiety. The various bases present in the nucleic acid and their corresponding nucleoside, mononucleotides and abbreviations are listed in the Table 1.4.

Table 1.4 Various bases, nucleoside, mononucleotides present in nucleic acid.

S. No.	Nitrogen base	Nucleoside	Mononucleotide	Abbreviation
A. Ribonucleotide				
1	Adenine (A)	Adenosine (Adenine + Ribose)	Adenosine-5'-monophosphate or adenylate (Adenosine + Phosphate)	AMP
2	Guanine (G)	Guanosine (Guanine + Ribose)	Guanosine-5'-monophosphate or guanylate (Guanosine + Phosphate)	GMP
3	Cytosine (C)	Cytidine (Cytosine + Ribose)	Cytidine-5'-monophosphate or cytidylate (Cytidine + Phosphate)	CMP
4	Uracil (U)	Uridine (Uracil + Ribose)	Uridine-5'-monophosphate or uridylate (Uridine + Phosphate)	UMP
B. Deoxyribonucleotide				
5	Adenine (A)	Deoxyadenosine (Adenine + 2-Deoxyibose)	Deoxyadenosine-5'-monophosphate or Deoxyadenylate (Deoxyadenosine + Phosphate)	dAMP
6	Guanine (G)	Deoxyguanosine (Guanine + 2-Deoxyibose)	Deoxyguanosine-5'-monophosphate or Deoxyguanylate (Deoxyguanosine + Phosphate)	dGMP
7	Cytosine (C)	Deoxycytidine (Cytosine + 2-Deoxyibose)	Deoxycytidine-5'-monophosphate or Deoxycytidylate (Deoxycytidine + Phosphate)	dCMP
8	Thymine (T)	Deoxythymidine (Thymine + 2-Deoxyibose)	Deoxythymidine-5'-monophosphate or Deoxythymidylate (Deoxythymidine + Phosphate)	dTMP

Binding of nucleotide components: The pentose sugars are bonded to nitrogen bases by N-glycosidic bonds. C-1′ of sugars are covalently attached to the N-9 of purine bases or N-1 of pyrimidine bases to form corresponding nucleosides. In nucleosides, the hydroxyl group present at C-5′ or C-3′ of sugar molecules is esterified with phosphates to produce corresponding 5′- or 3′- monophosphates (i.e., nucleotide). Generally, esterification takes place at C-5′, hence 5′ is usually omitted while writing names of nucleotides. In case if esterification takes place at C-3′ then 3′ is included while writing names of nucleotides. The structures of some nucleotides such as AMP & dTMP are given below.

Nucleoside di and triphosphates: Only one phosphate moiety is present in nucleoside monophosphates like AMP, GMP, CMP, UMP, dAMP, dGMP, dCMP and dTMP. When second or third phosphates are attached to nucleoside it produced nucleoside diphosphates like ADP, GDP, CDP, UDP, dADP, dGDP, dCDP and dTDP or nucleoside triphosphates like ATP, GTP, CTP, UTP, dATP, dGTP, dCTP and dTTP, respectively. The negative charges of the phosphate groups are responsible for anionic properties of nucleotides and nucleic acids.

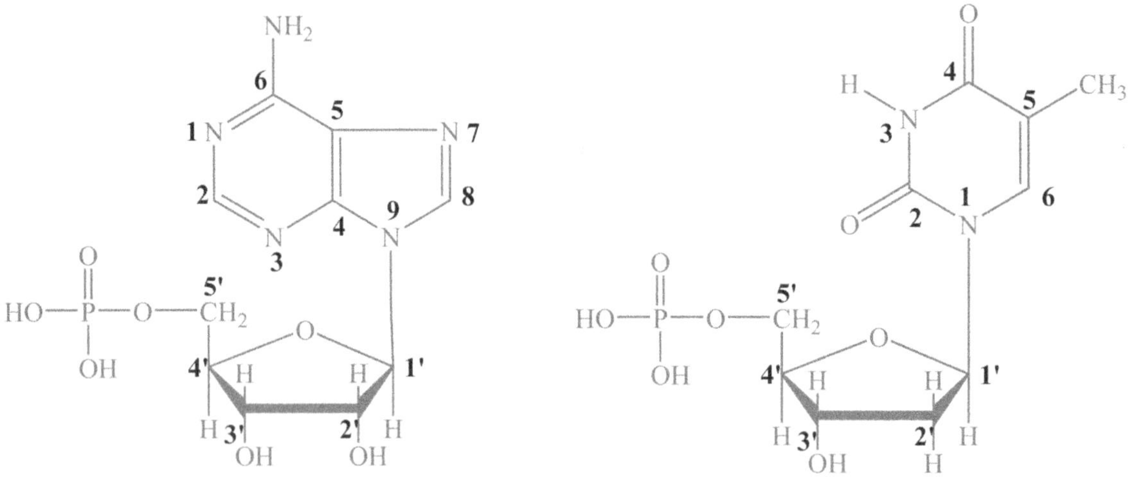

Adenosine monophosphate (AMP)

Deoxythymidine monophosphate (dTMP)

Biological Significance of Nucleic Acids

The various biological significance of nucleic acids are given under the following different headings.

(a) DNA

1. DNA is the chemical basis of heredity organized into genes. The fundamental unit of genetic information is gene.
2. DNA is regarded as the reserve bank of genetic information.
3. Over millions of years, identities of different species are maintained by DNA only.
4. In addition, DNA controls every aspect of cellular functions.
5. Through RNA mediation, gene controls the synthesis of proteins.
6. DNA is the precursor for the synthesis of RNA by a process called transcription.

(b) RNA

1. RNA is useful for the synthesis of protein by a process called translation.
2. To synthesize proteins, mRNA transfers genetic information from genes to ribosomes.
3. For protein synthesis, tRNA transfers amino acids to mRNA.
4. rRNA provides a structural framework for ribosomes.
5. hnRNA serves as a precursor for the synthesis of all RNAs including mRNA.
6. snRNA is involved in processing of mRNA.
7. snoRNA plays a major role in processing of rRNA.
8. scRNA is involved in the secretion of proteins for export.
9. In bacteria, tmRNA is mostly present and it facilitates the degradation of incorrectly synthesized proteins by adding short peptide tags to proteins.

(c) Ribozymes

Ribozymes are types of RNA which act as enzymes. Before the occurrence of protein enzymes during evolution, ribozymes were probably functioning as a catalyst. The following are the selected list of ribozymes and their corresponding biochemical reactions.

1. In protein synthesis rRNA is involved in peptide bond formation.
2. *Ribonuclease P (RNase P)* is a component of RNA and is a ribozyme containing protein. It is involved in cleavage of RNA particularly tRNA precursors to generate mature tRNA molecules. It is also involved in ligation.
3. Self-splicing RNA is involved in cleavage of DNA.
4. RNAs of spliceosome is involved in splicing of RNA.
5. *In vitro* selected RNAs are involved in RNA polymerization, RNA aminoacylation, RNA phosphorylation, redox reactions, glycoside bond formation and disulfide exchange.

(d) Nucleotides

1. Nucleotides are the monomeric unit or building blocks of nucleic acid.
2. Nucleotides are the structural components of some B-complex vitamin co-enzymes like FAD, NAD^+, etc.
3. ATP is one of the important nucleotides which is energy currency of the cell involved in energy reactions.
4. In addition, nucleotides also regulate the metabolic reactions.
5. Clinically some nucleotide analogs are used due to its pharmacological properties. They are,
   (a) Allopurinol is used in the treatment of gout and hyperuricemia.
   (b) Many nucleotide analogs are used in the treatment of cancers. **Example:** 6-Mercaptopurine, 5-fluorouracil, 3-deoxyuridine, 5-iodouracil, 5- or 6-azauridine, 5- or 6-azacytidine and arabinosylcytosine.
   (c) During transplantation azathioprine is used to suppress the immunological rejection of transplanted organs.
   (d) Neurological disease and viral encephalitis are treated by using arabinosyladenine.
   (e) Drugs like zidovudine, 3-azido-2′,3′-dideoxythymidine and didanosine are used in the treatment of AIDS.

Proteins

Proteins are the most abundant organic substances present in the living system. 50 % of the cellular dry weight is composed of proteins. Cell forms the fundamental basis of structure and functions of life. The term protein is obtained from Greek word "**proteios**" means "holding the first place (or) primary". In 1838, Dutch chemist Mulder used the term "protein" for high molecular weight nitrogen rich and most abundant substances present in plants and animals.

Proteins and peptides are polyamides composed of L-α-amino acids bonded in a head to tail manner through the carboxyl function of one amino acid with the amino function of other amino acid. The amide linkage is called a peptide bond. Hence, proteins are known as **polypeptides**. In other words, building blocks of peptides and proteins are composed of amino acids. By a variety of methods proteins undergo hydrolysis and cleaved i.e., hydrolyzed into their constituent amino acids. As proteins contain nitrogen also it acts as a major source of nitrogen to the biological system.

Peptide linkage (-CO-NH-) is formed when two or more amino acids are joined together, and a chain of many amino acids is called as polypeptide. One or more polypeptide molecules are present in proteins. Peptide bonds covalently link the amino acids. Every polypeptide contains two ends, in that one end is known as amino terminal or N-terminal which has a free amino group and conventionally it is present in the left-hand amino acid. The other end is known as carboxyl terminal or C-terminal which has a free carboxyl group and conventionally it is present in the right-hand amino acid. The above figure of tripeptide shows three amino acids linked by two peptide bonds.

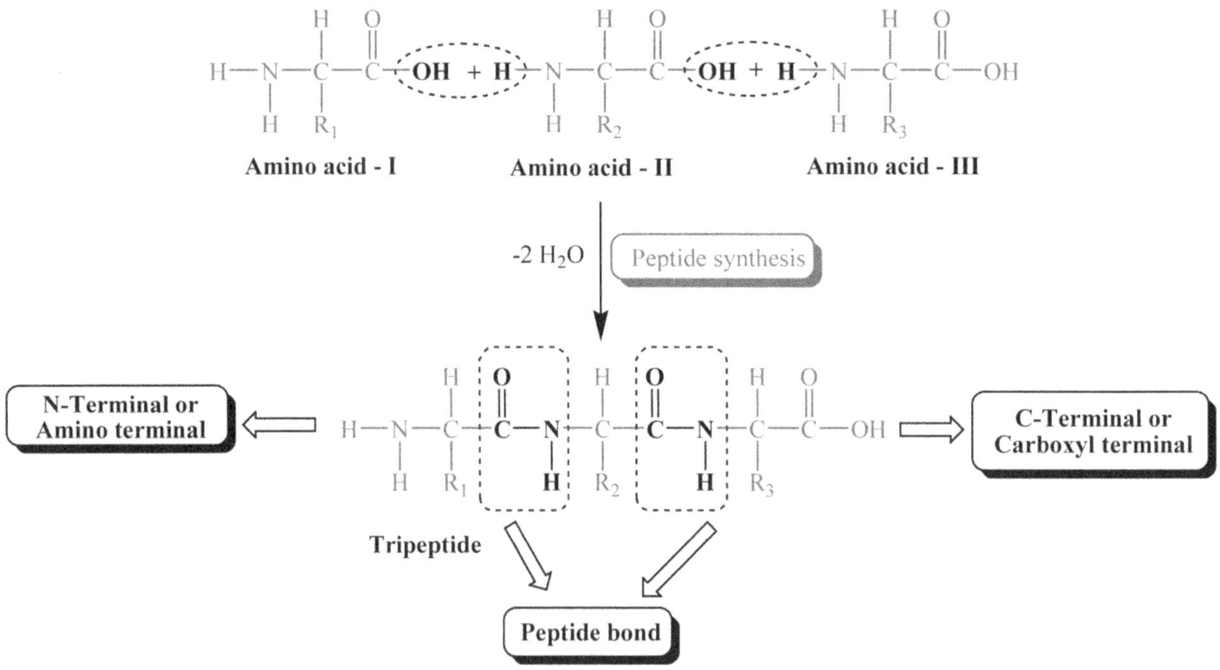

Amino acid - I   Amino acid - II   Amino acid - III

$-2\ H_2O$ Peptide synthesis

N-Terminal or Amino terminal   C-Terminal or Carboxyl terminal

Tripeptide

Peptide bond

Elemental composition of proteins: Five major elements are predominantly present in proteins. They are, a) Carbon (50 to 55 %), b) Hydrogen (6 to 7 %), c) Oxygen (19 to 24 %), d) Nitrogen (13 to 19 %), and e) Sulphur (0 to 4 %). The other elements such as phosphorous, iron, copper, iodine, magnesium, manganese, zinc, etc. are also present in proteins. On an average about 16 % nitrogen is present in proteins. Hence, Kjeldahl's method of nitrogen estimation in laboratory is used to estimate the amount of proteins present in biological fluids and foods.

Classification of Proteins

Proteins are classified in three different ways as follows,

1. Functional classification of proteins
2. Chemical nature and solubility classification of proteins
3. Nutritional classification of proteins

1. Functional Classification of Proteins

In this type of classification, proteins are broadly classified into nine different types according to its functions they perform. They are,

1. **Structural proteins:** These proteins are basis for cellular structure. **Example:** Keratin present in hair and nail, collagen present in bones, etc.
2. **Catalytic proteins or Enzyme proteins:** Proteins exhibit its function as enzyme comes in this category. **Example:** Almost all enzymes except ribosome, *glucokinase*, *pepsin*, etc.
3. **Transport proteins:** These proteins are useful for the transport of some compounds. **Example:** Hemoglobin used for transport of oxygen, serum albumin used for the transport of bilirubin, etc.
4. **Storage proteins:** Proteins are stored in one form in this type. **Example:** Ovalbumin is the storage form of protein in egg, glutelin is the storage form of protein in endosperm of certain seeds of the grass family, etc.
5. **Defense proteins:** These proteins perform defense function in biological system. **Example:** Snake venom is the defense protein of snake, immunoglobulin is the defense protein of human, etc.
6. **Hormonal proteins:** These proteins exhibit their function as hormones. **Example:** Insulin, growth hormone, etc.

7. **Receptor proteins:** Receptors are chemically proteins. **Example:** Receptors for hormones, receptors for viruses, etc.
8. **Genetic proteins:** These proteins involved in genetic functions. **Example:** Nucleoprotein.
9. **Contractile proteins:** This protein plays a role in muscle contraction. **Example:** Actin, myosin, etc.

2. **Chemical Nature and Solubility Classification of Proteins**

Proteins are classified into three major types on the basis of increasing complexity in their structure. They are,

1. Simple proteins
2. Conjugated or complex proteins and
3. Derived proteins

1. **Simple proteins:** These proteins on hydrolysis yield only α-amino acids. They are further classified into two major categories based on shape, solubility and digestion.
   A. Globular proteins
   B. Fibrous proteins

   A. **Globular proteins (Spheroproteins):** They are usually spherical or oval in shape, soluble in water and easily digestible. They are more highly branched and cross-linked condensation products of basic or acidic amino acids. As the globular proteins have diamino and dicarboxylic acids, branching and cross-linking takes place by the usual peptide linkage involving the second amino group of one amino acid and the second carboxyl group of another amino acid. The peptide chain is stabilized by intramolecular hydrogen bonds. They are further classified into several types based on their solubility.

   (i) **Albumins:** They are soluble in water, acids and alkalis and are coagulated by heat and precipitated by saturated solution of ammonium sulphate. These are usually deficient in glycine. **Example:** Serum albumin (blood), ovalbumin (egg white) and lactalbumin (milk).

   (ii) **Globulins:** They are insoluble in water, but soluble in dilute solutions of salt, strong inorganic acids and alkalis. They are coagulated by heat and precipitated by half saturating their solutions with ammonium sulphate. Generally, globulins contain glycine. **Example:** Serum globulin (blood), myosin (muscle), vitelline vegetable globulin and tissue globulin.

   (iii) **Glutelins:** They are insoluble in water and dilute salt solution, but soluble in dilute acids and alkalis. They are coagulated by heat, and are comparatively rich in arginine, proline and glutamic acid. **Example:** Glutenin (wheat) and oryzenin (rice).

   (iv) **Prolamins:** They are insoluble in water or salt solutions. But soluble in dilute acids, alkalis and 70-90 % ethyl alcohol. They contain large amounts of proline and are deficient in lysine. **Example:** Gliadin (wheat and rye), zein (corn), secaline (rye) and hordein (barley).

   (v) **Histones:** They are complex chemicals in nature, soluble in water or dilute acids but insoluble in dilute ammonia. They are not coagulated by heat. These are hydrolyzed by pepsin and trypsin. **Example:** Proteins of the nucleic acids and hemoglobin and thymus histones.

   (vi) **Globins:** These are also considered along with histones generally. However, globins are not basic proteins and are not precipitated by ammonium hydroxide.

   (vii) **Protamines:** They are soluble in water, dilute acids and dilute ammonia. These are more basic than the histones and have a simpler structure and found in sperm cells of certain fish. **Example:** Sturine (sturgeon), scombrine (mackerel), salmine (salmon) and clapeine (herring).

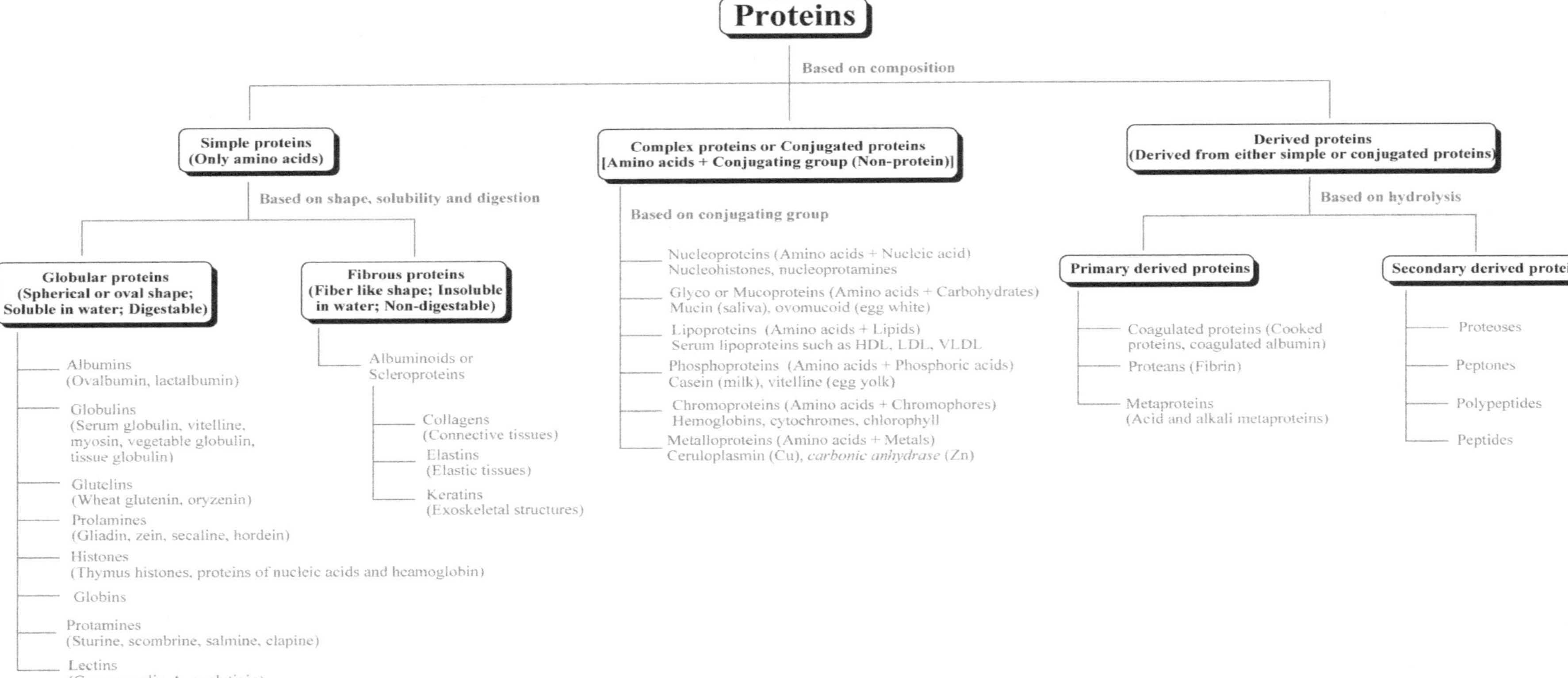
Proteins
Based on composition
Simple proteins (Only amino acids)
Complex proteins or Conjugated proteins [Amino acids + Conjugating group (Non-protein)]
Derived proteins (Derived from either simple or conjugated proteins)
Based on shape, solubility and digestion
Globular proteins (Spherical or oval shape; Soluble in water; Digestable)
Fibrous proteins (Fiber like shape; Insoluble in water; Non-digestable)
Albumins (Ovalbumin, lactalbumin)
Globulins (Serum globulin, vitelline, myosin, vegetable globulin, tissue globulin)
Glutelins (Wheat glutenin, oryzenin)
Prolamines (Gliadin, zein, secaline, hordein)
Histones (Thymus histones, proteins of nucleic acids and heamoglobin)
Globins
Protamines (Sturine, scombrine, salmine, clapine)
Lectins (Concanavalin-A, agglutinin)
Albuminoids or Scleroproteins
Collagens (Connective tissues)
Elastins (Elastic tissues)
Keratins (Exoskeletal structures)
Based on conjugating group
Nucleoproteins (Amino acids + Nucleic acid) Nucleohistones, nucleoprotamines
Glyco or Mucoproteins (Amino acids + Carbohydrates) Mucin (saliva), ovomucoid (egg white)
Lipoproteins (Amino acids + Lipids) Serum lipoproteins such as HDL, LDL, VLDL
Phosphoproteins (Amino acids + Phosphoric acids) Casein (milk), vitelline (egg yolk)
Chromoproteins (Amino acids + Chromophores) Hemoglobins, cytochromes, chlorophyll
Metalloproteins (Amino acids + Metals) Ceruloplasmin (Cu), carbonic anhydrase (Zn)
Based on hydrolysis
Primary derived proteins
Secondary derived proteins
Coagulated proteins (Cooked proteins, coagulated albumin)
Proteans (Fibrin)
Metaproteins (Acid and alkali metaproteins)
Proteoses
Peptones
Polypeptides
Peptides

(viii) **Lectins:** They are carbohydrate binding proteins and are involved in the interaction between cells and proteins. They help to maintain tissue and organ structures. In the laboratory they are used to purify carbohydrates by affinity chromatography. **Example:** Concanavalin-A and agglutinin.

B. **Fibrous proteins:** They are fiber like in shape, insoluble in water and resistant to digestion. They are formed by condensation of (neutral amino acids) monoamino monocarboxylic acids and there is a few or no branching. By intermolecular hydrogen bonds the linear protein chains are held together. Proteins that tend to be insoluble and strong play a structural role in organisms for support or protection. Scleroproteins or albuminoids are predominant group of fibrous proteins. They are insoluble in water and salt solution, but soluble in concentrated acids and alkalis. They are attacked by enzymes. **Example:** Keratin (from hair, nails, hooves, horns and feathers) and fibroin (silk). Albuminoids are sub-divided into three types.

(i) **Collagen:** It is the most common protein in the mammalian body. Found in skin, tendons and bones. They are attacked by pepsin and trypsin. When boiled with water, they form a water-soluble protein (gelatin).

(ii) **Elastin:** They are found in tendons, arteries and other elastic tissues. They are attacked slowly by trypsin.

(iii) **Keratins:** They are present in exoskeletal structures. **Example:** Hairs, nails and horns. Human hair contains as much as 14 % cysteine.

2. **Conjugated proteins:** Upon hydrolysis they yield α-amino acids and non-proteinous substances. They contain simple protein molecules linked with a non-protein substance. The non-proteinous moiety is referred as **prosthetic group.** On the basis of prosthetic group present in it, they are subdivided as follows.

A. **Nucleoproteins:** The prosthetic group present in nucleoprotein is a nucleic acid. **Example:** Nucleohistones and nucleoprotamines.

B. **Glycoproteins (mucoproteins):** They are produced by adding sugar residues through O-glycoside linkages to the hydroxyl groups of serine and threonine residues or via N -glycoside linkages to the amino group of asparagine. The prosthetic group present in glycoprotein is a carbohydrate or a derivative of carbohydrate. **Example:** Mucin of saliva and ovomucoid of egg white.

C. **Lipoproteins:** They have the phosphorylated hydroxyl groups of serine or threonine. The prosthetic group present in lipoprotein is phospholipid (a class of fat). **Example:** Lipoproteins of serum such as HDL, LDL and VLDL.

D. **Phosphoproteins:** The prosthetic group present in phosphoprotein is phosphoric acid. **Example:** Casein of milk and vitelline of egg yolk.

E. **Chromoproteins:** They contain colored prosthetic group, due to the presence of a metal in their structure. **Example:** Hemoglobin (in which heme is prosthetic group and globin is the protein), chlorophyll and cytochromes.

F. **Metalloproteins:** They contain metal ions such as Zn, Co, Fe, Mg, Cu, etc. as prosthetic group. **Example:** Copper in ceruloplasmin and zinc in *carbonic anhydrase.*

3. **Derived proteins:** These proteins are generally derived from either simple proteins or conjugated proteins. They are the products obtained by the action of heat, chemical or enzymatic agents on natural proteins. The derived proteins (intermediate hydrolysis products) are further classified on the basis of progressive cleavage into two major types.

A. Primary derived proteins

B. Secondary derived proteins

A. **Primary derived proteins:** These proteins are the first hydrolyzed products of either simple proteins or conjugated proteins. They are,

(i) **Coagulated proteins:** These are denaturated proteins. They are insoluble proteins, formed by the action of heat on proteins. **Example:** Cooked proteins and coagulated egg white albumin.

(ii) **Proteans:** These are the earliest products of protein hydrolysis by enzymes, dilute acids, alkalis, etc. These proteins are insoluble in water. **Example:** Fibrin obtained from fibrinogen.

(iii) **Metaproteins:** These are second stage products of protein hydrolysis obtained by treatment with slightly stronger acids and alkalis. They are insoluble in water, dilute salt solution and soluble in acids or alkalis. They are precipitated by half-saturation with ammonium sulphate. **Example:** Acid and alkali metaproteins.

B. **Secondary derived proteins:** These proteins are the progressive hydrolytic products of protein hydrolysis. **Example:** Proteoses, peptones, polypeptides and peptides.

3. **Nutritional Classification of Proteins**

Proteins are broadly classified into three major types based on their nutritive value as follows,

1. Complete proteins
2. Partially incomplete proteins
3. Incomplete proteins

1. **Complete proteins:**

Body required proportion of all ten essential amino acids are present in complete proteins. These proteins generally promote good growth in the body. **Example:** Egg albumin and milk casein.

2. **Partially incomplete proteins:**

One or more essential amino acids are partially lacking in these proteins. These proteins generally promote moderate growth in the body. **Example:** Rice proteins and wheat proteins which are partially lacking essential amino acids such as lysine and threonine.

3. **Incomplete proteins:**

One or more essential amino acids are completely lacking in these proteins. These proteins generally do not promote growth in the body. **Example:** Gelatin which completely lacks tryptophan and zein which completely lacks tryptophan and lysine.

Biological Significance of Proteins

Proteins possess diverse specialized and essential biological functions. These functions are broadly categorized into two categories as,

1. Structural or static function
2. Dynamic function

1. **Structural or static functions of proteins:**

Proteins play a major role in the structure and strength of the biological system due to their brick and mortar roles. **Example:** Some proteins like collagen and elastin in bone matrix, vascular system and other organs and keratin in epidermal tissues such as hair and nail act as biological structural materials.

2. **Dynamic functions of proteins:**

Dynamic functions of proteins are more diversified in nature. In general, the dynamic functions of proteins are approximately regarded as the working horses of the cell. The followings are the various dynamic functions performed by proteins.

1. Enzymes are made up of proteins, which catalyzes the biological reactions. **Example:** Almost all enzymes except ribosome, *glucokinase*, pepsin, etc.
2. Few proteins are useful for the transport of some compounds. **Example:** Hemoglobin used for transport of oxygen, serum albumin used for the transport of bilirubin, etc.
3. Proteins also performs storage function by stored in one form. **Example:** Ovalbumin is the storage form of protein in egg, glutelin is the storage form of protein in endosperm of certain seeds of the grass family, etc.
4. Some of the proteins perform defense function in biological system. **Example:** Snake venom is the defense protein of snake, immunoglobulin is the defense protein of human, etc.

5. Hormones are proteins which regulate various metabolic processes. **Example:** Insulin maintains blood sugar level and growth hormone maintains growth.
6. Receptors are chemically proteins. **Example:** Receptors for hormone, receptors for viruses, etc.
7. During cell division, genetic message is transmitted through nucleoproteins which is an important constituent of nucleic acids. **Example:** Nucleoproteins.
8. Some protein plays a role in muscle contraction. **Example:** Actin, myosin, etc.
9. Antibodies which makes immunity of the body for resistance to diseases are formed from blood proteins.
10. Blood clotting factors are protein in nature.
11. Immunoglobulins are also protein in nature and involved in immune functions.

Amino Acids

Amino acid is defined as a group of organic compounds possessing two functional groups namely carboxylic acid (COOH) and amino (NH_2) group. The amino group is attached at α-position of carboxylic acid or both carboxyl group and amino groups are attached to the same carbon, hence it is known as **α-amino acids**. The carboxylic acid group is acidic in nature and the amino group is basic in nature. General structure of amino acid is given below.

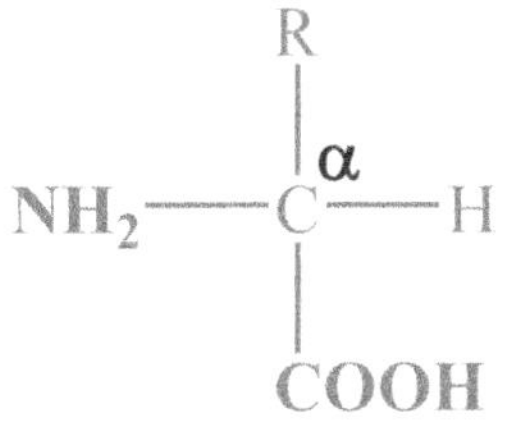

R
|
NH_2—C^{α}—H
|
COOH

General structure of L-α-amino acid

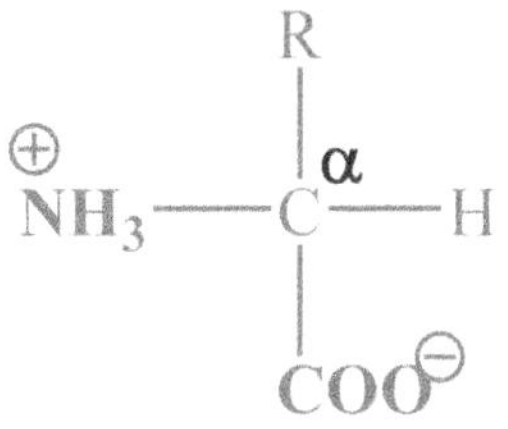

R
|
$\overset{\oplus}{NH_3}$—C^{α}—H
|
$COO^{\ominus}$

Amino acid exist as ion

Where α indicates position of amino group and L indicates configuration of amino acids [amino group present on left side]. If it is present on right side it is known as D-amino acid.

Classification of Amino Acids

Amino acids are classified in four different ways as follows,

1. Structural or chemical classification of amino acids
2. Nutritional classification of amino acids
3. Polarity classification of amino acids
4. Metabolic fate classification of amino acids

1. Structural or Chemical Classification of Amino Acids

It is one of the important classification method of amino acids. In this method twenty amino acids present in proteins are classified into seven different types based on its structure and chemical nature. A three letter or one letter symbol is assigned for each and every twenty amino acids present in proteins. In protein structure, these symbols are generally used to denote the amino acids (Table 1.5).

I. Aliphatic amino acids: These amino acids are chemically monoamino mono carboxylic acids. They are further divided into two types based on the presence of branching as follows.

(a) Un-branched aliphatic amino acids: No branch is present in aliphatic chain. **Example:** Glycine and alanine.

(b) Branched aliphatic amino acids: These amino acids contain branches in aliphatic chain. Leucine, isoleucine, and valine are sometimes called "branched-chain amino acids" (BCAA)

Table 1.5 Structural or chemical classification of amino acids.

S. No.	Name	Additional structural features present	Chemical structure	Reasoning for name	Three letters symbols	One letter symbol
I. Aliphatic amino acids						
1	Glycine	Un-branched aliphatic chain	$H—CH(NH_2)—COOH$	From the Greek word "Glukus" meaning sweet, because it was first isolated from gelatin	Gly	G
2	Alanine		$CH_3—CH(NH_2)—COOH$	"Al" is a shortening of aldehyde. The infix "an" was added to make it easier to pronounce	Ala	A
3	Valine	Branched aliphatic chain	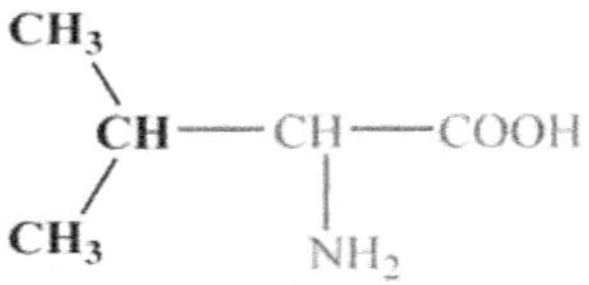 $(CH_3)_2CH—CH(NH_2)—COOH$	Named in 1906 after a type of acid that occurs in the roots of the "valerian" plant	Val	V
4	Leucine		$(CH_3)_2CH—CH_2—CH(NH_2)—COOH$	First used in 1826 by chemist William Henry comes from the Greek word "leukos" meaning "white"	Leu	L
5	Isoleucine		$CH_3—CH_2—CH(CH_3)—CH(NH_2)—COOH$	Named in 1904 by Felix Ehrlich, who observed that it was similar but not identical to leucine	Ile	I
II. Hydroxyl group containing amino acids						
6	Serine	Hydroxyl group	$CH_2(OH)—CH(NH_2)—COOH$	From the Latin word "sericum" meaning "silk", because it was first obtained from silk protein	Ser	S
7	Threonine		$CH_3—CH(OH)—CH(NH_2)—COOH$	Named in 1936 after threose, a type of monosaccharide that it was thought to resemble	Thr	T
	Tyrosine		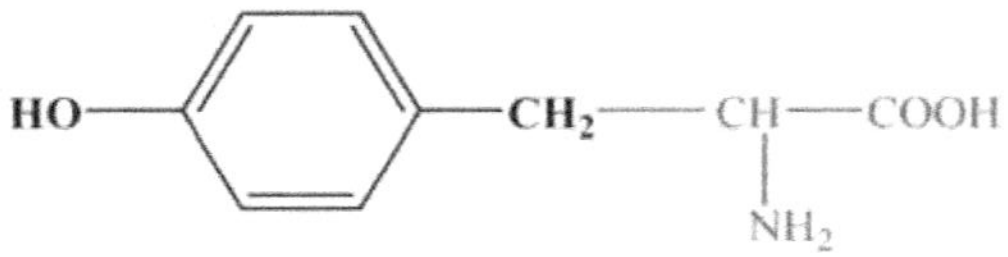 $HO—C_6H_4—CH_2—CH(NH_2)—COOH$	From Greek "tyros" meaning "cheese", because it was obtained from old cheese	Tyr	Y

Table 1.5 Contd...

S. No.	Name	Additional structural features present	Chemical structure	Reasoning for name	Three letters symbols	One letter symbol
III. Sulphur group containing amino acids						
8	Cysteine	Sulfhydryl group	$CH_2(SH)—CH(NH_2)—COOH$	Had an earlier spelling of cystine. That comes from the ancient Greek word for "bladder", "kustis"	Cys	C
	Cystine	Disulfide group	$CH_2—CH(NH_2)—COOH$ | S | S | $CH_2—CH(NH_2)—COOH$		-	-
9	Methionine	Thioether linkage	$CH_2(S—CH_3)—CH_2—CH(NH_2)—COOH$	Coined in 1926 by Barger and Coyne as a contraction of γ-methiol-α-aminobutyric acid	Met	M
IV. Acidic amino acids and their amides						
10	Aspartic acid	β-Carboxyl group	$\overset{\beta}{CH_2}(COOH)—\overset{\alpha}{CH}(NH_2)—COOH$	Named after asparagine, because it was first isolated from it by hydrolysis in 1827	Asp	D
11	Glutamic acid	γ-Carboxyl group	$\overset{\gamma}{CH_2}(COOH)—\overset{\beta}{CH_2}—\overset{\alpha}{CH}(NH_2)—COOH$	"Glut" refers how the compound was first isolated from gluten in 1866 by chemist Karl Rithausen	Glu	E
12	Asparagine	Amide group	$CH_2(CONH_2)—CH(NH_2)—COOH$	First extracted in 1806 from a sample of "asparagus" juice, after which it was named	Asn	N
13	Glutamine		$CH_2(CONH_2)—CH_2—CH(NH_2)—COOH$	Named before it was isolated, because it was hypothesized to be similar to glutamic acid	Gln	Q

Table 1.5 *Contd...*

S. No.	Name	Additional structural features present	Chemical structure	Reasoning for name	Three letters symbols	One letter symbol
V. Basic amino acids						
14	Lysine	ε-Amino group	ε: $CH_2(NH_2)$ — δ, γ, β: $(CH_2)_3$ — α: $CH(NH_2)$ — $COOH$	Named in 1889 from the ancient Greek word "lusis" meaning "loosening"	Lys	K
15	Arginine	Guanidino group	NH_2—C(=NH)—NH—$(CH_2)_3$—$CH(NH_2)$—$COOH$	From the Greek word "arginoeis" meaning "silver", due to the appearance of silver nitrate	Arg	R
16	Histidine	Imidazole ring	Imidazole ring (HN, N)—CH_2—$CH(NH_2)$—$COOH$	From Greek "histos" meaning "tissue", because it was thought to be important to tissue function	His	H
VI. Aromatic amino acids						
17	Phenylalanine	Phenyl ring	Benzene ring—CH_2—$CH(NH_2)$—$COOH$	Named by Erlenmeyer and Lipp in 1883 because it looks like alanine with a phenyl group	Phe	F
18	Tyrosine	Phenol analog	HO—benzene ring—CH_2—$CH(NH_2)$—$COOH$	From Greek "tyros" meaning "cheese", because it was obtained from old cheese	Tyr	Y
19	Tryptophan	Indole ring	Indole ring (N—H)—CH_2—$CH(NH_2)$—$COOH$	Traces to the Greek roots "tripsis" meaning "rubbing", and "phainein" meaning "to show"	Trp	W
VII. Imino acids						
20	Proline	Pyrrolidine ring	Pyrrolidine ring (N—H) with $COOH$	The name is a contraction of pyrrolidine, which makes up a side chain of the compound	Pro	P

because human beings cannot survive unless these amino acids are present in the diet. The combination of these three amino acids makes up approximately one-third of skeletal muscle in the human body. **Example:** Valine, leucine and isoleucine.

II. **Hydroxyl group containing amino acids:** These amino acids contain hydroxyl group in their structure. **Example:** Serine, threonine and tyrosine. In general, aromatic ring is present in tyrosine. Hence tyrosine is usually considered as aromatic amino acid and not as hydroxyl group containing amino acid.

III. **Sulphur containing amino acids:** These amino acids contain sulphur atom in their structure. **Example:** Cysteine (contain sulfhydryl group), cystine (formed by condensation of two molecules of cysteine and contain disulfide group) and methionine (contain thioether group).

IV. **Acidic amino acids and their amides:** These amino acids are generally dicarboxylic mono amino acids. They are highly acidic in character. These amino acids in general possess different codons for their incorporation into proteins. **Example:** Aspartic acid & glutamic acid are acidic amino acids and asparagine and glutamine are their corresponding amides.

V. **Basic amino acids:** These amino acids are generally dibasic monocarboxylic acids. They are highly basic in character. **Example:** Lysine and arginine (possess guanidine group) and histidine (possess imidazole ring).

VI. **Aromatic amino acids:** These amino acids are generally contains aromatic ring in their structure. **Example:** Phenylalanine and tyrosine (contain phenyl ring), tryptophan (contain indole ring) and histidine (contain imidazole ring).

VII. **Imino acids:** These amino acids generally contain imino group i.e., =NH instead of amino (NH_2) group in their structure. **Example:** Proline. Histidine, tryptophan and proline are considered as heterocyclic amino acids also as they have heterocyclic ring in their structure.

2. **Nutritional Classification of Amino Acids**

More than two hundred amino acids have been isolated and identified but only twenty-five are obtained from typical proteins, in turn only twenty amino acids are generally found in all proteins. Except other biological functions these twenty amino acids are needed for the synthesis of many proteins. But it is not necessary to take all these twenty amino acids in diet because some of the amino acids are biosynthesized in the biological system. Based on the dietary requirements of amino acids it is broadly classified into two major types as follows.

(a) **Essential amino acids:** Among the twenty amino acids, ten are called as essential amino acids. These amino acids **cannot be synthesized by the body** and must be supplied by dietary sources. They are also called as **indispensable amino acids.** Deficiency in any one of the essential amino acid prevents growth and may even cause death. Although there are ten essential amino acids to man, eight are more important, viz methionine, tryptophan, threonine, valine, isoleucine, leucine, phenylalanine and lysine. Two amino acids are less important namely arginine and histidine because it is partly synthesized by the body (To remember these ten essential amino acids, it can be mentioned as **MATT VIL PHLY** which corresponds to **M**ethionine, **A**rginine, **T**ryptophan, **T**heronine, **V**aline, **I**soleucine, **L**eucine, **P**henylalanine, **H**istidine and **LY**sine).

(b) **Non-essential amino acids:** The other ten amino acids are called as **non-essential amino acids** or **dispensable amino acids** and are **synthesized by the body.** Hence no need to take by dietary sources. The non-essential amino acids are alanine, asparagine, aspartic acid, cysteine, glutamine, glutamic acid, glycine, proline, serine and tyrosine.

3. **Polarity Classification of Amino Acids**

Based on their polarity, amino acids are broadly classified into four major types.

(a) **Non-polar amino acids:** Also known as hydrophobic amino acids because of its water hating property. These amino acids don't have any charge on "R" group. **Example:** Alanine, leucine, isoleucine, valine, methionine, phenylalanine, tryptophan and proline.

(b) **Polar amino acids with no charge on "R" group:** These amino acids don't have any charge on "R" group but having other polar groups such as hydroxyl, sulfhydryl and amide group leads to hydrogen bonding. **Example:** Glycine, serine, threonine, cysteine, glutamine, asparagine and tyrosine.

(c) **Polar amino acids with positive charge on "R" group:** These amino acids have positive charge on "R" group which makes them as polar. **Example:** Lysine, arginine and histidine.

(d) **Polar amino acids with negative charge on "R" group:** These amino acids have negative charge on "R" group which makes them as polar. **Example:** Aspartic acid and glutamic acid.

4. **Fate of Metabolism of Amino Acids Classification**

Amino acids are broadly classified into three types based on their fate of metabolism because the carbon skeleton of amino acids can serve as a precursor for the synthesis of carbohydrates (glucogenic) or fat (ketogenic) or both.

(a) **Glucogenic amino acids:** The amino acids serve as a precursor for the synthesis of carbohydrates such as glucose or glycogen are called as glucogenic amino acids. **Example:** Alanine, glycine, valine, serine, cysteine, methionine, arginine, threonine, histidine, aspartic acid, asparagine, glutamic acid, glutamine and proline.

(b) **Ketogenic amino acids:** The amino acids which serve especially as a precursor for the synthesis of fat are called as ketogenic amino acids. **Example:** Leucine and lysine.

(c) **Glucogenic and ketogenic amino acids:** The amino acids which serve as a precursor for the synthesis of both carbohydrates and fat are called as glucogenic and ketogenic amino acids. **Example:** Isoleucine, phenylalanine, tryptophan and tyrosine.

Nomenclature of Amino Acids

Trivial or common names are available for all the amino acids. These names are given some times based on the source from which they were first isolated. **Example:** Asparagine was first found in asparagus, glutamate in wheat gluten; tyrosine in cheese (In Greek *tyros*, means "cheese"). Sometime the names are given based on their taste. **Example:** Glycine (In Greek "*glykos*", means "sweet") was so named because of its sweet taste.

The amino acids are named in the IUPAC system, as amino derivatives of the corresponding acid with the position of the amino group defined by an appropriate number. The C-1 would be carboxyl carbon of an amino acid and the C-2 would be α-carbon, the C-3, C-4, C-5 and C-6 would be β, γ, δ and ε-carbon, respectively. The Greek lettering system is confusing in some cases, such as amino acids with heterocyclic R groups. Hence, generally the numbering system is used.

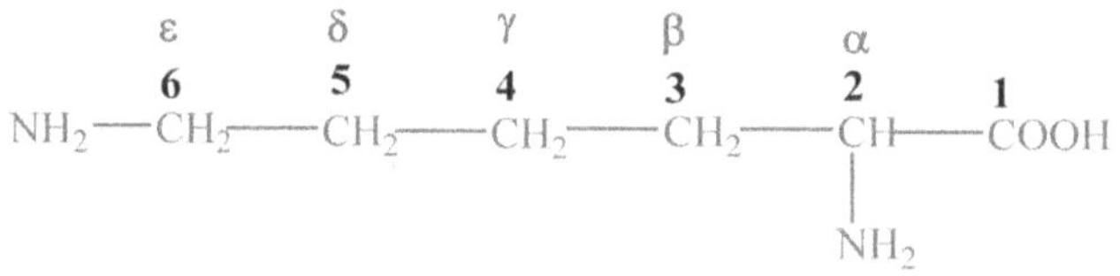

$$\overset{\varepsilon}{\underset{6}{}}\quad\overset{\delta}{\underset{5}{}}\quad\overset{\gamma}{\underset{4}{}}\quad\overset{\beta}{\underset{3}{}}\quad\overset{\alpha}{\underset{2}{}}\quad 1$$

$$NH_2-CH_2-CH_2-CH_2-CH_2-\underset{\underset{NH_2}{|}}{CH}-COOH$$

2, 6-Diamino heptanoic acid

Biological Significance of Amino Acids

Biological significance of amino acids explained under two sub divisions as follows.

(a) **Standard amino acids:**

The 20 amino acids present in proteins are known as standard amino acids which performs several biological functions as follows.

1. 4-Hydroxyproline and 5-hydroxylysine are the major constituents of the most abundant protein in mammals i.e., collagen.
2. Many methylated or acetylated or phosphorylated amino acids are present in the histones in association with DNA.
3. γ-Carboxyglutamic acid present in certain plasma protein is participated in blood clotting process.

(b) Non-standard amino acids:

There are several amino acids present in nature beyond 20 standard amino acids which are present in proteins. These amino acids are commonly known as non-standard amino acids or non-protein amino acids which performs some biologically important functions. They are,

1. Creatinine is derived from muscle and excreted in urine.
2. In biological system methyl group is donated by S-adenosylmethionine (SAM).
3. Thyroxine and triiodothyronine are thyroid hormones derived from tyrosine.
4. In the metabolism of threonine, aspartate and methionine, homoserine is the intermediate.
5. DOPA is a neurotransmitter which serves as a precursor for the synthesis of melanin pigment.
6. Ornithine, citrulline and arginosuccinate are intermediates in the urea biosynthesis.
7. Ovothiol is the sulphur containing amino acids found in fertilized eggs which acts as an antioxidant.
8. In methionine metabolism, homocysteine is the intermediate which is a risk factor for coronary heart diseases.
9. Azaserine is used as anticancer agent and cycloserine is used as antitubercular drug.
10. β-Alanine is the component of vitamins such as pantothenic acid and co-enzyme A.
11. The end product of pyrimidine metabolism is β-aminoisobutyric acid.
12. Taurine is found in association with bile acids.
13. From glutamic acid the neuro transmitter GABA is biosynthesized.
14. In the synthesis of porphyrin and heme, δ-aminolevulinic acid (ALA) is the intermediate.
15. D-Penicillamine effectively chelates copper and is chemically D-dimethylglycine. It is a metabolite of penicillin and is used in the chelation therapy of Wilson's disease.
16. N-Acetylcysteine is used in cystic fibrosis and chronic renal insufficiency due to its antioxidant property.
17. Gabapentin is chemically γ-aminobutyrate linked to cyclohexane used in the treatment of convulsion.

Bioenergetics (or) Biochemical Thermodynamics

Role of high energy compounds in biological process and basic knowledge of bioenergetics is very useful for better understanding of biological oxidation.

Study of energy changes (utilization and transfer) in biochemical reaction is termed as bioenergetics or biochemical thermodynamics. In bioenergetics mechanism of chemical reaction is not concerned but it concerned about the initial and final states of energy components of reactants. Based on energy released or consumed in biochemical reaction it was broadly classified into two types. They are,

1. **Exergonic reaction:** In this type biochemical reaction energy is released. ΔG^o value of this reaction is negative and the reactions will take place spontaneously. Almost all catabolic reactions are exergonic reactions. **Example:** Breakdown of ATP into ADP and inorganic phosphate liberates 7.3 Cal/mol energy.

$$ATP + H_2O \longrightarrow ADP + Pi \qquad (\Delta G^o = -7.3 \text{ Cal/mol})$$

2. **Endergonic reaction:** In this biochemical reaction energy is consumed or utilized by the reactants. It needs energy; hence, energy must be supplied. ΔG^o value of this reaction is positive and the reactions will not take place spontaneously. Almost all anabolic reactions, muscle contraction, nervous excitation, etc. are good examples for endergonic reactions. **Example:** Synthesis of ATP from ADP and inorganic phosphate. This reaction occurs only when 7.3 Cal/mol energy is supplied at least.

$$ADP + Pi \longrightarrow ATP + H_2O \quad (\Delta G^O = +7.3 \text{ Cal/mol})$$

Terms used in Bioenergetics

To understand the bioenergetics reactions, it is necessary to know about the following terms

1. Free energy
2. Enthalpy
3. Entropy

1. **Free energy:** It is defined as the energy actually available for utilization or to do work. The feasibility of chemical reaction is predicted valuably using changes in free energy and is represented by the symbol "ΔG". If the reaction is accompanied by decrease in free energy then the reaction can occur spontaneously.

   Standard free energy change: It is defined as the free energy change when the reactants or products are at a concentration of 1 mol/*l* at pH 7.0. This standard free energy is denoted by the symbol "ΔG°".

   The free energy change (ΔG) may be either,

   (a) **Negative free energy change:** In a chemical reaction if there is a loss of free energy then ΔG is represented by negative sign and the reaction is called as exergonic reaction and the reaction proceeds spontaneously. Free energy changes of almost all catabolic reactions possess negative sign only. **Example:** Breakdown of ATP into ADP and inorganic phosphate liberates 7.3 Cal/mol energy.

   $$ATP + H_2O \longrightarrow ADP + Pi \quad (\Delta G^\circ = -7.3 \text{ Cal/mol})$$

   (b) **Positive free energy change:** In a chemical reaction if free energy is supplied then the ΔG is represented by positive sign and the reaction is called as endergonic reaction and the reaction does not proceed spontaneously. Free energy changes of almost all anabolic reactions possess positive sign only. **Example:** Synthesis of ATP from ADP and inorganic phosphate and the reaction occurs only when 7.3 Cal/mol energy is supplied at least.

   $$ADP + Pi \longrightarrow ATP + H_2O \quad (\Delta G^\circ = +7.3 \text{ Cal/mol})$$

   (c) **Zero free energy change:** In a chemical reaction ΔG becomes zero when it is at equilibrium.

   $$A \rightleftharpoons B \quad (\Delta G^\circ = 0)$$

   The free energy change (ΔG) is generally dependent on the actual concentrations of reactants and products at a constant temperature and pressure. Consider the below reaction in which reactant "A" is converted to product "B".

   $$\underset{\text{(Reactant)}}{A} \longrightarrow \underset{\text{(Product)}}{B}$$

   The following mathematical relationship can be derived when the reactant "A" is converted to product "B".

   $$\Delta G = \Delta G^\circ + RT\, ln \frac{[B]}{[A]}$$

   Where,

   ΔG = Free energy change
   ΔG° = Standard free energy change
   R = 1.987 Cal / mol (Gas constant)
   T = Absolute temperature in Kelvin (273 + °C)

ln = Natural logarithm
[B] = Concentration of product
[A] = Concentration of reactant

When reaction is at equilibrium then the free energy change is zero i.e., $\Delta G = 0$. Substitute the value of ΔG in above equation.

$$0 = \Delta G^o + RT\ ln\frac{[B]_{eq}}{[A]_{eq}}$$

Therefore, $$\Delta G^o = -RT\ ln\frac{[B]_{eq}}{[A]_{eq}}$$

Where, K_{eq} = Equilibrium constant

The free energy change (ΔG) is an additive value for pathways. A series of reactions are often involved in biochemical pathways. In such reaction the free energy change (ΔG) is an additive value. Whether the particular pathway will proceed or not is crucially determined by the sum of the free energy change (ΔG). The pathway can operate when the sum of the free energy change (ΔG) is negative even though some of the individual reactions may have positive free energy change (ΔG).

2. **Enthalpy:** It is a measure of the change in the heat content of the reactants compared to products. It is denoted by the symbol "ΔH". During the thermodynamic reaction either the heat may be released or absorbed. Based on this the chemical reactions are broadly classified into two major types as,
   (a) **Exothermic reaction:** During a chemical reaction if the heat is released then the reaction is said to be exothermic reaction. **Example:** Sodium hydroxide dissolved in water.
   (b) **Endothermic reaction:** During a chemical reaction if the heat is absorbed then the reaction is said to be endothermic reaction. **Example:** Benedict's test, Fehling's test, etc.
3. **Entropy:** It is the change in the randomness or disorder of reactants and products. It is usually represented by "ΔS". When the reaction attains equilibrium, entropy attains a maximum. In general, temporary decrease in entropy was observed in the reactions of biological systems.

Relationship between the change of Free Energy, Enthalpy and Entropy

The relationship between the change of free energy, enthalpy and entropy is expressed in the below mentioned equation.

$$\Delta G = \Delta H - T\Delta S$$

Where,

ΔG = Free energy change

ΔH = Enthalpy

T = Absolute temperature in Kelvin (273 + °C)

ΔS = Entropy

Redox Potential

Redox potential is otherwise known as oxidation-reduction potential. A quantitative measure of the tendency of a redox pair to lose or gain electrons is known as redox potential. Specific standard redox potential (E_o Volts) is assigned to each redox pair based on their tendency to lose or gain electrons at 25 °C and pH 7.0. The redox potential (E_o) is directly related to the change in the free energy (ΔG^o).

The specific standard redox potential (E_o) may be either positive or negative. More negative redox potential (E_o Volts) indicates greater tendency of reductant to lose electrons and a more positive redox potential (E_o Volts) indicates greater tendency of oxidant to accept electrons. Generally, the electrons flow from a redox pair with more negative redox potential (E_o Volts) to another redox pair with more positive redox potential (E_o Volts). Specific standard redox potential (E_o volts) of various redox pair system is summarized in Table 1.6.

Table 1.6 Specific standard redox potential (E_o Volts) of various redox pair system.

S. No	Redox pair	E_o in Volts
1	Succinate / α-ketoglutarate	- 0.67
2	$2H^+ / H_2$	- 0.42
3	$NADH + H^+ / NAD^+$	- 0.32
4	$NADP^+ / NADP + H^+$	- 0.32
5	FMN / $FMNH_2$ (Enzyme bound)	- 0.30
6	Lipoate (ox / red)	- 0.29
7	FAD / $FADH_2$	- 0.22
8	Pyruvate / Lactate	- 0.19
9	Fumarate / succinate	+ 0.03
10	Cytochrome b (Fe^{3+} / Fe^{2+})	+ 0.07
11	Coenzyme Q (ox / red)	+ 0.10
12	Cytochrome c_1 (Fe^{3+} / Fe^{2+})	+ 0.23
13	Cytochrome c (Fe^{3+} / Fe^{2+})	+ 0.25
14	Cytochrome a (Fe^{3+} / Fe^{2+})	+ 0.29
15	½ O_2 / H_2O	+ 0.82

Energy Rich Compounds

It is otherwise known as high energy compounds or high energy phosphates. In the biological systems certain compounds on hydrolysis yield energy. Energy rich compounds or high energy compounds are substances which possess sufficient free energy to liberate at least 7 Cal/mol at pH 7.0. Energy rich compounds are otherwise known as high energy compounds. Compared to hydrolysis of ATP into ADP and inorganic phosphates, all the high energy compounds liberate more energy when undergo hydrolysis. High energy compounds except acetyl CoA generally contains phosphate group in their structure, hence it is also known as high energy phosphates. **Example:** Phosphoenol pyruvate, carbamoyl phosphate, cAMP, 1,3-bisphosphoglycerate, phosphocreatine, acetyl phosphate, S-adenosylmethionine (SAM), pyrophosphate (PPi), acetyl CoA and ATP.

Table 1.7 The standard free energy (ΔG°) liberated during hydrolysis of some important compounds.

S. No	Compounds Name	ΔG° (in Cal / mol)
High energy phosphates or High energy compounds		
1	Phosphoenol pyruvate	- 14.8
2	Carbamoyl phosphate	- 12.3
3	cAMP	- 12.0
4	1,3-Bisphosphoglycerate	- 11.8
5	Phosphocreatine	- 10.3
6	Acetyl phosphate	- 10.3
7	S-Adenosylmethionine (SAM; Sulfonium compound)	- 10.0
8	Pyrophosphate (PPi)	- 8.0
9	Acetyl CoA (Thioester)	- 7.7
10	ATP (Breakdown into ADP & inorganic phosphate)	- 7.3

Table 1.7 *Contd...*

S. No	Compounds Name	ΔG° (in Cal / mol)
Low energy phosphates or Low energy compounds		
11	ADP (Breakdown into AMP & inorganic phosphate)	- 6.6
12	Glucose-1-phosphate	- 5.0
13	Fructose-1-phosphate	- 3.8
14	Glucose-6-phosphate	- 3.3
15	Glycerol-3-phosphate	- 2.2

Compounds which liberate less than 7.0 Cal/mol (which is lower than hydrolysis of ATP into ADP and inorganic phosphate) are referred as low energy phosphates or low energy compounds. **Example:** ADP, glucose-1-phosphate, fructose-1-phosphate, glucose-6-phosphate and glycerol-3-phosphate. The standard free energy liberated during hydrolysis of some important compounds is summarized in Table 1.7.

Classification of High Energy Compounds

High energy compounds are broadly classified into five major types according to type of bonds present in their structure. They are,

1. Pyrophosphate
2. Acyl phosphate
3. Enol phosphate
4. Thioester or thiol ester
5. Phosphagens or guanidino phosphate

Acid anhydride bonds particularly phospho anhydride bonds are high energy bonds which are usually present in all high energy compounds. Condensation of two acidic groups or related compounds generally produces this acid anhydride bonds. These bonds liberate free energy when it undergoes hydrolysis; hence it is known as high energy bonds. The symbol '~' is used by Lipmann to represent high energy bonds. ATP is instantly written as AMP-P-P. The various examples and bonds present in different classes of high energy compounds are summarized in Table 1.8.

Table 1.8 High energy compounds.

S. No	Class	Type of bond present	Example
1	Pyrophosphate	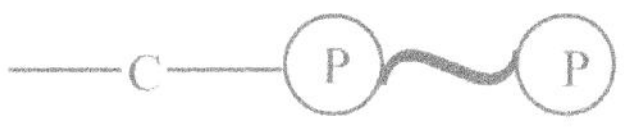 —C—(P)~(P)	Pyrophosphate, ATP
2	Acyl phosphate	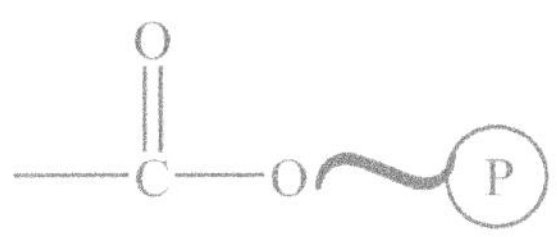 —C(=O)—O~(P)	Carbamoyl phosphate, 1,3-bisphosphoglycerate, acetyl phosphate
3	Enol phosphate	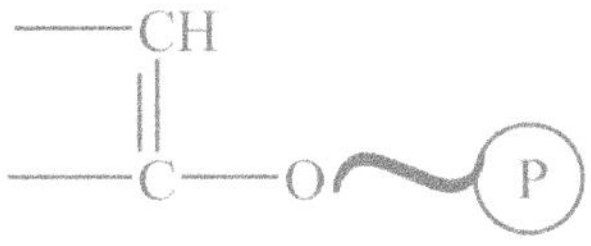 —CH=C—O~(P)	Phosphoenol pyruvate
4	Thioester or thiol ester	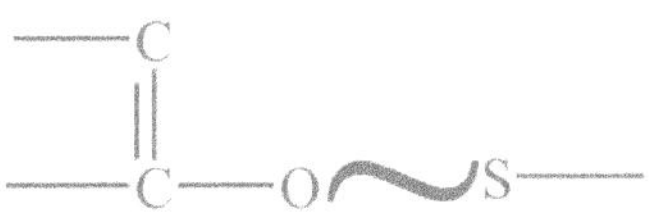 —C=C—O~S—	Acetyl CoA, acyl CoA
5	Phosphagens or guanidino phosphate	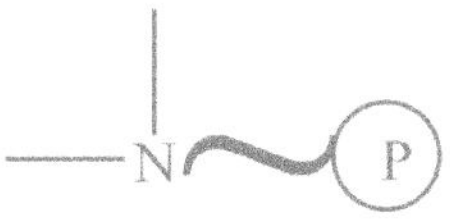 —N(—)~(P)	Phosphocreatine, phosphoarginine

Adenosine Triphosphate (ATP)

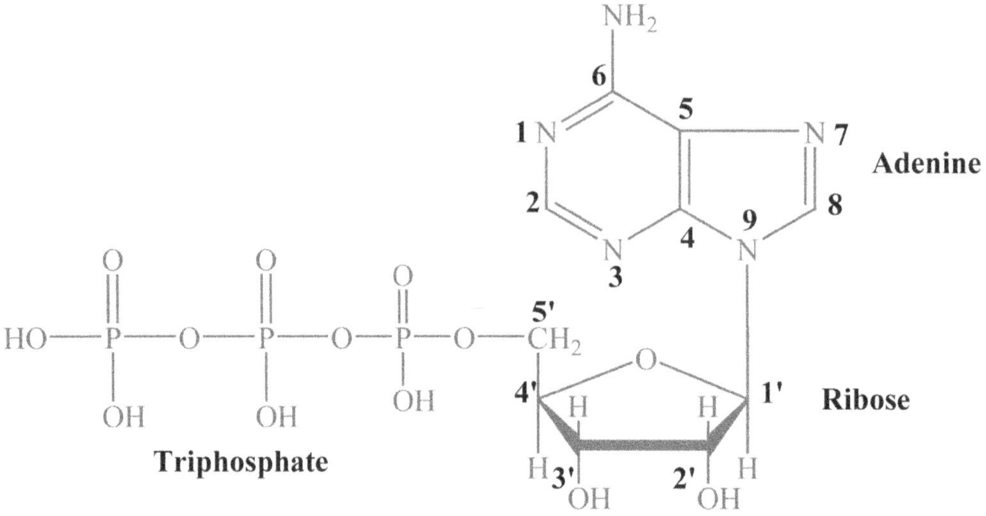

Adenosine triphosphate (ATP)

In living cells, the most important high energy molecule present is adenosine triphosphate (ATP). It is a nucleotide and composed of

1. Adenine (nitrogen base)
2. Ribose (sugar) and
3. A triphosphate groups.

In the triphosphate moiety of ATP, it contains two phospho anhydride bonds, hence ATP is a high energy compounds. ATP-ADP cycle evidences that ATP is the energy currency of the cell.

ATP-ADP Cycle

Large amount of energy (7.3 Cal/mol) is released when ATP is hydrolyzed to ADP and inorganic phosphate.

$$ATP + H_2O \longrightarrow ADP + Pi \qquad (\Delta G^\circ = -7.3\ Cal/mol)$$

Several processes in the biological systems such as muscle contraction, active transport, biosynthesis, etc. utilizes the energy liberated from the ATP when it breaks. In addition, energy rich compounds are biosynthesized from low energy compounds by reacting with high energy phosphates which is donated by ATP. Whilst, the compounds possessing higher free energy content donates high energy phosphates to ADP in order to produce ATP. ATP-ADP cycle is represented in Figure 1.1.

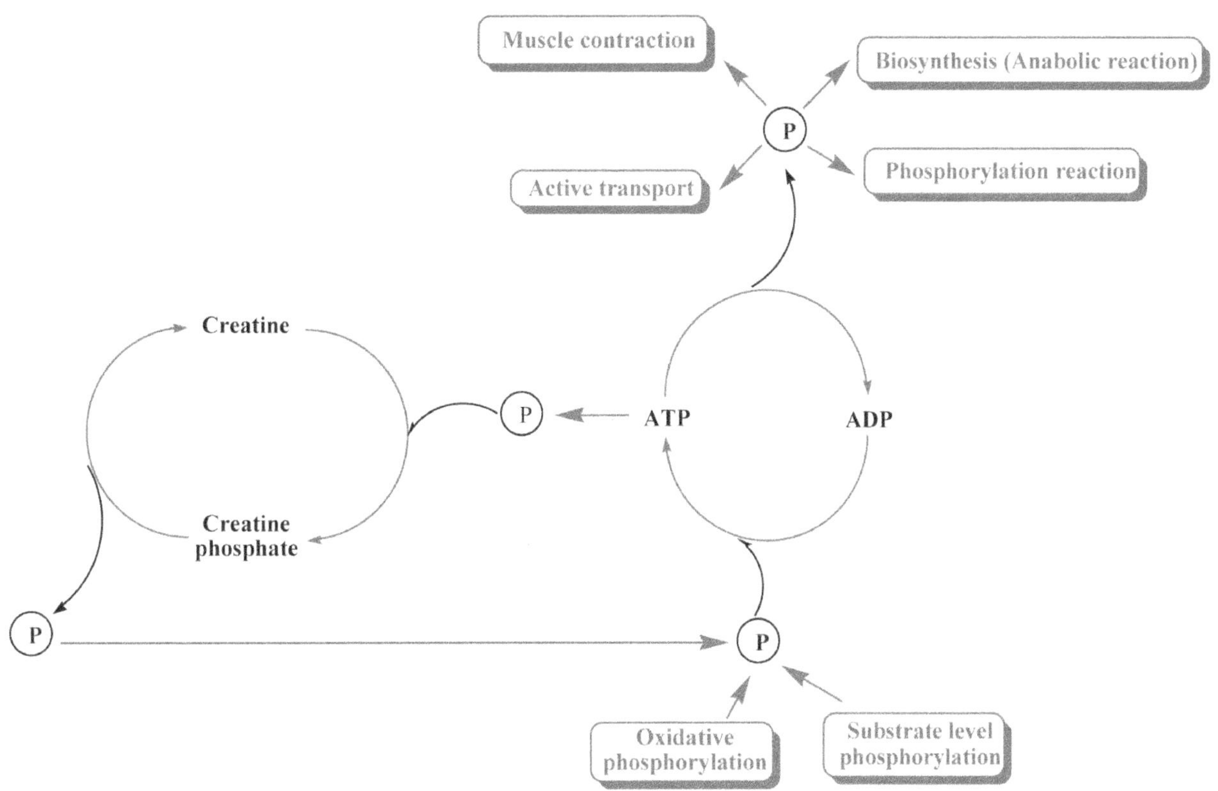

Figure 1.1 ATP-ADP cycle along with formation and breakdown of ATP (Phosphate will not exist free in biological system. It is only transferred).

Biological Significance of ATP

1. ATP is the short-term energy store of the cell.
2. Universally for all living things ATP is the energy currency of cell.
3. ATP is the source of phosphate moiety for phosphorylation reaction.
4. In addition, ATP can also donate pyrophosphate (PPi) and adenosine monophosphate (AMP) to other suitable acceptor for the formation of important biological compounds.
5. It easily participates in many biological reactions.
6. ATP is necessary for muscle contraction.
7. ATP is useful for nerve impulse transmission.
8. ATP is important for normal growth and development.
9. ATP is necessary for active transport.
10. ATP is also useful for homeostasis.
11. ATP is needed for all anabolic reactions.
12. ATP is helpful for intracellular signaling.
13. ATP is useful for the synthesis of nucleic acid.
14. ATP also plays a role in synthesis of proteins for the activation of amino acids.

Cyclic Adenosine Monophosphate (cAMP)

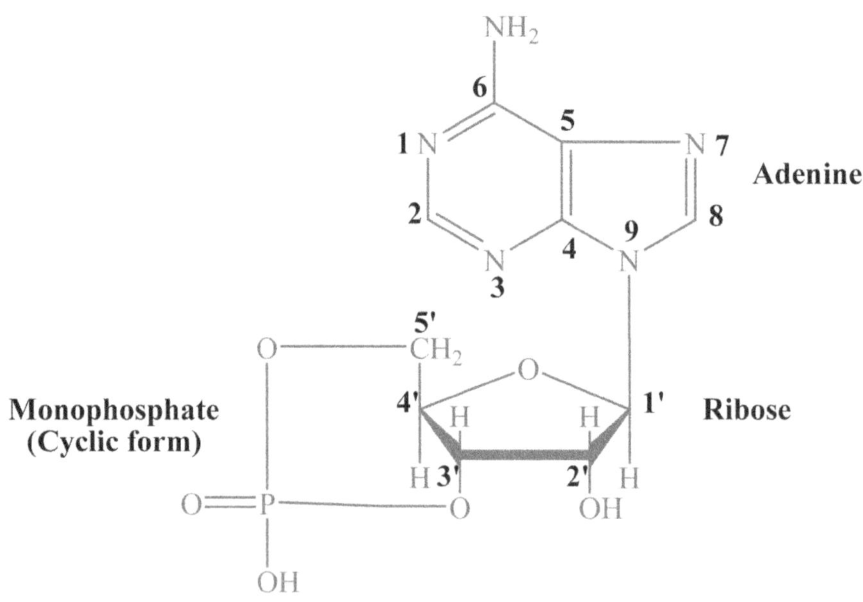

Cyclic adenosine monophosphate (*c*AMP)

In living cells, another important high energy molecule present is cyclic adenosine monophosphate (cAMP). The prefix 'cyclic' indicates the cyclic structure formed between phosphate moiety present at C-5 of ribose and hydroxyl group present at C-3 of ribose molecule.

It is a nucleotide and composed of

1. Adenine (nitrogen base)
2. Ribose (sugar) and
3. A monophosphate group.

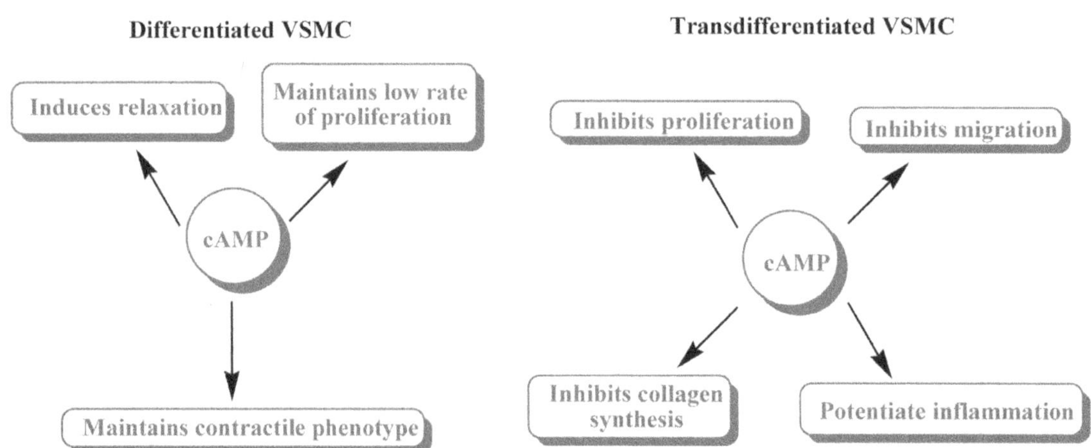

Biological Significance of cAMP

1. It is the intracellular secondary messenger present in many biological processes.
2. It is used for signal transduction intracellularly.
3. cAMP plays an important key regulatory role in most type of cells.
4. *Adenyl cyclase* particularly alters cAMP and this cAMP regulates the enzyme called *phosphodiesteraeses*.
5. cAMP mediates some short-term aspects of synaptic transmission. In addition, some rapid actions of certain neurotransmitter on ion channels that do not involve ligand gated channels are mediated through cAMP.
6. Along with other intracellular messenger, cAMP plays a central role in mediating other aspects of synaptic transmission.
7. Virtually all other effects of neurotransmitter on target neuron functioning both short and long term are achieved through intracellular messengers.

PROBABLE QUESTIONS

PART - A: Multiple Choice Questions

1. ____________ are the building blocks of lipids.
   (a) Fatty acid (b) Glycerol
   (c) Both a & b (d) None of the above
2. If enthalpy change for a reaction is zero, then $\Delta G°$ equals to ____________
   (a) $-T\Delta S°$ (b) $T\Delta S°$
   (c) $-\Delta H°$ (d) $\ln k_{eq}$
3. $\Delta G°$ is defined as the ____________
   (a) Residual energy present in the reactants at equilibrium
   (b) Residual energy present in the products at equilibrium
   (c) Difference in the residual energy of reactants and products at equilibrium
   (d) Energy required in converting one mole of reactants to one mole of products
4. For a reaction if $\Delta G°$ is positive, then ____________
   (a) The products will be favored
   (b) The reactants will be favored
   (c) The concentration of the reactants and products will be equal
   (d) All of the reactant will be converted to products
5. The study of energy relationships and conversions in biological systems is called as ____________
   (a) Biophysics (b) Biotechnology
   (c) Bioenergetics (d) Microbiology
6. Which of the following statement is false?
   (a) The reaction tends to go in the forward direction if ΔG is large and positive
   (b) The reaction tends to move in the backward direction if ΔG is large and negative
   (c) The system is at equilibrium if $\Delta G = 0$
   (d) The reaction tends to move in the backward direction if ΔG is large and positive
7. Anabolism and catabolism are chemically linked in the form of __________
   (a) ADP (b) ATP
   (c) Phosphodiester linkage (d) ASP

8. Which of the following statements is false about ATP hydrolysis?
   (a) It is highly exergonic
   (b) Activation energy is relatively high
   (c) ΔG^{o} = -30.5 kJ/mol
   (d) ΔG^{o} = 30.5 kJ/mol
9. An endergonic reaction ___________
   (a) Proceeds spontaneously
   (b) Does not require activation energy
   (c) Releases energy
   (d) Requires energy
10. An exergonic reaction ___________
   (a) Proceeds spontaneously
   (b) Does not require activation energy
   (c) Releases energy
   (d) Requires energy
11. Phosphoryl groups are derivatives of ___________
   (a) Phosphorous acid
   (b) Phosphoric acid
   (c) Acetic acid
   (d) Citric acid
12. Water does a nucleophilic attack on phosphate monoester by producing ___________
   (a) Phosphorous chloride
   (b) Phosphorous sulfide
   (c) Inorganic phosphate
   (d) Organic phosphate
13. Which is an example of chemical to osmotic energy conversion that occurs in living organisms?
   (a) ATP-driven muscle contraction
   (b) ATP-dependent photon emission in fireflies
   (c) Light-induced electron flow in chloroplasts
   (d) ATP-driven active transport across a membrane
14. Which of the following statements about redox potential is false?
   (a) NADH/NAD^+ redox pair has the least redox potential
   (b) Oxygen/H_2O redox pair has the highest redox potential
   (c) The components of the electron transport chain are organized in terms of their redox potential
   (d) The redox potential of a system is usually compared with the potential of the hydrogen electrode
15. Which out of the following has the highest redox potential?
   (a) NAD^+
   (b) FMN
   (c) FAD
   (d) O_2
16. Which one out of the following is not a NAD^+ requiring enzyme?
   (a) *Lactate dehydrogenase*
   (b) *Pyruvate dehydrogenase* complex
   (c) *Malate dehydrogenase*
   (d) *Acyl CoA dehydrogenase*
17. Which of the following enzyme catalyzes the direct transfer and incorporation of O_2 into a substrate molecule is
   (a) *Reductase*
   (b) *Oxidase*
   (c) *Oxygenase*
   (d) *Peroxidase*
18. Loss of electrons can be termed as ___________
   (a) Metabolism
   (b) Anabolism
   (c) Oxidation
   (d) Reduction
19. Gain of electrons can be termed as ___________
   (a) Metabolism
   (b) Anabolism
   (c) Oxidation
   (d) Reduction

20. Name the compound with the greatest free energy
    (a) ATP (b) Phosphocreatine
    (c) Cyclic AMP (d) Phosphoenolpyruvate
21. 1,3-Bisphosphoglycerate is a example for which type of high energy compound?
    (a) Acyl phosphate (b) Enol phosphate
    (c) Pyrophosphate (d) Guanidino phosphate
22. In general, high energy compounds contain which type bond in its structure?
    (a) Peptide (b) Glycoside
    (c) Acid anhydride (d) Covalent
23. What happened to free energy changes when a reaction is at equilibrium?
    (a) Maximum (b) Minimum
    (c) Average (d) Zero
24. Standard redox potential of NAD^+/NADH pair is ________ volts.
    (a) - 0.67 (b) - 0.22
    (c) +0.29 (d) - 0.32
25. Which of the following is the general formula for polysaccharides?
    (a) $(C_6H_{10}O_5)n$ (b) $(C_6H_{12}O_5)n$
    (c) $(C_6H_{10}O_6)n$ (d) $(C_6H_{12}O_6)n$
26. Out of the following polysaccharide which one is homopolysaccharide?
    (a) Inulin (b) Heparin
    (c) Hyaluronic acid (d) Keratan sulfate
27. Which of the following one is aldose sugar?
    (a) Glycerose (b) Ribulose
    (c) Erythrulose (d) Dihydoxyacetone
28. Which of the following one is a triose sugar?
    (a) Glycerose (b) Ribose
    (c) Erythrose (d) Fructose
29. Which of the following one is a pentose sugar?
    (a) Dihydroxyacetone (b) Ribulose
    (c) Erythrose (d) Glucose
30. How many isomers are possible for glucose?
    (a) 2 (b) 4
    (c) 8 (d) 16
31. ______________ are compounds having the same structural formula but differing in spatial configuration.
    (a) Stereoisomers (b) Anomers
    (c) Optical isomers (d) Epimers
32. In semen which sugar is present abundant?
    (a) Glucose (b) Lactose
    (c) Galactose (d) Fructose
33. In solution, glucose is present predominantly in which form.
    (a) Acyclic form (b) Glucopyranose
    (c) Glucofuranose (d) Hydrated acyclic form

34. Which of the following sugars are not an oligosaccharide?

(P) Raffinose (Q) Stachyose
(R) Glucoheptose (S) Sedoheptulose.

Choose the correct option.

(a) P and Q (b) R and S
(c) P and S (d) Q and S

35. Which of the following sugar does not form osazone?

(a) Maltose (b) Sucrose
(c) Lactose (d) Glucose

36. Which is a sweetener used in sugarless gums and candies?

(a) Sorbitol (b) Ribitol
(c) Myoinositol (d) Xylitol

37. Esters of fatty acids with alcohols other than glycerol are commonly known by which of the following name? P) Fats Q) Oils R) Waxes S) Phospholipids. Choose the correct option.

(a) P & Q (b) R & S
(c) P only (d) R only

38. Which of the following fatty acids are hydroxy fatty acids? P) β-Hydroxy butyric acid Q) Cerebronic acid R) Recinoleic acid S) Linolenic acid. Choose the correct option.

(a) Both P, Q & R (b) Both Q, R & S
(c) Both R, S & P (d) Both S, P & Q

39. Which of the following are glycolipids? P) Lecithin Q) Cephalin R) Cerebrosides S) Gangliosides. Choose the correct option.

(a) Both P & Q (b) Both R & S
(c) Both Q & R only (d) Both P & S

40. Spingomyelin is comes under which of the following class of complex lipid? P) Phospholipid Q) Glycolipid R) Lipoprotein S) Sulpholipid. Choose the correct option.

(a) Only P (b) Only S
(c) Both Q & R only (d) Both P & S

41. In short hand representation of fatty acids, second digit indicates what?

(a) Number of carbons (b) Number of double bonds
(c) Position of double bonds (d) Number of oxygens

42. Which of the following fatty acids are known as essential fatty acids? P) Palmitic acid Q) Linoleic acid R) Oleic acid S) Linolenic acid. Choose the correct option.

(a) Both P & Q (b) Both R & S
(c) Both P & R (d) Both Q & S

43. Which of the following is important for the synthesis & transport of lipoproteins and reverse transport of cholesterol?

(a) Phospholipid (b) Glycolipid
(c) Lipoprotein (d) Sulpholipid

44. The following substance(s) is(are) ketogenic

(a) Fatty acids (b) Leucine
(c) Lysine (d) All of them

45. Which of the following compounds possessing characteristics of lipids? P) Carotenoids Q) Squalene R) Pentacosane S) Alkaloids. Choose the correct option.
   (a) Both P & Q (b) Both R & S
   (c) Both P, Q & R (d) Both Q, R & S
46. Which lipoprotein possess the highest quantity of phospholipid.
   (a) HDL (b) LDL
   (c) VLDL (d) Chylomicrons
47. Which of the following is not a non-drying oil?
   (a) Almond oil (b) Peanut oil
   (c) Olive oil (d) Castor oil
48. Which of the following is example for semi-drying oil?
   (a) Olive oil (b) Mustard oil
   (c) Poppy seed oil (d) Almond oil
49. Which of the following is not on drying oil?
   (a) Linseed oil (b) Poppy seed oil
   (c) Cotton seed oil (d) Hemp oil
50. Cocoa butter is an example for what type of lipids?
   (a) Simple lipid (b) Complex lipid
   (c) Derived lipid (d) Miscellaneous lipid
51. Which of the following statement is not correct with respect to lipid functions?
   (a) It is as a concentrated fuel reserve of the body
   (b) It acts as an insulating material
   (c) It serve as a source of fat-soluble vitamins
   (d) It is not responsible for the shape and smooth appearance to the body
52. Which of the following fatty acid is not an even carbon fatty acid?
   (a) Valeric acid (b) Oleic acid
   (c) Palmitic acid (d) Stearic acid
53. Which of the following fatty acids are not an essential fatty acid?
   (a) Linoleic acid (b) Linolenic acid
   (c) Palmitic acid (d) Arachidonic acid
54. Proteins are the polymer of which of the following?
   (P) D-α-Amino acids (Q) D-β-Amino acids
   (R) L-α-Amino acids (S) L-β-Amino acids
   Choose the correct option.
   (a) Only R (b) Only S
   (c) Both R & S (d) Both P & Q
55. Which of the following function of a protein is regarded as "The working horses" of the cell?
   (a) Structural functions (b) Dynamic functions
   (c) Both a & b (d) None of the above
56. Which of the following amino acids are essential amino acids?
   (P) Alanine (Q) Methionine
   (R) Tyrosine (S) Lysine

Choose the correct option.

(a) P & S (b) Q & R

(c) P & R (d) Q & S

57. Which of the following one is wrong with respect to peptide bond?

(P) Rigid & planar (Q) Partial double bond character

(R) Covalent bond (S) Weak bond.

Choose the correct option.

(a) P, Q & R is correct; S is wrong (b) Q, R & S is correct; P is wrong

(c) P, Q & S is correct; R is wrong (d) P, R & S is correct; Q is wrong

58. Which of the following is true in peptide chain?

(P) C-terminal residue at the left (Q) N-terminal residue at the left

(R) N-terminal residue at the right (S) C-terminal residue at the right.

Choose the correct option.

(a) Both P & Q (b) Both P & R

(c) Both P & S (d) Both Q & S

59. For naming peptides which of the following suffix is added by replacing existing suffix with the exception of C-terminal amino acid?

(a) -ine (b) -yl

(c) -ane (d) –ate

60. Which of the following bond is not present in the protein structure?

(a) Covalent bond (b) Non-covalent bond

(c) Hydrogen bond (d) Co-ordinate covalent bond

61. Which of the followings are not globular proteins?

(P) Collagens (Q) Prolamines

(R) Histones (S) Keratins

Choose the correct option.

(a) Both Q & R (b) Both P & S

(c) Both R & S (d) Both P & Q

62. Casein present in milk & vitelline present in egg yolk are comes under which of the following category?

(a) Glycoprotein (b) Nucleoprotein

(c) Phosphoprotein (d) Lipoprotein

63. Hydroxyl group is not present in which of the following amino acid?

(a) Proline (b) Tyrosine

(c) Threonine (d) Serine

64. Which of the following amino acids are both glucogenic and ketogenic in nature?

(P) Phenylalanine (Q) Isoleucine

(R) Tryptophan (S) Tyrosine

Choose the correct option.

(a) P, Q & R (b) Q, R & S

(c) P, R & S (d) P, Q, R & S

65. Which of the following amino acids is not a polar with positive R group in structure?
    (a) Arginine (b) Lysine
    (c) Alanine (d) Histidine
66. Which of the following amino acid was first identified as essential amino acid.
    (a) Valine (b) Cystine
    (c) Cysteine (d) Tryptophan
67. Which of the following sulphur containing amino acid is participated in transmethylation reactions?
    (a) Methionine (b) Cysteine
    (c) Cystine (d) Glutathione
68. Which of the following amino acid is not a branched chain amino acid?
    (a) Leucine (b) Isoleucine
    (c) Alanine (d) Valine
69. Nucleotide contains which of the following?
    (a) Nitrogen base (b) Sugar
    (c) Phosphate group (d) All of them
70. Numbering of purine follows which pattern?
    (a) Anti-clockwise (b) Clockwise
    (c) Either (a) or (b) (d) Both (a) and (b)
71. Which of the following is not a pyrimidine base?
    (a) Uracil (b) Guanine
    (c) Orotate (d) Thymine
72. Which of the following is not a purine base?
    (a) Orotate (b) Guanine
    (c) Xanthine (d) Uric acid

Key for Multiple Choice Questions

1 (c)	2 (a)	3 (d)	4 (b)	5 (c)
6 (d)	7 (b)	8 (d)	9 (d)	10 (c)
11 (b)	12 (c)	13 (d)	14 (a)	15 (d)
16 (d)	17 (c)	18 (c)	19 (d)	20 (d)
21 (a)	22 (c)	23 (d)	24 (d)	25 (a)
26 (a)	27 (a)	28 (a)	29 (b)	30 (d)
31 (a)	32 (d)	33 (b)	34 (b)	35 (b)
36 (d)	37 (d)	38 (a)	39 (b)	40 (a)
41 (b)	42 (d)	43 (a)	44 (d)	45 (c)
46 (a)	47 (d)	48 (b)	49 (c)	50 (a)
51 (d)	52 (a)	53 (c)	54 (a)	55 (b)
56 (d)	57 (a)	58 (d)	59 (b)	60 (d)
61 (b)	62 (c)	63 (a)	64 (d)	65 (c)
66 (d)	67 (a)	68 (c)	69 (d)	70 (a)
71 (b)	72 (a)			

PART – B: Short Answers

1. What is free energy and free energy change?
2. What is energy rich compounds?
3. What are the main reasons for the ATP acts as universal energy currency molecule?
4. Write a brief account on ATP cycle.
5. Write about the biological significance of ATP & cAMP.
6. Explain redox potential & free energy constant.
7. Explain the biological significance of ATP.
8. Define and classify carbohydrates with suitable examples.
9. Write a note on structural aspects of carbohydrates.
10. Write a note on chemical nature of carbohydrates.
11. Write a note on biological significance of carbohydrates.
12. Write short notes on a) Epimer, b) Anomer.
13. Explain optical activity and D- & L-isomer of monosaccharides.
14. Define and classify lipids with suitable examples.
15. Define and classify fatty acid with suitable examples.
16. List out various biological significance of cholesterol.
17. Note on biological functions of lipids.
18. Explain the various biological importance of fatty acids.
19. What is the difference between glucogenic and ketogenic amino acids?
20. Explain about complete proteins.
21. What is conjugated protein?
22. List out the biological importance of amino acids.
23. List out nitrogen bases present in nucleic acid and draw the chemical structure of any one nitrogen base.
24. Write a note on nomenclature of nucleotides.
25. What is the importance of DNA & RNA?
26. What is nucleotide?
27. What are nucleosides?

PART – C: Long Answers

1. Write a detailed note on bioenergetics.
2. Define free energy, enthalpy and entropy. Explain the relationship between free energy, enthalpy and entropy.
3. Define and classify energy rich compounds. Explain any one compound in detail with chemical structure.
4. Write short notes on cyclic AMP.
5. Write briefly on: a) biological significance of ATP, b) Free energy, c) Energy rich compounds.
6. Write an account of high energy compounds metabolism.
7. Define carbohydrates and explain its various structural aspects with special emphasize on anomer and mutarotation.
8. Define and list out various types of protein classification. Explain any one classification in detail with suitable examples?
9. Write a detailed note on chemical nature and solubility classification of proteins.
10. Explain the biological significance of proteins.

11. Define and list out various types of amino acid classification. Explain any one classification in detail with suitable examples?
12. How amino acids are classified based on their chemical structure? Explain with suitable structure of amino acids.
13. Explain the biological significance of amino acids.
14. Explain the composition of nucleic acid.

UNIT 2

Carbohydrate Metabolism and Biological Oxidation

Carbohydrate Metabolism

All major pathways of carbohydrate metabolism relate to glucose. Hence, glucose is the central molecule of carbohydrate metabolism. The various other important monosaccharides involved in carbohydrate metabolism are fructose, galactose and mannose. Overview of carbohydrate metabolism is presented in Figure 2.1 & Table 2.1.

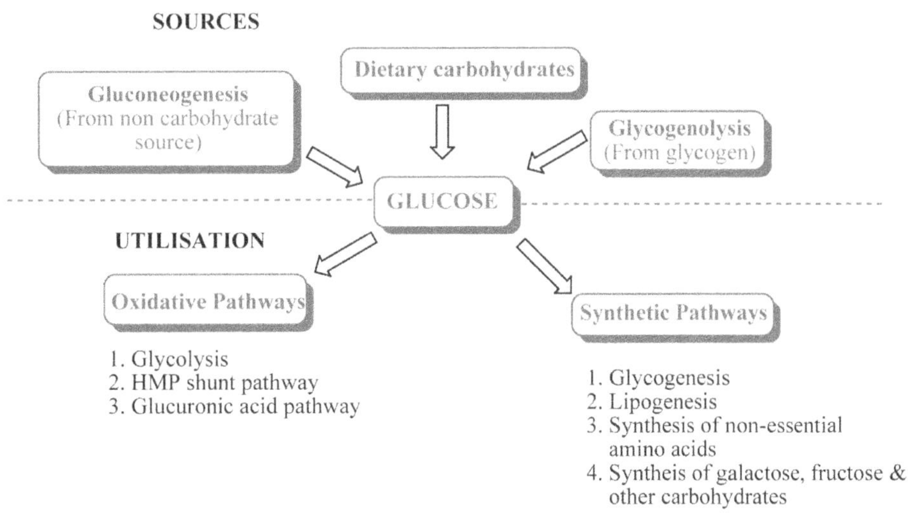

Figure 2.1 Overview of carbohydrate metabolism.

Transport of Glucose

Compared to blood glucose concentration (< 100 mg/dl), cell glucose concentration is very low. Even though, glucose is not entered the cell by simple diffusion (Movement from high concentrated area to low concentrated area without energy and carrier molecule). Glucose is transported into the cell by the following two specific transport system.

1. **Insulin independent transport system:** This transport system of glucose is not dependent on hormone insulin. This transport system comes under the category of facilitated diffusion (Movement from high concentrated area to low concentrated area without energy using specific carrier molecule i.e., glucose transporters or GLUT). There are five different glucose transporters (GLUT-1, GLUT-2, GLUT-3, GLUT-4 and GLUT-5) identified in cell membranes. In hepatocytes, brain and erythrocytes, glucose is transported by this transport system. In erythrocytes, GLUT-1 is abundantly present.
2. **Insulin dependent transport system:** This transport system of glucose is dependent on hormone insulin. This transport system also comes under the category of facilitated diffusion like insulin

independent transport system. In muscles and adipose tissue, glucose is transported by this transport system. In skeletal muscle and adipose tissue, GLUT-4 is abundantly present. In skeletal muscle and adipose tissue, insulin increases and promotes the activity of GLUT-4. Transport of glucose in cell by facilitated diffusion is presented in Figure 2.2.

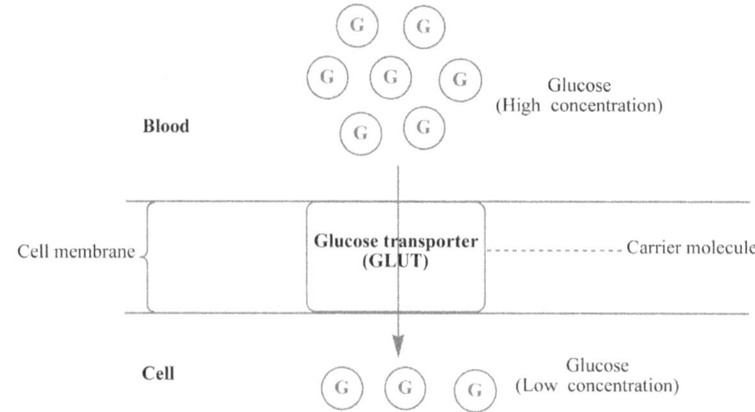

Figure 2.2 Transport of glucose in cell by facilitated diffusion.

Table 2.1 Overview of carbohydrate metabolism.

S. No.	Name of the pathway	Definition	Schematic representation
1.	Glycolysis or Embden Meyerhof pathway or EM pathway	Oxidation of glucose or glycogen into pyruvate or lactate with the production of ATP	Glucose / Glycogen → (Oxidation) → Pyruvate / Lactate + n ATP
2.	Kreb's cycle or Citric acid cycle or Tri carboxylic acid cycle or TCA cycle	Oxidation of acetyl CoA to carbon dioxide with the production of ATP	Acetyl CoA → (Oxidation) → CO_2 + n ATP
3.	Glycogenesis	Formation of glycogen from glucose	Glucose + n ATP → (Synthesis) → Glycogen

Table 2.1 *Contd...*

S. No.	Name of the pathway	Definition	Schematic representation
4.	Glycogenolysis	Breakdown of glycogen into glucose and then glucose undergoes glycolysis to produce pyruvate or lactate	Glycogen → (Breakdown) → Glucose + Glucose-1-phosphate
5.	Gluconeogenesis	Synthesis of glucose from non-carbohydrate sources such as lactate, pyruvate, propionate, glycerol and glucogenic amino acids	Non-carbohydrate sources (Lactate, pyruvate, propionate, glycerol and glucogenic amino acids) → (Synthesis) → Glucose
6.	Hexose mono phosphate pathway or HMP shunt or Pentose phosphate pathway or Direct oxidative pathway	Glucose is directly oxidized into carbon dioxide	Glucose → (Direct oxidation) → CO_2
7.	Uronic acid pathway or glucuronic acid pathway	Glucose is converted into glucuronic acid, pentoses and in some animals to ascorbic acid	Glucose → (Oxidation) → Glucuronic acid / Pentoses / In some animal ascorbic acid
8.	Galactose metabolism	Conversion of galactose to glucose and synthesis of lactose	Galactose → (Synthesis) → Lactose; Galactose → (Epimerization) → Glucose

Table 2.1 *Contd...*

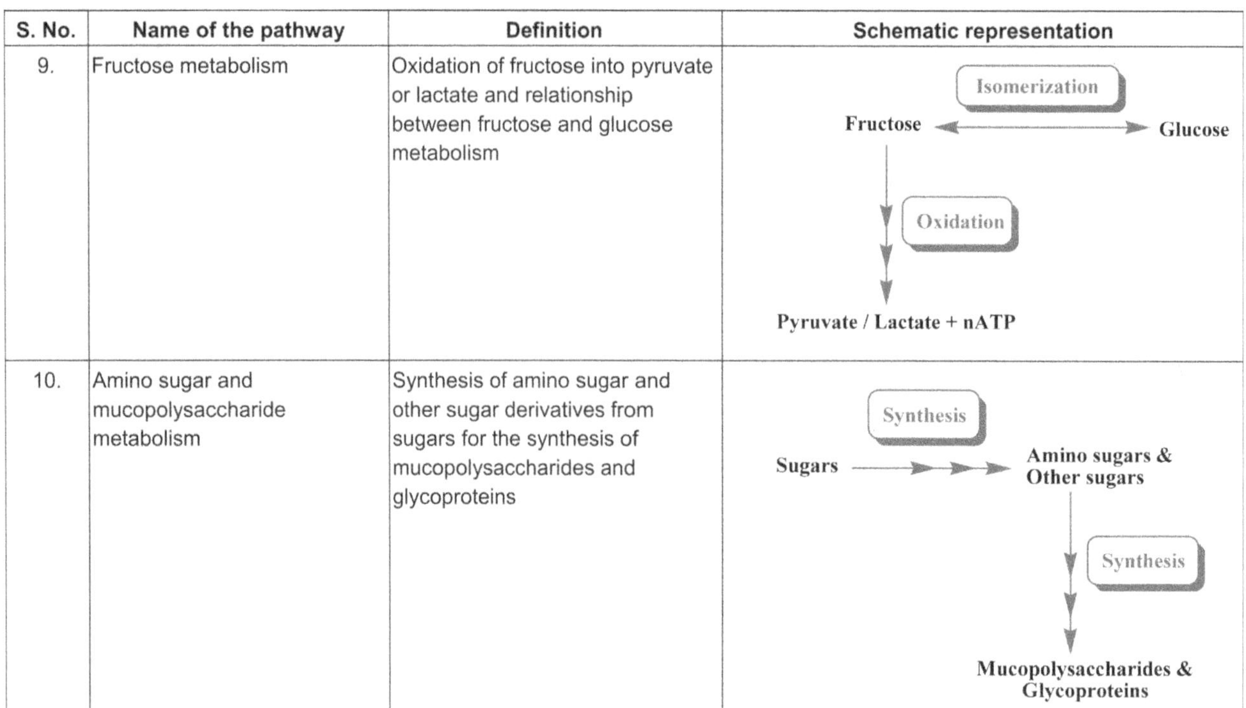

S. No.	Name of the pathway	Definition	Schematic representation
9.	Fructose metabolism	Oxidation of fructose into pyruvate or lactate and relationship between fructose and glucose metabolism	Fructose ⟷ Glucose (Isomerization); Fructose → Pyruvate / Lactate + nATP (Oxidation)
10.	Amino sugar and mucopolysaccharide metabolism	Synthesis of amino sugar and other sugar derivatives from sugars for the synthesis of mucopolysaccharides and glycoproteins	Sugars → Amino sugars & Other sugars (Synthesis); Amino sugars & Other sugars → Mucopolysaccharides & Glycoproteins (Synthesis)

Glycolysis

Definition: In Greek glycose means "sugar or sweet" and lysis means "dissolution or breakdown". Hence glycolysis means "breakdown or dissolution of sugar or sweet". It is also known as *Embden–Meyerhof pathway* or EM pathway. **Glycolysis is defined as "A series of chemical reactions taking place in biological system which converts glucose or glycogen into pyruvate or lactate with the production of energy".**

$$\text{Glucose or Glycogen} \xrightarrow{\text{Biological System}} \text{Pyruvate or Lactate} + n\,\text{ATP}$$

Glycolysis takes place in all the cells of the body and the necessary enzymes are present in cytosol fraction of the cell. Various intermediates produced in glycolysis are useful for the synthesis of several non-essential amino acids and glycerol (which is useful for formation of fat). Glucose can be synthesized from lactate or pyruvate (Reverse of glycolysis) by making alternate arrangements at three irreversible steps of glycolysis and the process is known as gluconeogenesis.

Types: Glycolysis can take place either in the presence or in the absence of oxygen. Based on this there are two different types of glycolysis.

1. **Aerobic glycolysis:** It takes place in presence of oxygen and the end product is pyruvate. The aerobic glycolysis can be summarized as follows.

$$\textbf{Glucose} + 2\,NAD^+ + 2\,ADP + 2\,Pi \longrightarrow \textbf{2 Pyruvate} + 2\,NADH + 2\,H^+ + 2\,ATP$$

2. **Anaerobic glycolysis:** It takes place in absence of oxygen and the end product is lactate. The anaerobic glycolysis can be summarized as follows.

$$\textbf{Glucose} + 2\,ADP + 2\,Pi \longrightarrow \textbf{2 Lactate} + 2\,ATP$$

Pathway:

There are three important stages in glycolysis as a) Priming stage or Energy investment stage, b) Splitting stage c) Energy generation stage.

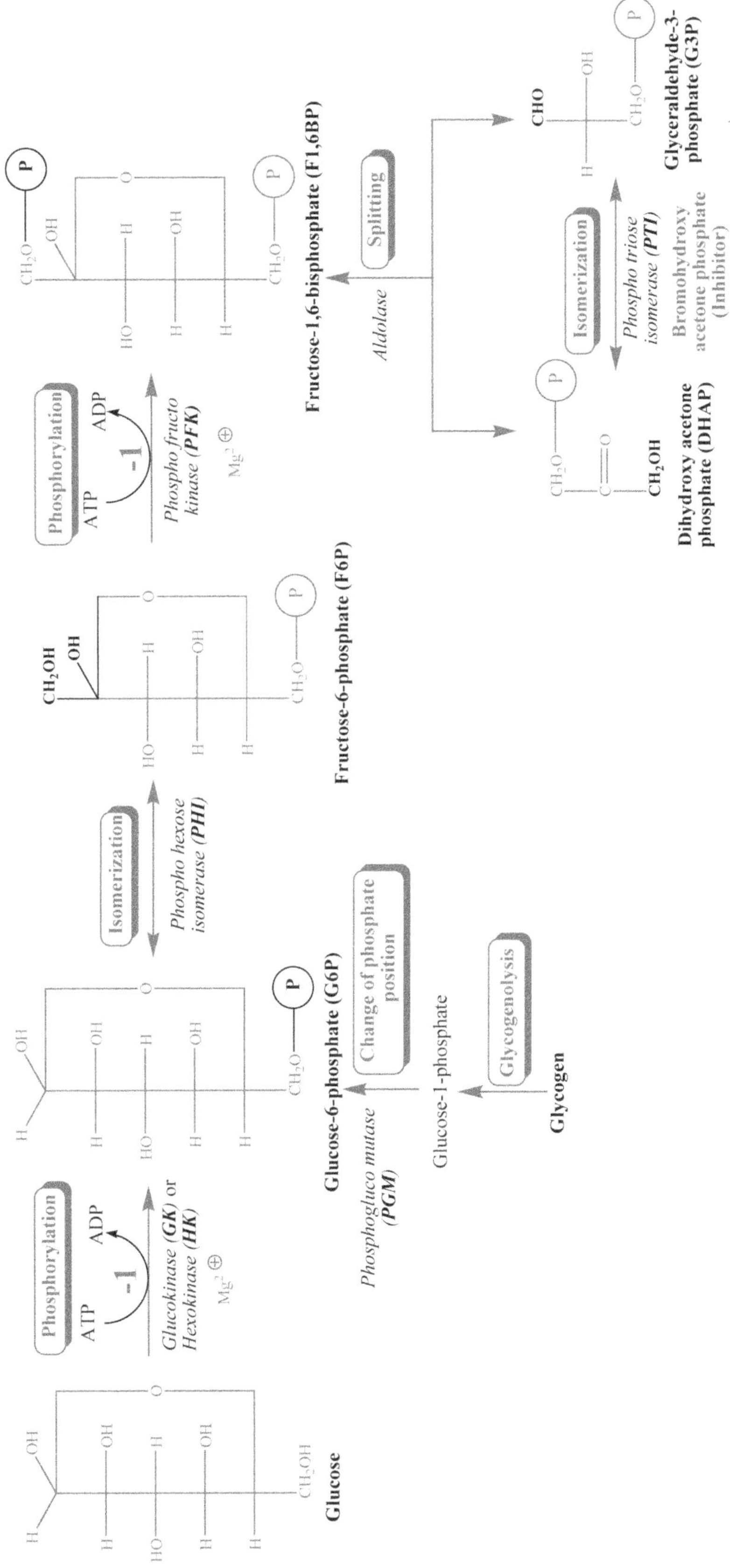
Glucose
Phosphorylation
ATP
ADP
-1
Glucokinase (GK) or Hexokinase (HK)
Mg2+
Glucose-6-phosphate (G6P)
Phosphogluco mutase (PGM)
Change of phosphate position
Glucose-1-phosphate
Glycogenolysis
Glycogen
Isomerization
Phospho hexose isomerase (PHI)
Fructose-6-phosphate (F6P)
Phosphorylation
ATP
ADP
-1
Phospho fructo kinase (PFK)
Mg2+
Fructose-1,6-bisphosphate (F1,6BP)
Aldolase
Splitting
Dihydroxy acetone phosphate (DHAP)
Isomerization
Phospho triose isomerase (PTI)
Bromohydroxy acetone phosphate (Inhibitor)
Glyceraldehyde-3-phosphate (G3P)

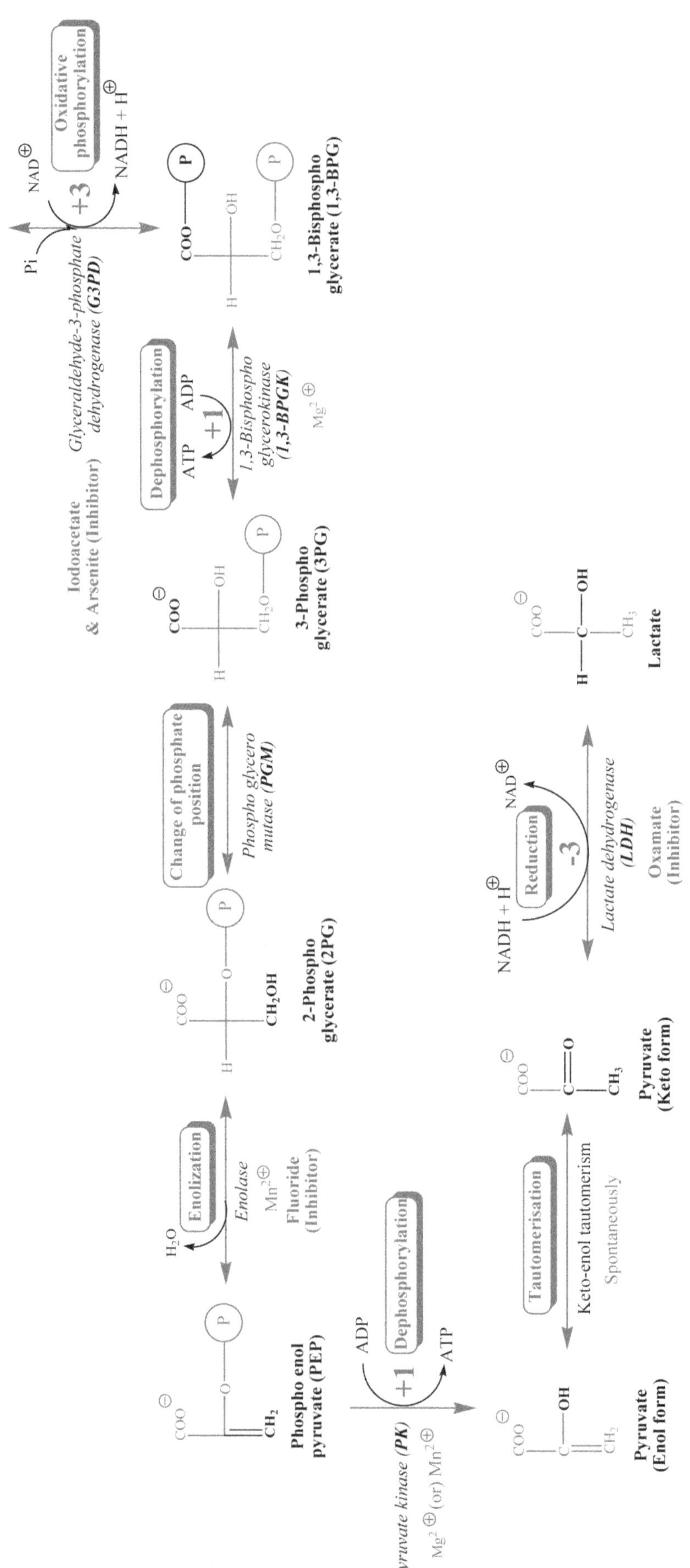
Pi
NAD⊕
+3
Oxidative phosphorylation
NADH + H⊕
Glyceraldehyde-3-phosphate dehydrogenase (G3PD)
Iodoacetate & Arsenite (Inhibitor)
1,3-Bisphospho glycerate (1,3-BPG)
Dephosphorylation
ATP
ADP
+1
1,3-Bisphospho glycerokinase (1,3-BPGK)
Mg2⊕
3-Phospho glycerate (3PG)
Change of phosphate position
Phospho glycero mutase (PGM)
2-Phospho glycerate (2PG)
H2O
Enolization
Enolase
Mn2⊕
Fluoride (Inhibitor)
Phospho enol pyruvate (PEP)
Pyruvate kinase (PK)
Mg2⊕ (or) Mn2⊕
ADP
+1
Dephosphorylation
ATP
Pyruvate (Enol form)
Tautomerisation
Keto-enol tautomerism
Spontaneously
Pyruvate (Keto form)
NADH + H⊕
Reduction
-3
NAD⊕
Lactate dehydrogenase (LDH)
Oxamate (Inhibitor)
Lactate

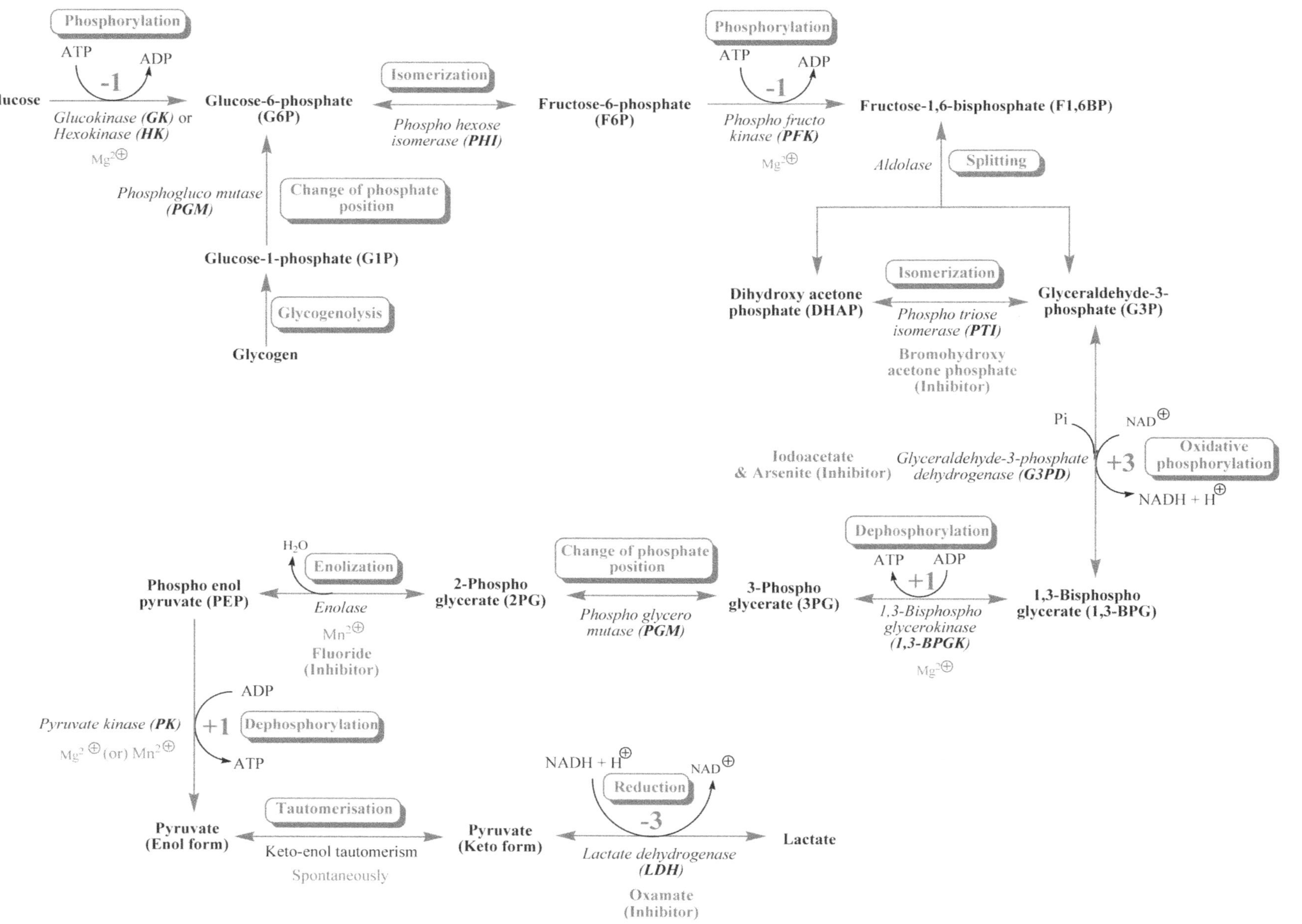

Phosphorylation
ATP
ADP
-1
Glucose
Glucokinase (GK) or
Hexokinase (HK)
Mg2⊕
Glucose-6-phosphate (G6P)
Isomerization
Phospho hexose isomerase (PHI)
Fructose-6-phosphate (F6P)
Phosphorylation
ATP
ADP
-1
Phospho fructo kinase (PFK)
Mg2⊕
Fructose-1,6-bisphosphate (F1,6BP)
Aldolase
Splitting
Phosphogluco mutase (PGM)
Change of phosphate position
Glucose-1-phosphate (G1P)
Glycogenolysis
Glycogen
Dihydroxy acetone phosphate (DHAP)
Isomerization
Phospho triose isomerase (PTI)
Bromohydroxy acetone phosphate (Inhibitor)
Glyceraldehyde-3-phosphate (G3P)
Pi
NAD⊕
Iodoacetate & Arsenite (Inhibitor)
Glyceraldehyde-3-phosphate dehydrogenase (G3PD)
+3
Oxidative phosphorylation
NADH + H⊕
Dephosphorylation
ATP
ADP
+1
3-Phospho glycerate (3PG)
1,3-Bisphospho glycerokinase (1,3-BPGK)
Mg2⊕
1,3-Bisphospho glycerate (1,3-BPG)
H2O
Enolization
Phospho enol pyruvate (PEP)
Enolase
Mn2⊕
Fluoride (Inhibitor)
2-Phospho glycerate (2PG)
Change of phosphate position
Phospho glycero mutase (PGM)
ADP
Pyruvate kinase (PK)
+1
Dephosphorylation
Mg2⊕ (or) Mn2⊕
ATP
NADH + H⊕
NAD⊕
Reduction
-3
Tautomerisation
Pyruvate (Enol form)
Keto-enol tautomerism
Spontaneously
Pyruvate (Keto form)
Lactate dehydrogenase (LDH)
Oxamate (Inhibitor)
Lactate

(a) Priming stage or Energy investment stage:

1. The first step in glycolysis is a simple phosphorylation reaction. In this step glucose is phosphorylated at 6th position in the presence of enzyme called "*hexokinase* (*HK*) or *glucokinase* (*GK*)" (In ATP / GTP involved reactions, the enzymes acted are "*kinase*" and the substrate is "glucose" which is a "hexose" sugar) and produces glucose-6-phosphate (G6P). *Kinase* enzyme needs magnesium ion (Mg^{2+}) as co-factor for its activity. **This step is the first irreversible step of glycolysis.** In this step one ATP is converted into ADP **(1 ATP is utilized)**.
2. Glucose-1-phosphate (G1P) is the product of glycogenolysis obtained from glycogen. Further, phosphate group present in 1st position of glucose-1-phosphate is shifted to 6th position and produces glucose-6-phosphate (G6P). The enzyme responsible is *phospho gluco mutase* (*PGM*) (In change of position of phosphate group involved reactions, the enzymes acted are "*mutase*" and the substrate is "glucose-1-phosphate").
3. In the next step glucose-6-phosphate (G6P) is isomerized into fructose-6-phosphate (F6P) by "*phospho hexose isomerase* (*PHI*)" (glucose-6-phosphate and fructose-6-phosphate are "phospho hexose sugar" and the reaction involved is "isomerization").
4. **This is the second irreversible step of glycolysis.** Like first step, fructose-6-phosphate (F6P) undergoes phosphorylation at 1st position and produces fructose-1,6-bisphosphate (F1,6BP) in the presence of "*phospho fructo kinase* (*PFK*)" (In ATP / GTP involved reactions, the enzymes acted are "*kinase*" and the substrate is "fructose-6-phosphate"). One ATP is converted into ADP in this step **(1 ATP utilized).**

(b) Splitting stage:

5. Dihydroxy acetone phosphate (DHAP) and glyceraldehyde-3-phosphate (G3P) are formed from fructose-1,6-bisphosphate (F1,6BP) by splitting reaction using "*aldolase*" enzyme. In this step 6 carbon fructose-1,6-bisphosphate is broken into two 3 carbon containing compounds (Dihydroxy acetone phosphate (DHAP) and glyceraldehyde-3-phosphate (G3P)). DHAP and G3P are functional isomers like glucose and fructose. These two are interconvertible by "*phospho triose isomerase* (*PTI*)" enzyme (Dihydroxy acetone phosphate (DHAP) and glyceraldehyde-3-phosphate (G3P) are "phospho triose sugar" and the reaction involved is "isomerization") There is no role for dihydroxy acetone phosphate (DHAP) except its conversion into glyceraldehyde-3-phosphate (G3P).

(c) Energy generation stage:

6. Glyceraldehyde-3-phosphate (G3P) undergoes oxidative phosphorylation by reacting with inorganic phosphate and produces 1,3-bisphospho glycerate (1,3BPG). *Glyceraldehyde-3-phosphate dehydrogenase* (*G3PD*) enzyme (In NAD^+ / $NADP^+$ / FAD involved reactions, the enzymes acted are "*dehydrogenase*" and the substrate is "glyceraldehyde-3-phosphate") catalyzes this step. During this reaction one molecule of NAD^+ is reduced to NADH + H^+ **(3 ATP generated)**.
7. In the next step 1,3-bisphospho glycerate (1,3BPG) produced 3-phospho glycerate (3PG) by dephosphorylation reaction in presence of *phospho glycero kinase* (*PGK*) (In ATP / GTP involved reactions, the enzymes acted are "*kinase*" and the substrate is "1,3-bisphospho glycerate"). One ADP is converted into ATP in this step **(1 ATP generated)**.
8. Further, phosphate group present in 3rd position of 3-phospho glycerate (3PG) is shifted to 2nd position and produces 2-phospho glycerate (2PG). The enzyme responsible is *phospho glycero mutase* (*PGM*) (In change of position of phosphate group involved reactions, the enzymes acted are "*mutase*" and the substrate is "3-phospho glycerate").
9. In the succeeding step, 2-phospho glycerate (2PG) produces phospho enol pyruvate (PEP) by enolization reaction in the presence of *enolase* (In reverse reaction, "enol" is the substrate and type of reaction is "hydrolysis"). *Enolase* needs magnesium ion (Mg^{2+}) as co-factor for its activity.
10. In the next step phospho enol pyruvate (PEP) undergoes dephosphorylation and produces pyruvate in enol form in the presence of *pyruvate kinase* (*PK*) (In ATP / GTP involved reactions,

the enzymes acted are "*kinase*" and the product formed is "pyruvate"). One ADP is converted into ATP in this step **(1 ATP generated). This step is the third irreversible step of glycolysis.**

11. Spontaneously pyruvate is converted into its keto form by keto-enol tautomerism from enol form. Pyruvate is the end product of aerobic glycolysis.
12. In absence of oxygen, pyruvate is converted into lactate with the help of *lactate dehydrogenase* (*LDH*) (In NAD^+ / $NADP^+$ / FAD involved reactions, the enzymes acted are "*dehydrogenase*" and the product is "lactate"). During this reaction one molecule of NADH + H^+ is oxidized to NAD^+ **(3 ATP utilized)**. Lactate is the end product of anaerobic glycolysis.

Regulation:

The three irreversible steps regulate glycolysis i.e., *hexokinase* (*HK*) or *glucokinase* (*GK*), *phospho fructo kinase* (*PFK*) and *pyruvate kinase* (*PK*). These three enzymes are rate limiting enzymes of glycolysis. Bromohydroxy acetone phosphate inhibits *phospho triose isomerase* (*PTI*); iodo acetate and arsenite inhibits *glyceraldehyde-3-phosphate dehydrogenase* (*G3PD*); fluoride inhibits *enolase* and oxamate inhibits *lactate dehydrogenase* (*LDH*).

Importance / Significance:

1. In the absence of oxygen, glycolysis is an emergency energy yielding pathway to the cells.
2. It is an important pathway which synthesizes ATP in the tissue lacking mitochondria (**Example:** Erythrocyte, cornea and lens).
3. Glycolysis is also significant for ATP synthesis in some other tissues having a smaller number of mitochondria (**Example:** Kidneys, testes and leucocytes).
4. Glycolysis occurrence is pre-requisite for the aerobic oxidation of carbohydrates which later takes place in the cells having mitochondria.
5. Glycolysis is very essential for brain because it is dependent on glucose for its energy demand. Glucose present in the brain must undergo glycolysis before it is oxidized into carbon dioxide.

Energetics:

Energetic of aerobic and aerobic glycolysis are summarized in Table 2.2.

Table 2.2 Energetic of glycolysis.

S. No	Enzyme responsible	Conversion takes place	No. of moles involved	No. of ATP generated or utilized
1	*Hexokinase (HK)* or *glucokinase (GK)*	One ATP is converted into ADP	1	- 1
2	*Phospho fructo kinase (PFK)*	One ATP is converted into ADP	1	- 1
3	*Glyceraldehyde-3-phosphate dehydrogenase (G3PD)*	One NAD^+ is reduced to NADH + H^+ (One NADH + H^+ is equals to 3 ATP)	2	+ 6
4	*Phospho glycero kinase (PGK)*	One ADP is converted into ATP	2	+ 2
5	*Pyruvate kinase (PK)*	One ADP is converted into ATP	2	+ 2
	Net ATP generated in aerobic glycolysis (-1 -1 + 6 + 2 + 2)			**8**
6	*Lactate dehydrogenase (LDH)*	One NADH + H^+ is oxidized to NAD^+ (One NADH + H^+ is equals to 3 ATP)	2	- 6
	Net ATP generated in anaerobic glycolysis (8-6)			**2**

Metabolic disorders:

1. **Pasteur effect:** It is defined as the process of inhibition of glycolysis by oxygen (aerobic condition). It is due to the inhibition of *phospho fructo kinase* (*PFK*) enzyme.
2. **Crabtree effect:** Crabtree effect is basically opposite to Pasteur effect. It is defined as the phenomenon of inhibition of oxygen consumption by the addition of glucose to tissues having high aerobic glycolysis. This effect is due to increased competition of glycolysis for inorganic phosphate and NAD^+ which limits the availability for phosphorylation and oxidation.

Conversion of Pyruvate to Acetyl CoA

Pyruvate dehydrogenase (*PDH*) (In NAD^+ / $NADP^+$ / FAD involved reactions, the enzymes acted are "*dehydrogenase*" and the substrate is "pyruvate") is an enzyme which converts pyruvate in to acetyl CoA by oxidative decarboxylation (Both oxidation and decarboxylation takes place). Decarboxylation of pyruvate produces acetaldehyde which on further oxidation produces acetic acid. Finally, acetic acid reacts with coenzyme A and produced acetyl CoA by esterification. One molecule of NAD^+ is reduced to NADH + H^+ during this reaction (**3 ATP generated**).

$$CH_3-\overset{O}{\overset{\|}{C}}-COO^{\ominus}$$

Pyruvate

CoASH → *Pyruvate dehydrogenase* (***PDH***) → CO_2, H_2O

$NAD^{\oplus}$ → +3 **Oxidative decarboxylation** → NADH + $H^{\oplus}$

$$CH_3-\overset{O}{\overset{\|}{C}}-SCoA$$

Acetyl CoA

Cardiac muscle and kidney contain high concentration of *PDH*. It is found only in mitochondria. It is a very good example for multi enzyme complex which requires the following five co-factors for its activity. 1) TPP (Thiamine pyrophosphate); 2) Lipoamide; 3) FAD; 4) Co-enzyme A and 5) NAD^+. Lactic acidosis is observed in patients with inherited deficiency of *PDH* usually after glucose load. Arsenic and mercuric ion binds with sulfhydryl (-SH) groups of lipoic acid; hence it inhibits *PDH* activity.

Citric Acid Cycle

Other Names:

1) TCA (tricarboxylic acid) cycle (First few compounds formed are tricarboxylic acid derivatives like citrate, cis-aconitate, isocitrate and oxalosuccinate), 2) Krebs cycle (In 1937, Hans Adolf Krebs proposed this cycle based on studies of oxygen consumption in pigeon breast muscle. He got noble prize in 1953 in physiology and medicine for this discovery).

Definition: Citric acid cycle is defined as a process of oxidation of acetyl CoA into carbon dioxide with the production of 12 ATPs in a cyclic manner. The first product formed in this cycle is citrate; hence this cycle is known as citric acid cycle.

$CH_3COSCoA + 3\ NAD^+ + FAD + GDP + Pi + 3\ H_2O$

Acetyl CoA

↓ **Oxidation**

$2\ CO_2 + 3\ NADH + 3\ H^+ + FADH_2 + GTP + CoASH$

Carbon dioxide

Pathway:

Glycolysis and TCA cycle are linked by oxidative decarboxylation of pyruvate to acetyl CoA. The enzymes necessary for citric acid cycle are present very near to ETC in mitochondrial part of cell. In this pathway a two-carbon acetyl CoA reacts with four-carbon oxaloacetate and produced six-carbon citrate. During pathways, two carbons are oxidized into carbon dioxide and oxaloacetate is regenerated and utilized again. Hence, **oxaloacetate is considered to play catalytic role in TCA cycle**.

1. In the first step, acetyl CoA reacts with oxaloacetate by aldol condensation like reaction and produced tricarboxylic acid citrate with the removal of co-enzyme A. *Citrate synthase* (*CS*) enzyme (The product formed is "citrate" and the type of reaction is "synthesis") catalyzed this step.
2. In the next step, citrate loses one molecule of water (-OH from C-2 and -H from C-1) and produced cis-aconitate by dehydration in presence of *cis-aconitase* (*CA*) (It is reversible reaction. In reverse reaction, substrate is "cis-aconitate" and the type of reaction is "hydrolysis").
3. Further, the cis-aconitate undergoes hydrolysis in the presence of same *cis-aconitase* (*CA*) enzyme and forms isocitrate (In citrate the position of -OH group is C-2; whereas in isocitrate it is C-1. Hence, it is good example for positional isomer).
4. Oxalosuccinate is produced when isocitrate (IC) reacts with reducing equivalent NAD^+ by dehydration reaction. *Isocitrate dehydrogenase* (*ICDH*) (In NAD^+ / $NADP^+$ / FAD involved reactions, the enzymes acted are "*dehydrogenase*" and the substrate is "isocitrate") catalyzes this reaction. During this reaction one molecule of NAD^+ is reduced to NADH + H^+ **(3 ATP generated)**.
5. This step is also catalyzed by *isocitrate dehydrogenase* only. It is a decarboxylation reaction in which C-2 carboxylic (-COOH) group of oxalosuccinate is removed as carbon dioxide and results in formation of α-ketoglutarate **(First carbon dioxide is produced)**.
6. α-Ketoglutarate (α-KG) undergoes oxidative decarboxylation reaction and produces succinyl CoA in presence of *α-ketoglutarate dehydrogenase* (*α-KGDH*) (In NAD^+ / $NADP^+$ / FAD involved reactions, the enzymes acted are "*dehydrogenase*" and the substrate is "α-ketoglutarate"). This reaction is similar to pyruvate to acetyl CoA catalyzed by *pyruvate dehydrogenase* (*PDH*). Like *pyruvate dehydrogenase* (PDH), *α-ketoglutarate dehydrogenase* (*α-KGDH*) also needs five co-factors such as 1) TPP (Thiamine pyrophosphate); 2) Lipoamide; 3) FAD; 4) Co-enzyme A and 5) NAD^+ for its activity. During this reaction one molecule of NAD^+ is reduced to NADH + H^+ **(3 ATP generated and second carbon dioxide is produced)**.
7. In the next step succinyl CoA is hydrolyzed into succinate with loss of co-enzyme A. The reaction is catalyzed by *succinate thiokinase* (*STK*) enzyme (In ATP / GTP involved reactions, the enzymes acted are "*kinase*", sulphur atom of CoA is involved and the product formed is "succinate"). One GDP is converted into GTP in this step by reacting with inorganic phosphate **(1 ATP generated)**.
8. Succinate is reduced to fumarate in the succeeding step by *succinate dehydrogenase* (*SDH*) (In NAD^+ / $NADP^+$ / FAD involved reactions, the enzymes acted are "*dehydrogenase*" and the substrate is "succinate"). During this reaction one molecule of FAD is reduced to $FADH_2$ **(2 ATP generated)**.
9. In presence of *fumarase* (Substrate is "fumarate" and the type of reaction is "hydrolysis"), maleate is produced from fumarate by hydrolysis reaction with one mole of water.
10. In the last step, oxaloacetate is regenerated from maleate by simple reduction with the involvement of NAD^+. *Maleate dehydrogenases* (*MDH*) enzyme (In NAD^+ / $NADP^+$ / FAD involved reactions, the enzymes acted are "*dehydrogenase*" and the substrate is "maleate") catalyze this reaction. During this reaction one molecule of NAD^+ is reduced to $NADH^+$ H^+ **(3 ATP generated)**.

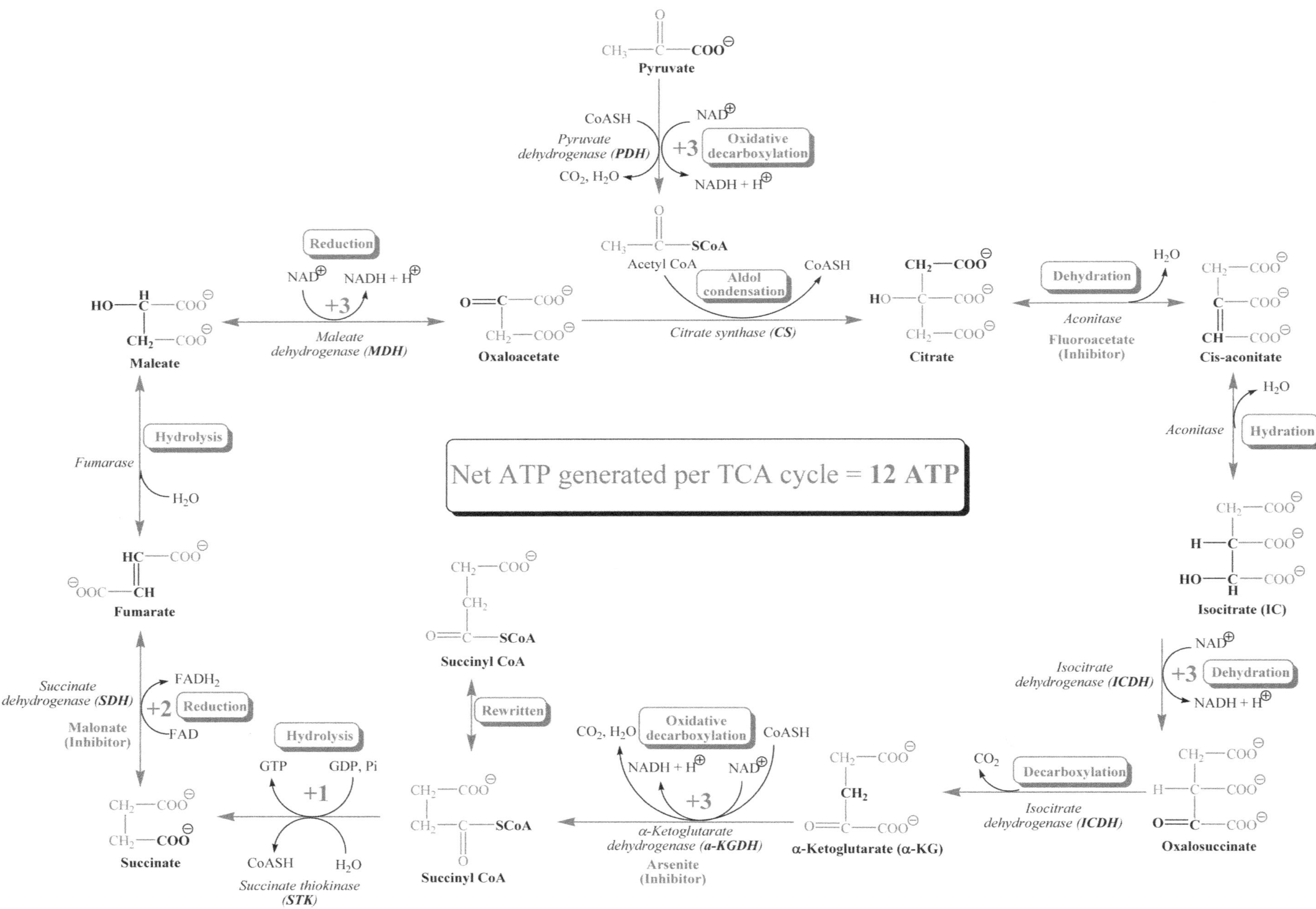
Pyruvate
CoASH
$NAD^{\oplus}$
Pyruvate dehydrogenase (PDH)
+3
Oxidative decarboxylation
CO_2, H_2O
$NADH + H^{\oplus}$
Acetyl CoA
Aldol condensation
CoASH
Citrate synthase (CS)
Oxaloacetate
Reduction
$NAD^{\oplus}$
$NADH + H^{\oplus}$
+3
Maleate dehydrogenase (MDH)
Maleate
Citrate
Dehydration
H_2O
Aconitase
Fluoroacetate (Inhibitor)
Cis-aconitate
H_2O
Aconitase
Hydration
Isocitrate (IC)
$NAD^{\oplus}$
Isocitrate dehydrogenase (ICDH)
+3
Dehydration
$NADH + H^{\oplus}$
Oxalosuccinate
CO_2
Decarboxylation
Isocitrate dehydrogenase (ICDH)
α-Ketoglutarate (α-KG)
CO_2, H_2O
Oxidative decarboxylation
CoASH
$NADH + H^{\oplus}$
$NAD^{\oplus}$
+3
α-Ketoglutarate dehydrogenase (α-KGDH)
Arsenite (Inhibitor)
Succinyl CoA
Rewritten
Succinyl CoA
Hydrolysis
GTP
GDP, Pi
+1
CoASH
H_2O
Succinate thiokinase (STK)
Succinate
Succinate dehydrogenase (SDH)
Malonate (Inhibitor)
$FADH_2$
+2
Reduction
FAD
Fumarate
Fumarase
Hydrolysis
H_2O
Net ATP generated per TCA cycle = 12 ATP

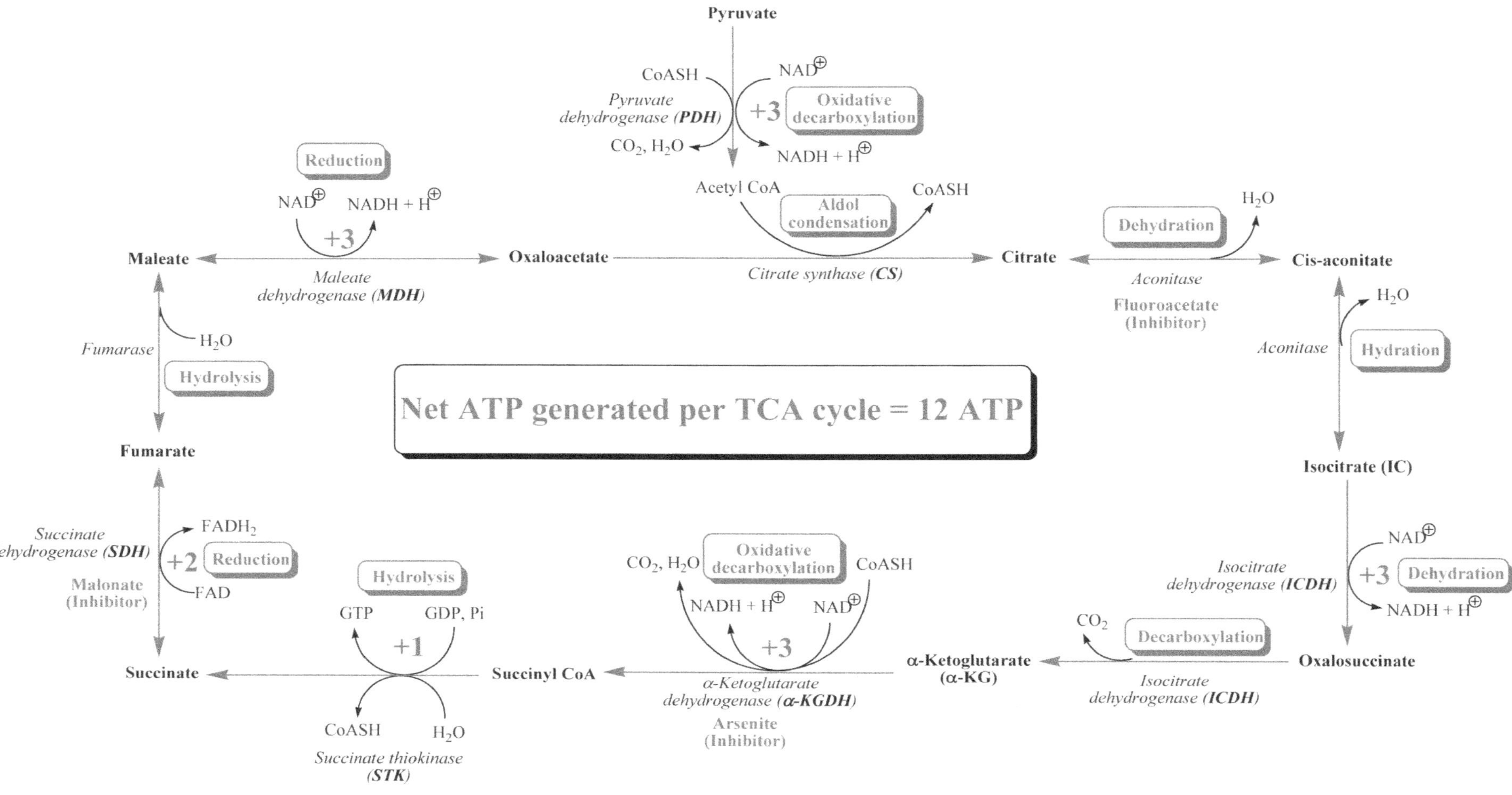

Pyruvate
CoASH
NAD⊕
Pyruvate dehydrogenase (PDH)
+3
Oxidative decarboxylation
CO_2, H_2O
NADH + H⊕
Reduction
NAD⊕
NADH + H⊕
+3
Acetyl CoA
Aldol condensation
CoASH
H_2O
Dehydration
Maleate
Oxaloacetate
Citrate
Cis-aconitate
Maleate dehydrogenase (MDH)
Citrate synthase (CS)
Aconitase
Fluoroacetate (Inhibitor)
H_2O
Fumarase
Hydrolysis
Aconitase
Hydration
Net ATP generated per TCA cycle = 12 ATP
Fumarate
Isocitrate (IC)
Succinate dehydrogenase (SDH)
$FADH_2$
+2
Reduction
FAD
Malonate (Inhibitor)
Hydrolysis
GTP
GDP, Pi
+1
CO_2, H_2O
Oxidative decarboxylation
CoASH
NADH + H⊕
NAD⊕
+3
NAD⊕
Isocitrate dehydrogenase (ICDH)
+3
Dehydration
NADH + H⊕
CO_2
Decarboxylation
Succinate
Succinyl CoA
α-Ketoglutarate (α-KG)
Oxalosuccinate
CoASH
H_2O
Succinate thiokinase (STK)
α-Ketoglutarate dehydrogenase (α-KGDH)
Arsenite (Inhibitor)
Isocitrate dehydrogenase (ICDH)

Importance / Significance:

1. It is the final common oxidative pathway for carbohydrates, proteins and lipids.
2. About 65-70 % of total ATPs are synthesized in citric acid cycle. Hence, it is important metabolic pathway for the supply of energy.
3. About 2/3 of the oxygen consumed by the biological system is utilized by this cycle.
4. It is the most important central pathway because it connects either directly or indirectly almost all other individual metabolic pathway.
5. In addition to energy supply, TCA cycle also produces many intermediates necessary for the synthesis of glucose, amino acids, heme, etc.
6. Krebs cycle is amphibolic because it is both catabolic (breakdown of acetyl CoA to carbon dioxide) and anabolic (produces many intermediates necessary for the synthesis of glucose, amino acids, heme, etc.) in nature.
7. It is a cyclic process but not the closed one. It is open chain cycle i.e., several compounds may enter and leave the cycle at different stages.
8. Presence of oxygen is necessary for TCA cycle, even though oxygen is not directly participated. Because for the regeneration of reducing equivalent NAD^+ and FAD from NADH+ H^+ and $FADH_2$ in ETC needs oxygen.
9. Citric acid cycle will not take place in the absence of oxygen (anaerobic condition).

Regulation:

Citric acid cycle is regulated by the following three enzymes such as 1) *Citrate synthase* (*CS*), 2) *Isocitrate dehydrogenase* (*ICDH*) and 3) α-*Ketoglutarate dehydrogenase* (α-*KGDH*). ADP availability is the most important one because accumulation of NADH and $FADH_2$ inhibits the above rate limiting enzymes of TCA cycle. Fluoroacetate and arsenite non-competitively inhibits *aconitase* and α-*ketoglutarate dehydrogenase* (α-*KGDH*), respectively; whereas malonate competitively inhibits *succinate dehydrogenase* (*SDH*).

Energetic:

Energetic of citric acid cycle are summarized in Table 2.3.

Table 2.3 Energetic of citric acid cycle.

S. No.	Enzyme responsible	Conversion takes place	No. of moles involved	No. of ATP generated or utilized
1	*Isocitrate dehydrogenase (ICDH)*	One NAD^+ is reduced to NADH + H^+ (One NADH + H^+ is equals to 3 ATP)	1	+ 3
2	*α-Ketoglutarate dehydrogenase (α-KGDH)*	One NAD^+ is reduced to NADH + H^+ (One NADH + H^+ is equals to 3 ATP)	1	+ 3
3	*Succinate thiokinase (STK)*	One GDP is converted into GTP	1	+ 1
4	*Succinate dehydrogenase (SDH)*	One FAD is reduced into $FADH_2$	1	+ 2
5	*Maleate dehydrogenase (MDH)*	One NAD^+ is reduced to NADH + H^+ (One NADH + H^+ is equals to 3 ATP)	1	+ 3
6	**Net ATP generated in TCA cycle for one acetyl CoA**			**12**

Energetic of glucose oxidation

(a) Aerobic condition

Energetic of complete oxidation of one glucose molecule in presence of oxygen is summarized in Table 2.4.

(b) Anaerobic condition

Energetic of complete oxidation of one glucose molecule in absence of oxygen is summarized in Table 2.5.

Table 2.4 Energetic of aerobic glucose oxidation.

S. No.	Pathway name	Conversion takes place	No. of ATP generated or utilized
1	Aerobic glycolysis	One glucose into 2 pyruvate	+ 8
2	Connecting link	2 Pyruvate to 2 acetyl CoA (For one mole of pyruvate 3 ATP generated. Hence for 2 pyruvate it is 6)	+ 6
3	TCA cycle	2 Acetyl CoA to 4 CO_2 (For one acetyl CoA 12 ATP generated. Hence for 2 acetyl CoA it is 24)	+ 24
4	**Net ATP generated for complete oxidation of one glucose molecule in aerobic condition**		**+ 38**

Table 2.5 Energetic of anaerobic glucose oxidation.

S. No.	Pathway name	Conversion takes place	No. of ATP generated or utilized
1	Anaerobic glycolysis	One glucose into 2 lactate (Lactate is not undergoing any further oxidative pathways and it is excreted in urine)	+ 2
2	**Net ATP generated for complete oxidation of one glucose molecule in anaerobic condition**		**+ 2**

Gluconeogenesis

Definition: Gluco means "glucose / glycogen", in Greek neo means "new (other than carbohydrates)" and genesis means "synthesis". **Gluconeogenesis is defined as the process of synthesising glucose or glycogen from non-carbohydrate sources such as lactate, pyruvate, propionate, glycerol and glucogenic amino acids**.

Pathway:

Gluconeogenesis is the reverse of glycolysis. The three irreversible steps of glycolysis are modified / reversed by specific alternate enzymes. The enzymes are mainly present in cytosol even though few precursors are synthesized in mitochondria. Mostly gluconeogenesis takes place in liver and to small extent in kidney also,. The enzymes involved in three irreversible steps of glycolysis are "1) *Gluco kinase* (*GK*) or *hexo kinase* (*HK*), 2) *Phospho fructo kinase* (*PFK*) and 3) *Pyruvate kinase* (*PK*)". The alternative for these enzymes in gluconeogenesis are "1) *Glucose-6-phosphatase* (*G6Pase*), 2) *Fructose-1,6-bisphosphatase* (*F1,6BPase*), and 3) *Phospho enol pyruvate carboxy kinase* (*PEPCK*)".

1. ***Glucose-6-phosphatase* (*G6Pase*):** This step is the final step of gluconeogenesis. This enzyme directly reverses the reaction catalyzed by *gluco kinase* (*GK*) or *hexo kinase* (*HK*). *Glucose-6-phosphatase* (Substrate is "glucose-6-phosphate" and the type of reaction is "hydrolysis") hydrolyses glucose-6-phosphate (G6P) into glucose with removal of one molecule of inorganic phosphate. *Glucose-6-phosphatase* (*G6Pase*) is mainly present in liver and kidney but not present in muscle, brain and adipose tissue.
2. ***Fructose-1,6-bisphosphatase (F1,6BPase):*** This enzyme directly reverses the reaction catalyzed by *phospho fructo kinase* (PFK). *Fructose-1,6-bisphosphatase* (Substrate is "fructose-1,6-bisphosphate" and the type of reaction is "hydrolysis") hydrolyses fructose-1,6-bisphosphate (F1,6BP) into fructose-6-phosphate (F6P) with removal of one molecule of inorganic phosphate. *Fructose-1,6-bisphosphatase* (*F1,6BPase*) is not present in smooth muscle and heart muscle.

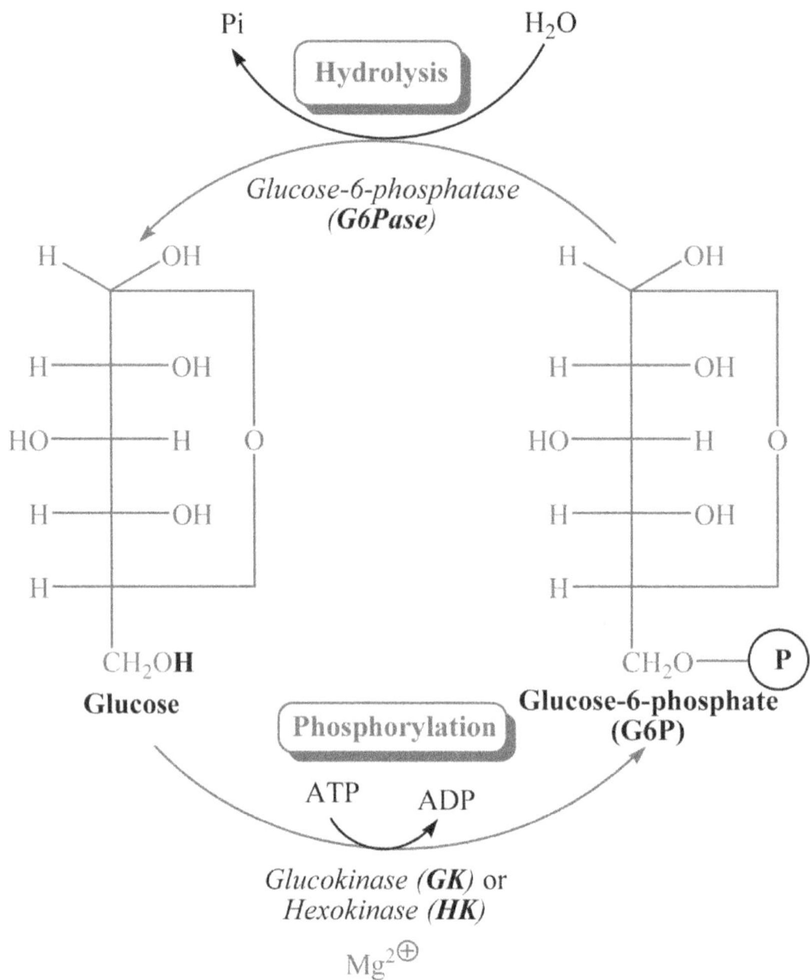

3. ***Phospho enol pyruvate carboxy kinase* (PEPCK):** This enzyme reverses the reaction catalyzed by *pyruvate kinase* (*PK*) but not directly. Pyruvate from cytosol enters into mitochondria where it reacts with carbon dioxide and get converted to oxaloacetate by carboxylation reaction in the presence of *pyruvate carboxylase* (*PC*) ("Pyruvate" is the substrate and the type of reaction is "carboxylation"). The energy for this anabolic reaction is obtained from the breakdown of ATP into ADP and inorganic phosphate **(1 ATP utilized)**. Later, oxaloacetate undergoes oxidation with the involvement of NADH and produces maleate. *Maleate dehydrogenase* (*MDH*) (In NAD^+ / $NADP^+$ / FAD involved reactions, the enzymes acted are "*dehydrogenase*" and the product is "maleate") catalyze this reaction. During this reaction one molecule of NADH + H^+ is oxidized to NAD^+ **(3 ATP utilized)**. Later maleate is transported from mitochondria to cytosol. In cytosol maleate produces oxaloacetate in the presence of *maleate dehydrogenase* (*MDH*) (Same reaction but in reverse manner i.e. reversible reaction) **(Hence, 3 ATP generated)**. Finally, oxaloacetate undergoes decarboxylated phosphorylation and produces phospho enol pyruvate (PEP). The enzyme responsible is *phospho enol pyruvate carboxy kinase* (*PEPCK*) (Product is "phospho enol pyruvate", the type of reaction is "carboxylation" (reverse reaction) and in ATP / GTP involved reactions, the enzymes acted are "*kinase*"). One GTP is converted into GDP in this step by donating one inorganic phosphate to substrate **(1 ATP utilized)**. Totally 2 ATP are utilized for the conversion of pyruvate to phospho enol pyruvate (PEP). But only one ATP is generated when phospho enol pyruvate (PEP) is converted into pyruvate.

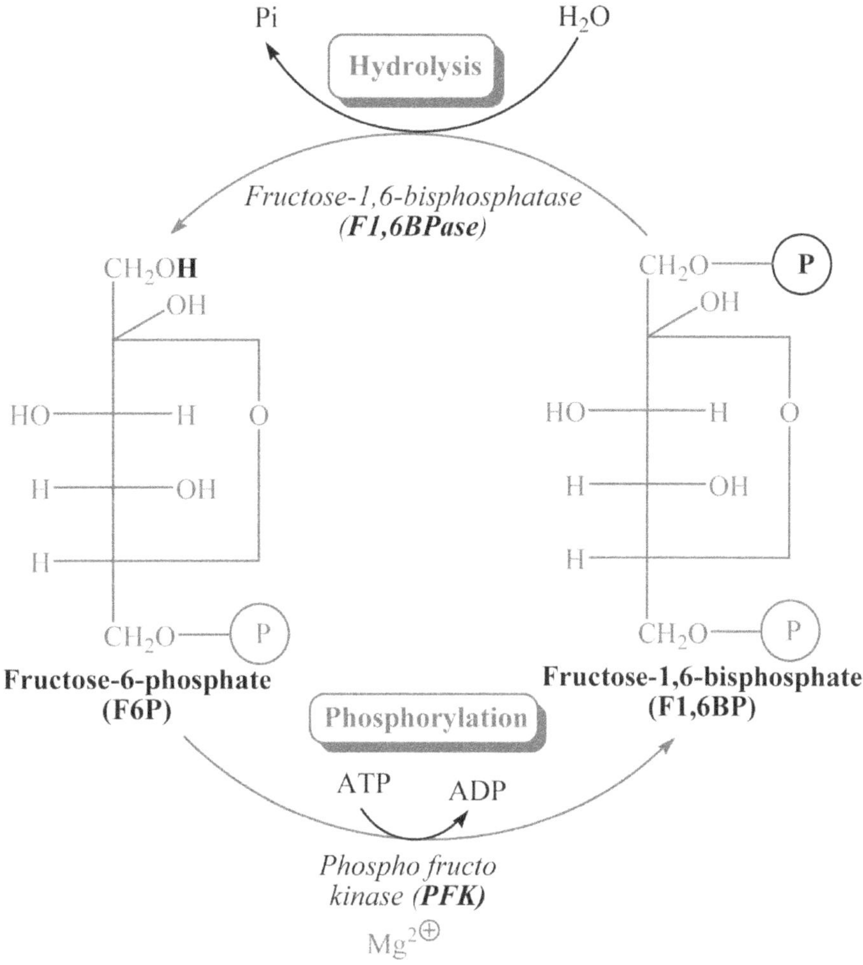

The overall reaction of pyruvate to glucose are summarized as follows,

$$2\ \text{Pyruvate} + 4\ \text{ATP} + 2\ \text{GTP} + 2\ \text{NADH} + 2\ H^+ + 6\ H_2O$$

$$\downarrow$$

$$\textbf{Glucose} + 4\ \text{ADP} + 2\ \text{GDP} + 6\ \text{Pi} + 2\ \text{NAD}^+$$

Due to lack of *glucose-6-phosphatase* (*G6Pase*) and *fructose-1,6-bisphosphatase* (*F1,6BPase*) in muscle, it can't utilize lactate or pyruvate to produce glucose. But through "Cori cycle" lactate present in muscle is transported to liver where glucose is synthesized by gluconeogenesis followed by transport of glucose into muscle.

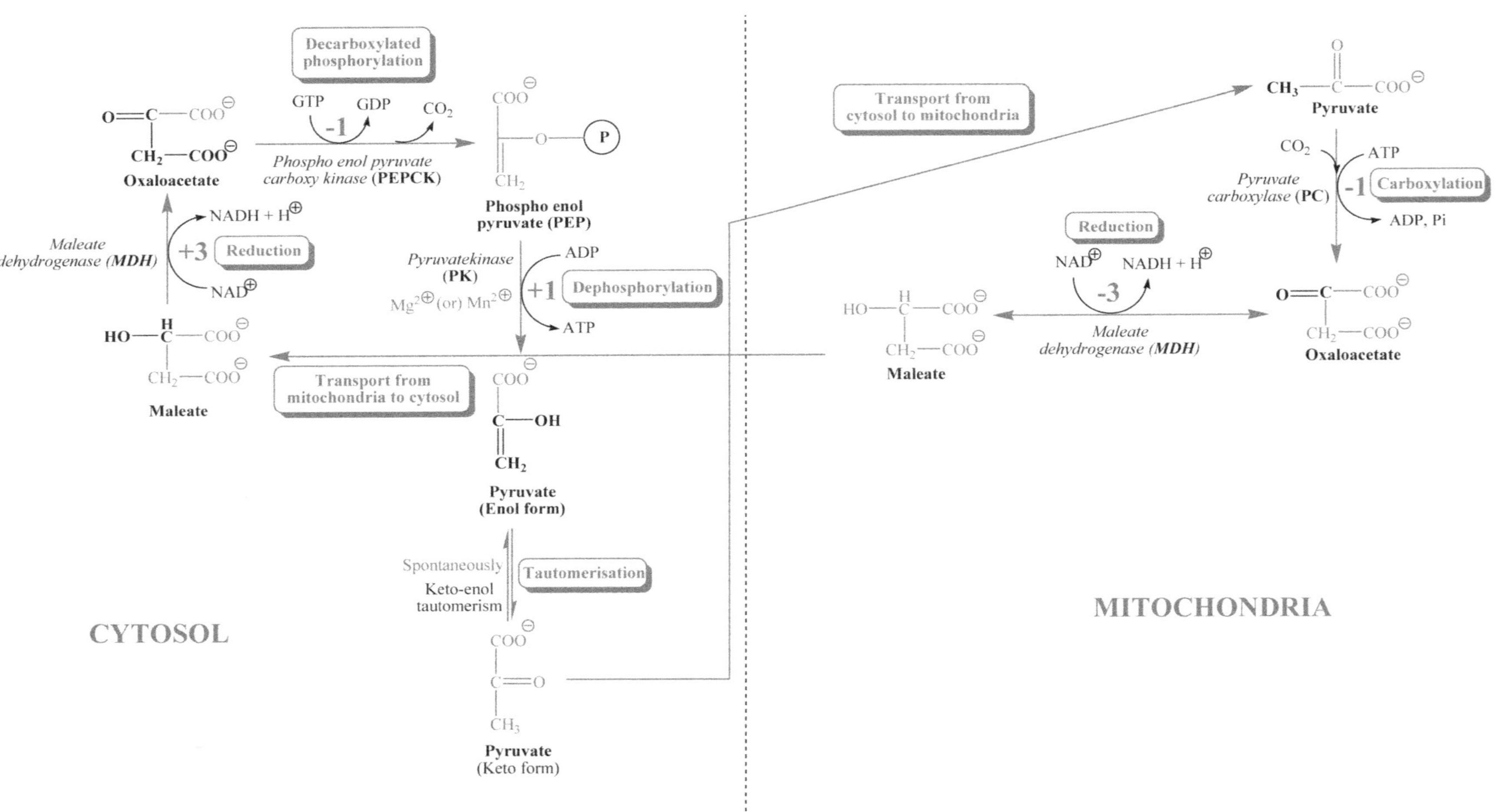
Decarboxylated phosphorylation
GTP
GDP
CO2
-1
Oxaloacetate
Phospho enol pyruvate carboxy kinase (PEPCK)
Phospho enol pyruvate (PEP)
NADH + H⊕
Maleate dehydrogenase (MDH)
+3
Reduction
NAD⊕
Pyruvatekinase (PK)
Mg2⊕ (or) Mn2⊕
ADP
+1
Dephosphorylation
ATP
Maleate
Transport from mitochondria to cytosol
Pyruvate (Enol form)
Spontaneously
Keto-enol tautomerism
Tautomerisation
CYTOSOL
Pyruvate (Keto form)
Transport from cytosol to mitochondria
Pyruvate
CO2
ATP
Pyruvate carboxylase (PC)
-1
Carboxylation
ADP, Pi
Reduction
NAD⊕
NADH + H⊕
-3
Maleate
Maleate dehydrogenase (MDH)
Oxaloacetate
MITOCHONDRIA

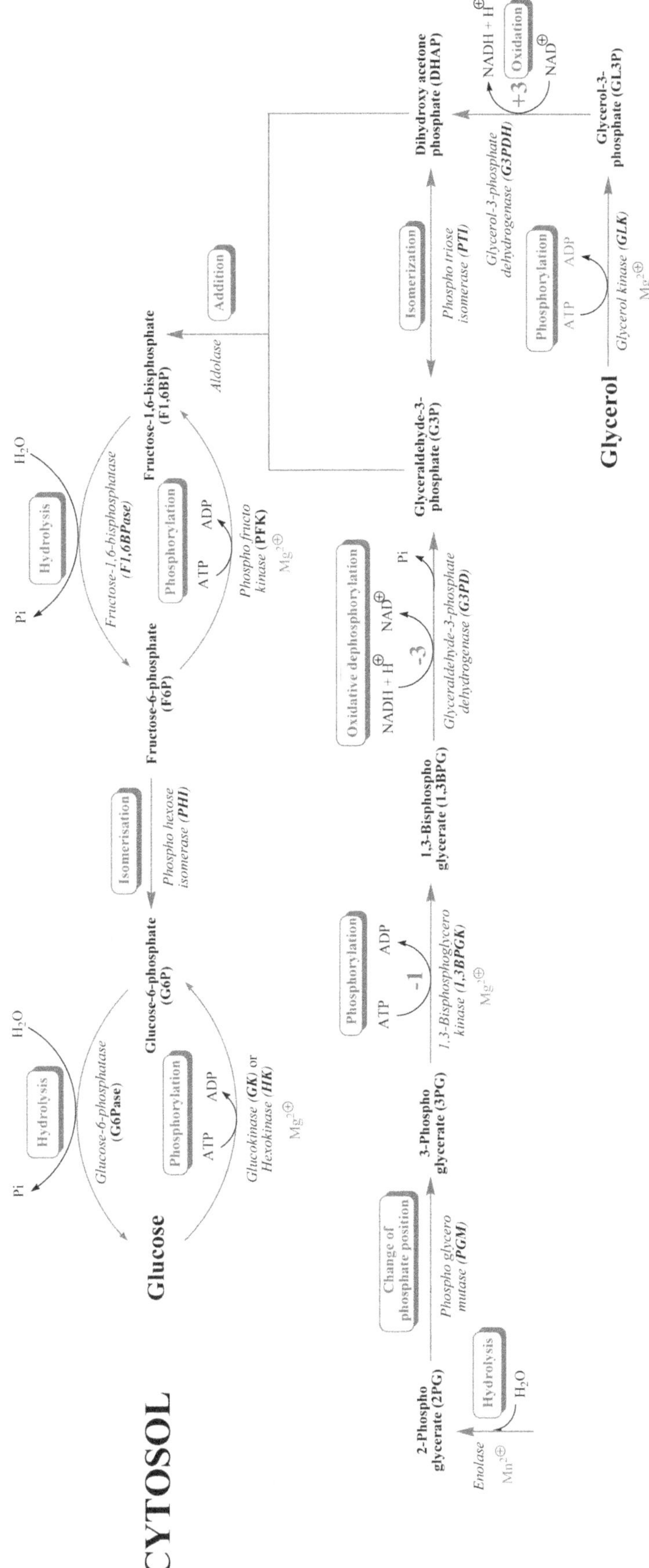
CYTOSOL
Glucose
Hydrolysis
Pi
H_2O
Glucose-6-phosphatase (G6Pase)
Phosphorylation
ATP
ADP
Glucokinase (GK) or Hexokinase (HK)
$Mg^{2\oplus}$
Glucose-6-phosphate (G6P)
Isomerisation
Phospho hexose isomerase (PHI)
Fructose-6-phosphate (F6P)
Hydrolysis
Pi
H_2O
Fructose-1,6-bisphosphatase (F1,6BPase)
Phosphorylation
ATP
ADP
Phospho fructo kinase (PFK)
$Mg^{2\oplus}$
Fructose-1,6-bisphosphate (F1,6BP)
Aldolase
Addition
Glyceraldehyde-3-phosphate (G3P)
Isomerization
Phospho triose isomerase (PTI)
Dihydroxy acetone phosphate (DHAP)
Glycerol-3-phosphate dehydrogenase (G3PDH)
Oxidation
+3
$NADH + H^{\oplus}$
$NAD^{\oplus}$
Glycerol-3-phosphate (GL3P)
Phosphorylation
ATP
ADP
Glycerol kinase (GLK)
$Mg^{2\oplus}$
Glycerol
Oxidative dephosphorylation
$NADH + H^{\oplus}$
$NAD^{\oplus}$
-3
Pi
Glyceraldehyde-3-phosphate dehydrogenase (G3PD)
1,3-Bisphospho glycerate (1,3BPG)
Phosphorylation
ATP
ADP
-1
1,3-Bisphosphoglycero kinase (1,3BPGK)
$Mg^{2\oplus}$
3-Phospho glycerate (3PG)
Change of phosphate position
Phospho glycero mutase (PGM)
2-Phospho glycerate (2PG)
Hydrolysis
H_2O
Enolase
$Mn^{2\oplus}$

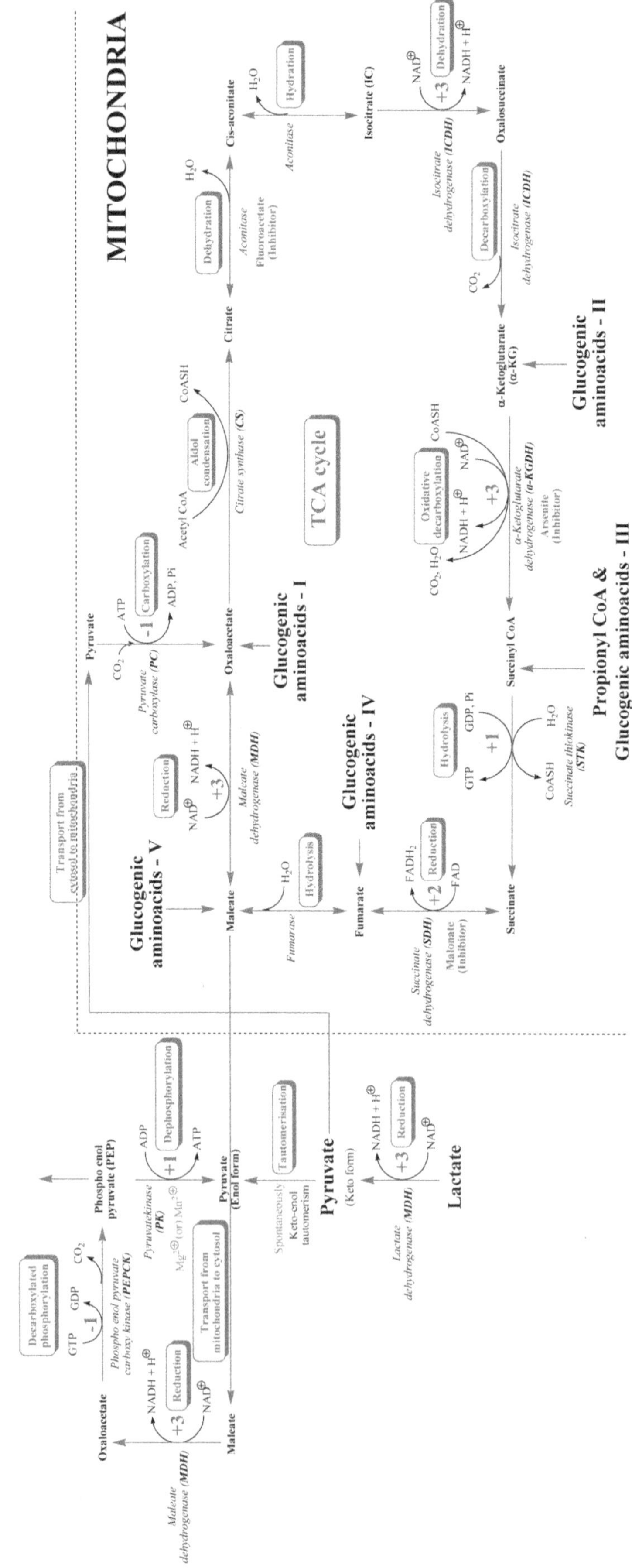

MITOCHONDRIA
TCA cycle
Pyruvate
Pyruvate carboxylase (PC)
Carboxylation
ATP
ADP, Pi
CO_2
Oxaloacetate
Acetyl CoA
Aldol condensation
CoASH
Citrate synthase (CS)
Citrate
Dehydration
H_2O
Aconitase
Fluoroacetate (Inhibitor)
Cis-aconitate
Hydration
Isocitrate (IC)
Isocitrate dehydrogenase (ICDH)
Dehydration
NADH + H⊕
Oxalosuccinate
Decarboxylation
α-Ketoglutarate (α-KG)
Glucogenic aminoacids - II
Oxidative decarboxylation
CO_2, H_2O
α-Ketoglutarate dehydrogenase (α-KGDH)
Arsenite (Inhibitor)
Succinyl CoA
Propionyl CoA & Glucogenic aminoacids - III
Hydrolysis
GTP
GDP, Pi
CoASH
Succinate thiokinase (STK)
Succinate
Reduction
FAD
$FADH_2$
Succinate dehydrogenase (SDH)
Malonate (Inhibitor)
Fumarate
Glucogenic aminoacids - IV
Hydrolysis
Fumarase
Maleate
Reduction
Malate dehydrogenase (MDH)
Glucogenic aminoacids - I
Glucogenic aminoacids - V
Transport from cytosol to mitochondria
Oxaloacetate
Malate dehydrogenase (MDH)
Decarboxylated phosphorylation
GTP
GDP
Phospho enol pyruvate carboxy kinase (PEPCK)
Transport from mitochondria to cytosol
Phospho enol pyruvate (PEP)
Pyruvatekinase (PK)
Mg^{2+} (or) Mn^{2+}
Dephosphorylation
ADP
ATP
Pyruvate (Enol form)
Tautomerisation
Spontaneously Keto-enol tautomerism
Pyruvate
(Keto form)
Lactate dehydrogenase (MDH)
Lactate

List of glucogenic amino acids:

The followings are the list of various glucogenic amino acids entered into citric acid cycle at various stages and produces glucose through gluconeogenesis.

1. Glucogenic amino acids – I: Alanine, glycine, serine, cysteine, threonine and tryptophan
2. Glucogenic amino acids – II: Asparagine and aspartate
3. Glucogenic amino acids – III: Glutamate, glutamine, arginine, histidine and proline
4. Glucogenic amino acids – IV: Isoleucine, methionine and valine
5. Glucogenic amino acids – V: Phenyl alanine and tyrosine

Significance:

1. Continuous supply of glucose is very essential for the biological systems as it occupies a major position in metabolism.
2. For continuous supply of energy, organs like brain, CNS, erythrocytes, testes and kidney medulla is dependent on glucose. Per day 160 g of glucose is needed for the whole body. Out of this around 120 g is utilized by brain only.
3. Under aerobic condition glucose only supplies energy to the skeletal muscle.
4. Other carbohydrates such as lactose, amino sugars, etc. are bio-synthesized from glucose only.
5. Glucose is also utilized for the synthesis of fat by converting into glycerol.
6. In fasting condition more than a day, gluconeogenesis is essential for the survival of animals in order to meet the basal requirements of the biological systems for glucose and to maintain intermediate of TCA cycle.
7. Gluconeogenesis effectively clears some metabolites like lactate, glycerol, propionate, etc. produced in tissues which will accumulate in blood.

Regulation:

Gluconeogenesis is regulated by the hormone glucagon (hormone secreted by α-cells of islets of pancreas). Glucagon stimulates gluconeogenesis by inactivating *pyruvate kinase (PK)*, inhibiting *phospho fructo kinase (PFK)* and activating *fructose-1,6-bisphosphatase (F1,6BPase)*. In addition, glucogenic amino acids and acetyl CoA stimulate gluconeogenesis as it allosterically activates *pyruvate carboxylase (PC)*. *Glucose-6-phosphatase (G6Pase), fructose-1,6-bisphosphatase (F1,6BPase)*, and *phospho enol pyruvate carboxy kinase (PEPCK)* are the **rate limiting enzymes of gluconeogenesis**. Hence it also regulates gluconeogenesis.

Hexose Mono Phosphate (HMP) Shunt

Other Names: Pentose phosphate pathway or Phospho gluconate pathway

Definition: For oxidation of glucose, HMP shunt is an alternative oxidative pathway for glycolysis and citric acid cycle. This pathway is concerned with the biosynthesis of pentose sugars and reducing equivalent NADPH; hence it is more anabolic in nature. **HMP pathway is defined as direct complete oxidation of glucose into carbon dioxide with the production of NADPH + H⁺.** Out of 6 moles of glucose-6-phosphate (G6P) entered in HMP shunt, one mole is completely oxidized into carbon dioxide and the rest of five moles are regenerated.

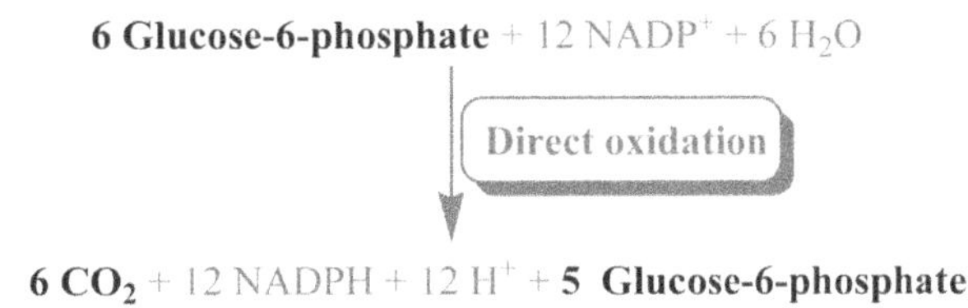

Pathway: HMP shunt takes place in tissues like liver, adipose tissue, testes, erythrocyte, adrenal gland and lactating mammary gland which are involved in the synthesis of steroids and fatty acids. The necessary enzymes are present in cytosol fraction of the cell. HMP shunt pathway is divided into two different phases as (a) oxidative phase and (b) non-oxidative phase.

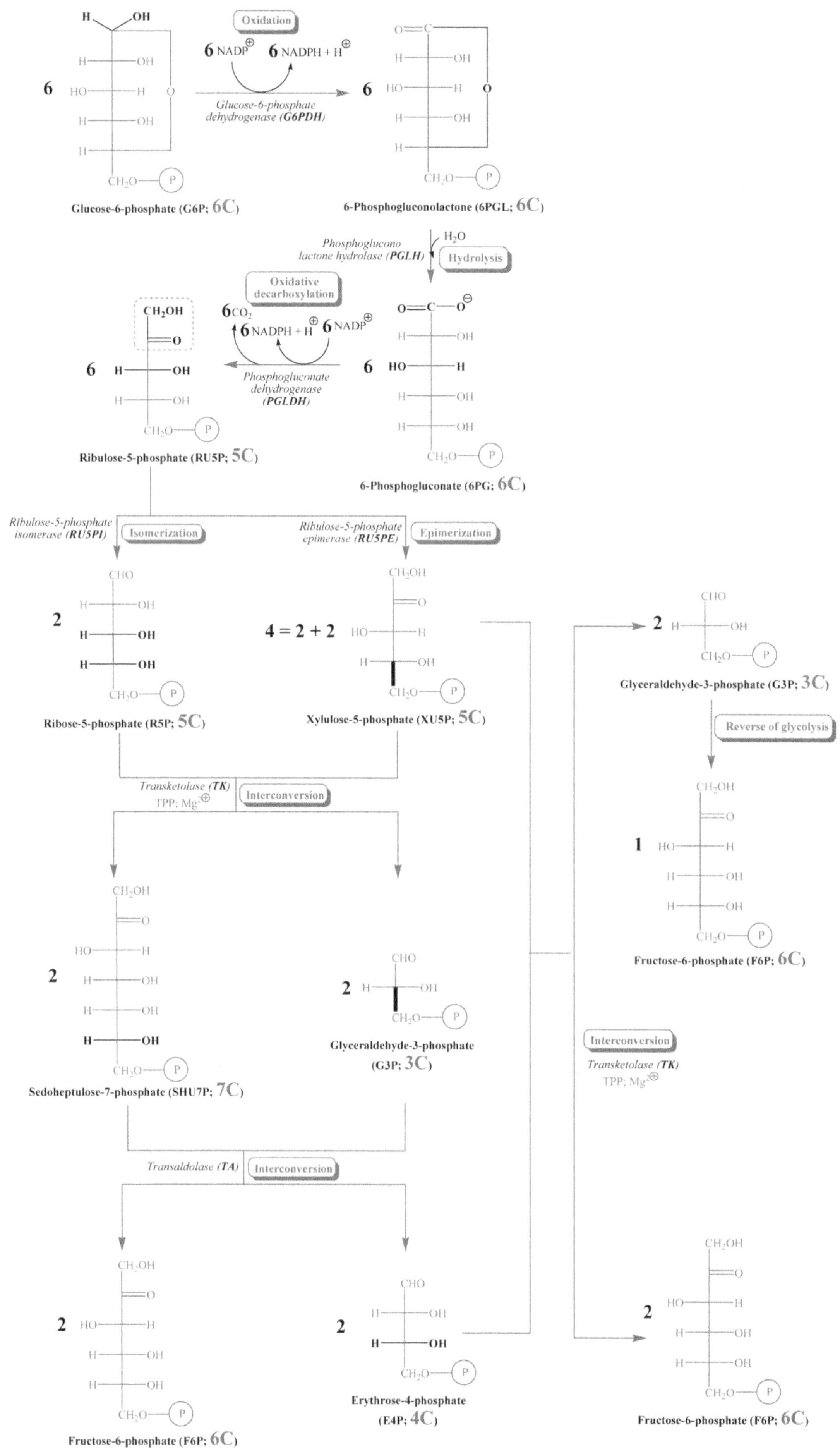

Oxidation
6 NADP⊕
6 NADPH + H⊕
Glucose-6-phosphate dehydrogenase (G6PDH)
Glucose-6-phosphate (G6P; 6C)
6-Phosphogluconolactone (6PGL; 6C)
Phosphoglucono lactone hydrolase (PGLH)
H_2O
Hydrolysis
Oxidative decarboxylation
6CO_2
6 NADPH + H⊕
6 NADP⊕
Phosphogluconate dehydrogenase (PGLDH)
Ribulose-5-phosphate (RU5P; 5C)
6-Phosphogluconate (6PG; 6C)
Ribulose-5-phosphate isomerase (RU5PI)
Isomerization
Ribulose-5-phosphate epimerase (RU5PE)
Epimerization
4 = 2 + 2
Ribose-5-phosphate (R5P; 5C)
Xylulose-5-phosphate (XU5P; 5C)
Glyceraldehyde-3-phosphate (G3P; 3C)
Reverse of glycolysis
Transketolase (TK)
TPP; $Mg^{2⊕}$
Interconversion
Fructose-6-phosphate (F6P; 6C)
Sedoheptulose-7-phosphate (SHU7P; 7C)
Glyceraldehyde-3-phosphate (G3P; 3C)
Interconversion
Transketolase (TK)
TPP; $Mg^{2⊕}$
Transaldolase (TA)
Interconversion
Fructose-6-phosphate (F6P; 6C)
Erythrose-4-phosphate (E4P; 4C)
Fructose-6-phosphate (F6P; 6C)

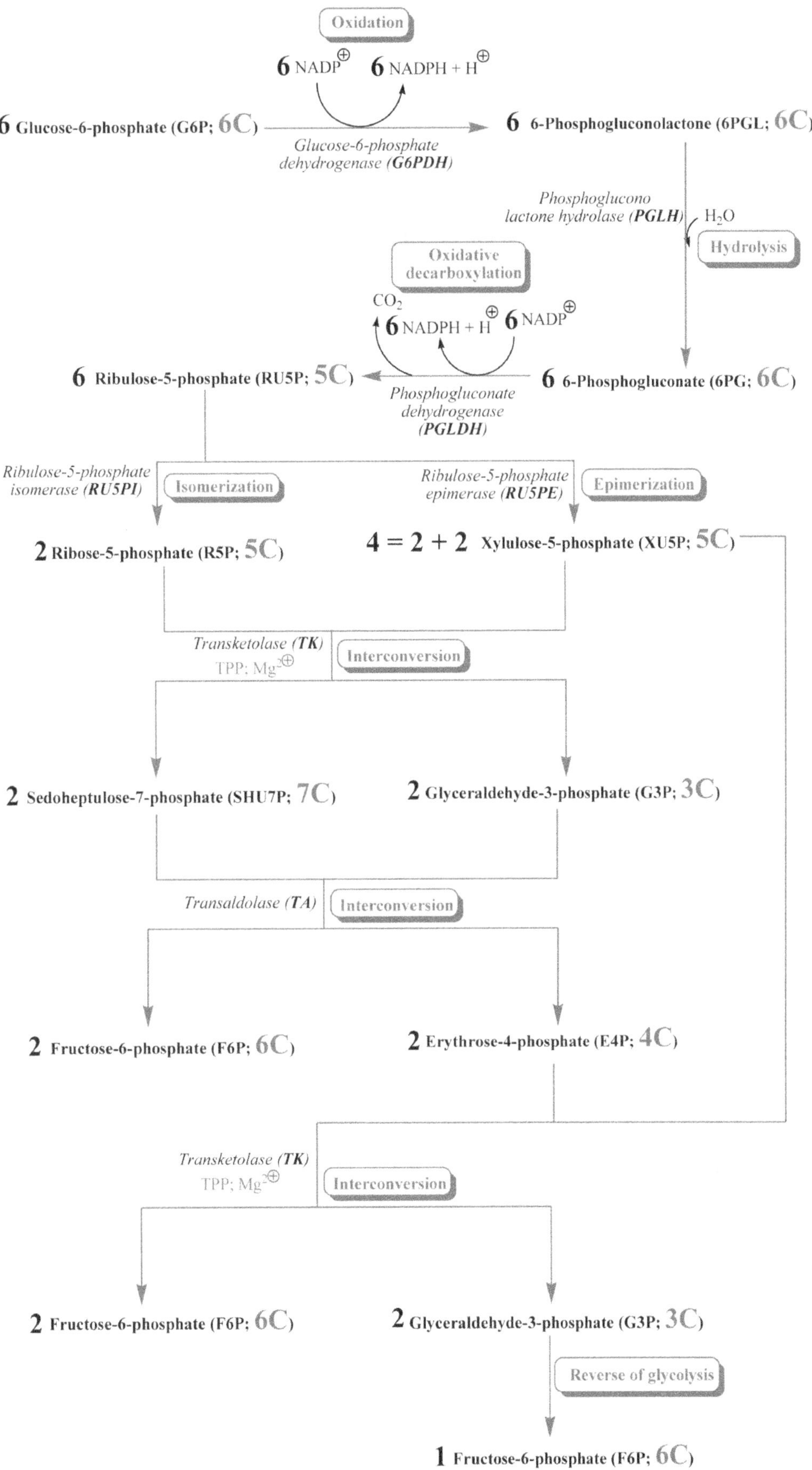
Oxidation
6 NADP⊕
6 NADPH + H⊕
6 Glucose-6-phosphate (G6P; 6C)
Glucose-6-phosphate dehydrogenase (G6PDH)
6 6-Phosphogluconolactone (6PGL; 6C)
Phosphoglucono lactone hydrolase (PGLH)
H2O
Hydrolysis
Oxidative decarboxylation
CO2
6 NADPH + H⊕
6 NADP⊕
6 Ribulose-5-phosphate (RU5P; 5C)
Phosphogluconate dehydrogenase (PGLDH)
6 6-Phosphogluconate (6PG; 6C)
Ribulose-5-phosphate isomerase (RU5PI)
Isomerization
Ribulose-5-phosphate epimerase (RU5PE)
Epimerization
2 Ribose-5-phosphate (R5P; 5C)
4 = 2 + 2 Xylulose-5-phosphate (XU5P; 5C)
Transketolase (TK)
TPP; Mg2⊕
Interconversion
2 Sedoheptulose-7-phosphate (SHU7P; 7C)
2 Glyceraldehyde-3-phosphate (G3P; 3C)
Transaldolase (TA)
Interconversion
2 Fructose-6-phosphate (F6P; 6C)
2 Erythrose-4-phosphate (E4P; 4C)
Transketolase (TK)
TPP; Mg2⊕
Interconversion
2 Fructose-6-phosphate (F6P; 6C)
2 Glyceraldehyde-3-phosphate (G3P; 3C)
Reverse of glycolysis
1 Fructose-6-phosphate (F6P; 6C)

(a) **Oxidative phase:** This phase starts from glucose-6-phosphate (G6P) and ends in the formation of ribose-5-phosphate (R5P). During this phase, compounds undergo oxidation in presence of reducing equivalent $NADP^+$.

1. Initially, glucose-6-phosphate (G6P) is oxidized at C-1 and produced 6-phosphogluconolactone (6PGL) by *glucose-6-phosphate dehydrogenase (G6PDH)* (In NAD^+ / $NADP^+$ / FAD involved reactions, the enzymes acted are "*dehydrogenase*" and the substrate is "glucose-6-phosphate"). **During this reaction one molecule of $NADP^+$ is reduced to NAPH + H^+.**
2. The formed 6-phosphogluconolactone (6PGL) undergoes hydrolysis by reacting with water in presence of *phosphoglucono lactone hydrolase (PGLH)* (Substrate is "6-phosphogluconolactone" and the type of reaction is "hydrolysis") results in formation of 6-phosphogluconate (6PG).
3. Oxidative decarboxylation of 6-phosphogluconate (6PG) produces pentose sugar ribulose-5-phosphate (RU5P). **One mole of carbon dioxide is eliminated** in the presence of *phosphogluconate dehydrogenase (PGLDH)* (In NAD^+ / $NADP^+$ / FAD involved reactions, the enzymes acted are "*dehydrogenase*" and the substrate is "6-phosphogluconate"). **During this reaction one molecule of $NADP^+$ is reduced to NAPH + H^+.**
4. In the next step, ribulose-5-phosphate (RU5P) is isomerized into ribose-5-phosphate (R5P) by "*ribulose-5-phosphate isomerase (RU5PI)*" (Substrate is "ribulose-5-phosphate" and the type of reaction is "isomerization"). In another way, ribulose-5-phosphate (RU5P) is epimerized into xylulose-5-phosphate (XU5P) by "*ribulose-5-phosphate epimerase (RU5PE)*" (Substrate is "ribulose-5-phosphate" and the type of reaction involved is "epimerization"). In HMP shunt, ribulose-5-phosphate (RU5P) undergoes isomerization and epimerization reaction in the ratio of 1:2.

(b) **Non-oxidative phase:** This phase starts from ribose-5-phosphate (R5P) and ends in the formation of fructose-6-phosphate (F6P). During this phase compounds do not undergo oxidation and only inter conversion of 3, 4, 5 and 7 carbon sugar molecules takes place.

1. 5 Carbon ribose-5-phosphate (R5P) reacts with 5 carbon xylulose-5-phosphate (XU5P) in the presence of *transketolase (TK)* (Transfer takes place from aldose to ketose sugar) and produces 7 carbon sedoheptulose-7-phosphate (SHU7P) and 3 carbon glyceraldehyde-3-phosphate (G3P). *Transketolase* (TK) needs thiamine pyrophosphate (TPP) and magnesium ion as co-enzyme for activity.
2. Later, 7 carbon sedoheptulose-7-phosphate (SHU7P) reacts with 3 carbon glyceraldehyde-3-phosphate (G3P) in the presence of *transaldolase (TA)* (Transfer takes place from ketose to aldose sugar) and produces 6 carbon fructose-6-phosphate (F6P) and 4 carbon erythrose-4-phosphate (E4P). Unlike *transketolase (TK)* enzymes, *transaldolase (TA)* do not need any co-enzyme for its activity.
3. The formed 4 carbon erythrose-4-phosphate (E4P) reacts with another mole of 5 carbon xylulose-5-phosphate (XU5P; earlier synthesized in oxidative phase) and produces 6 carbon fructose-6-phosphate (F6P) and 3 carbon glyceraldehyde-3-phosphate (G3P) in presence of *transketolase (TK)* (Transfer takes place from aldose to ketose sugar).
4. Glyceraldehyde-3-phosphate (G3P) produces fructose-6-phosphate (F6P) by gluconeogenesis pathway (2 mole of glyceraldehyde-3-phosphate (G3P) produce one mole of fructose-6-phosphate (F6P)).
5. Fructose-6-phosphate (F6P) and glyceraldehyde-3-phosphate (G3P) can be further catabolized through glycolysis and TCA cycle. Alternatively, glucose may also be synthesized from these two compounds.

Significance:

1. As such in HMP shunt pathway ATP is neither synthesized nor utilized directly which is uniqueness of this pathway.
2. Several inter convertible substances are produced in HMP shunt and these compounds may proceed in different directions in metabolic reactions. This is another uniqueness of HMP shunt pathway.
3. In this pathway 3, 4, 5 and 7 carbon sugar molecules undergo inter conversion.

4. Out of 6 moles of glucose-6-phosphate (G6P) entered in HMP shunt, one mole is completely oxidized into carbon dioxide and the rest of five moles are regenerated.
5. Two important compounds are biosynthesized in HMP shunt pathway namely pentose sugar and NADPH.
6. **Pentose sugar:** Three pentose sugars such as ribulose-5-phosphate (RU5P), ribose-5-phosphate (R5P) and xylulose-5-phosphate (XU5P) are biosynthesized in pentose phosphate pathway. Among this ribose-5-phosphate (R5P) is more important because this pentose or its derivatives are used for the synthesis of nucleic acid (RNA and DNA) and many nucleotides like ATP, NAD^+, FAD and co-enzyme A. For the synthesis of pentoses through HMP shunt, complete pathway may not be required. Hence, pentoses are synthesized in skeletal muscle even though it contains only first few enzymes of pathway.
7. **NADPH:** Reductive biosynthesis of steroids and fatty acids are dependent on NADPH. *Glutamate dehydrogenase* (GDH) is an enzyme useful for the synthesis of certain amino acid also needs NADPH for its activity. In anti-oxidant reactions, NADPH is necessary for the conversion of hydrogen peroxide (damages DNA, unsaturated lipids and proteins) into water molecule. Cytochrome P_{450} (It is a microsomal enzyme involved in oxidation reactions for detoxification of foreign compounds) are dependent on NADPH. It is also necessary for phagocytosis (engulfment of foreign particles including micro-organism). Reduced form of glutathione (necessary for the maintenance of integrity of RBC) in RBC was maintained by NADPH only. It also prevents the accumulation of methemoglobin by maintaining ferrous ion of hemoglobin in reduced form.

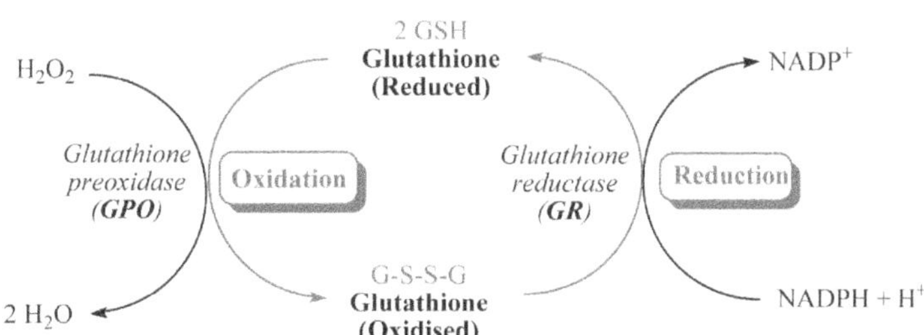

Metabolic disorder:

1. ***Glucose-6-phosphate dehydrogenase* (G6PD) deficiency or Hemolysis:** Deficiency of *G6PD* results in decreased synthesis of NADPH in RBC. Hence, peroxides and methemoglobins are accumulated in erythrocytes results in hemolysis. Severe conditions may lead to hemolytic anemia. In these patients hemolytic jaundice is produced by drugs like primaquine, sulfamethoxazole and acetanilide. *Glucose-6-phosphate dehydrogenase* (*G6PD*) deficiency is associated with resistance to *plasmodium falciparum* caused malaria because these micro-organisms are dependent on HMP shunt for reduced form of glutathione which is needed for their optimum growth in RBC.
2. **Wernicke-Korsakoff syndrome:** It is due to one tenth of reduced affinity of thiamine pyrophosphate (TPP) with *transketolase* (*TK*). Mental disorder, partial paralysis and loss of memory are the symptoms of this syndrome. Symptoms are manifested in alcoholics whose diet is vitamin deficient. Erythrocyte *transketolase* (*TK*) activity is increased in pernicious anemia.

Regulation: Glucose-6-phosphate dehydrogenase (*G6PD*) which catalyzes irreversible step is a **rate limiting enzymes** of HMP shunt pathway. Consequently, it regulates the HMP pathway. Moreover, NADPH competitively inhibits *glucose-6-phosphate dehydrogenase* (*G6PD*). Hence, the flux of cycle is determined by the ratio of NADPH / $NADP^+$.

Glycogen Metabolism

Glycogen: Glycogen is the storage form of glucose in animals like starch in plants. Glycogen is mainly stored in liver (6-8 %) and muscles (1-2 %); but the quantity of glycogen stored in muscle (250 g) is approximately 3 times more than liver glycogen (75 g) due to more muscle mass. Liver glycogen maintains or regulates blood glucose level particularly between meals whereas muscle glycogen is utilized for ATP supply during muscle contraction.

Glycogen is composed of α-D-glucose (Approximately 1,00,000 residues/molecules). Glucose molecules are attached to another glucose molecules by 1,4-α-glycosidic linkage. After every 8-10 glucose molecules branching takes place. In the branching point the glucose molecules are linked by 1,6-α-glycosidic linkage. Glycogen is stored as granules in cytosol where most of the enzymes of glycogen synthesis and breakdown are present. Glycogen metabolism includes two pathways namely,

1. Glycogenesis (Anabolic pathway - Synthesis of glycogen)
2. Glycogenolysis (Catabolic pathway - Breakdown of glycogen).

Glycogenesis

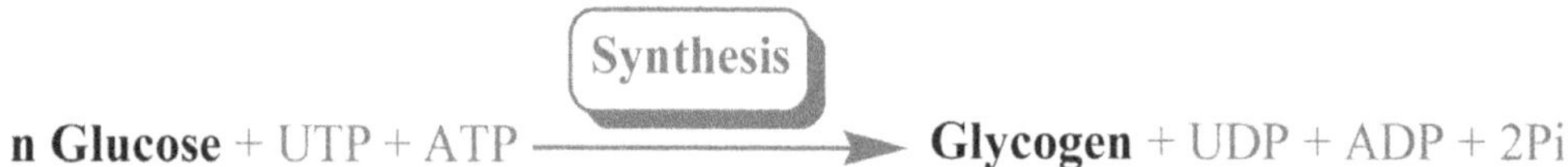

Definition: Glyco indicates "glycogen" and in Greek genesis means "synthesis / production". **It is defined as synthesis of glycogen from glucose with utilization of ATP and UTP**. It takes place in cytosol fraction of the cell.

Pathway:

1. The first step in glycogenesis is a simple phosphorylation reaction. In this step glucose is phosphorylated at 6th position in presence of enzyme called "*hexokinase (HK)* or *glucokinase (GK)*" (In ATP / GTP involved reactions, the enzymes acted are "*kinase*" and the substrate is "glucose' which is a "hexose sugar") and produces glucose-6-phosphate (G6P). *Kinase* enzyme needs magnesium ion as co-factor for its activity. In this step one ATP is converted into ADP **(1 ATP is utilized)**.
2. Further, the phosphate group present in 6th position of glucose-6-phosphate (G6P) is shifted to 1st position and produces glucose-1-phosphate (G1P). The enzyme responsible is *phospho gluco mutase (PGM)* (In change of position of phosphate group involved reactions, the enzymes acted are "*mutase*" and the substrate is "glucose-1-phosphate). **These two steps are similar to glycolysis first two steps.**
3. In the next step, glucose-1-phosphate (G1P) reacts with UTP and produces glucose carrier molecule uridine diphosphate glucose (UDPG) in presence of *UDP-glucose pyrophosphorylase (UDPGPP)* (The product is "UDP-glucose (UDPG)" and "pyrophosphate" is removed). The pyrophosphate is immediately broken into two inorganic phosphate by *pyrophosphatase (PPase)* (Substrate is "pyrophosphate" and type of reaction is "hydrolysis") through hydrolysis reaction. Otherwise the backward reaction takes place because it is reversible reaction.
4. A small fragment of pre-existing glycogen must act as a "primer" to initiate glycogen synthesis. Glycogen primer is necessary for initiation of glycogen synthesis. In case, if it is not available it is synthesized from UDP-glucose (UDPG) by reacting with tyrosine moiety of glycogenin with the removal of UDP in presence of *glycogen initiator synthase (GIS)* (Product formed is "glycogen" and the type of reaction is "synthesis initiation"). UDP can be converted to UTP by *nucleoside diphosphate kinase (NDPK)* (In ATP / GTP involved reactions, the enzymes acted are "*kinase*" and the substrate is "UDP" which is "nucleoside diphosphate") **(1 ATP is utilized)**.
5. In the next step, glycogen primer was reacted with more UDP-glucose (UDPG) in presence of *glycogen synthase (GS)* (Product is "glycogen" and the type of reaction is "synthesis") with a loss of UDP. The glucose molecules are linked to each other by 1,4-α-glycosidic linkage. The reaction will continue up to 16 glucose molecules in chain. Later, *glycogen synthase* is not able to increase the chain length.
6. After every 8 to 10 glucose molecules branching takes place by *branching enzyme (BE)* (Type of reaction is "branch production"). *Branching enzymes (BE)* otherwise known as "*glucosyl-α-4,6-transferase (G4,6T)* or *amylo-α-1,4 to α-1,6-transglucosidase (A1,4T1,6TG)* (Glucose is transferred from "α-1,4 linkage to α-1,6 linkage") transfer a small fragment of 5-8 glucose residues from non-reducing end of

glycogen chain to another glucose residue where it is linked by 1,6-α-glycosidic linkage. Only in the branching point the type of linkage is α-1,6-glycosidic linkage; whereas in rest of case it is α-1,4-glycosidic linkage.

7. Later, the chain length is increased by "*glycogen synthase (GS)*" and more branching are formed by *branching enzymes* (*BE*) which results in formation of homopolysaccharide "glycogen".
8. Totally 2 ATP are consumed for the attachment of single glucose residue. Out of these two, one ATP is needed for phosphorylation of glucose and another one is needed for conversion of UDP to UTP. The overall reactions of glycogenesis are summarized as follows

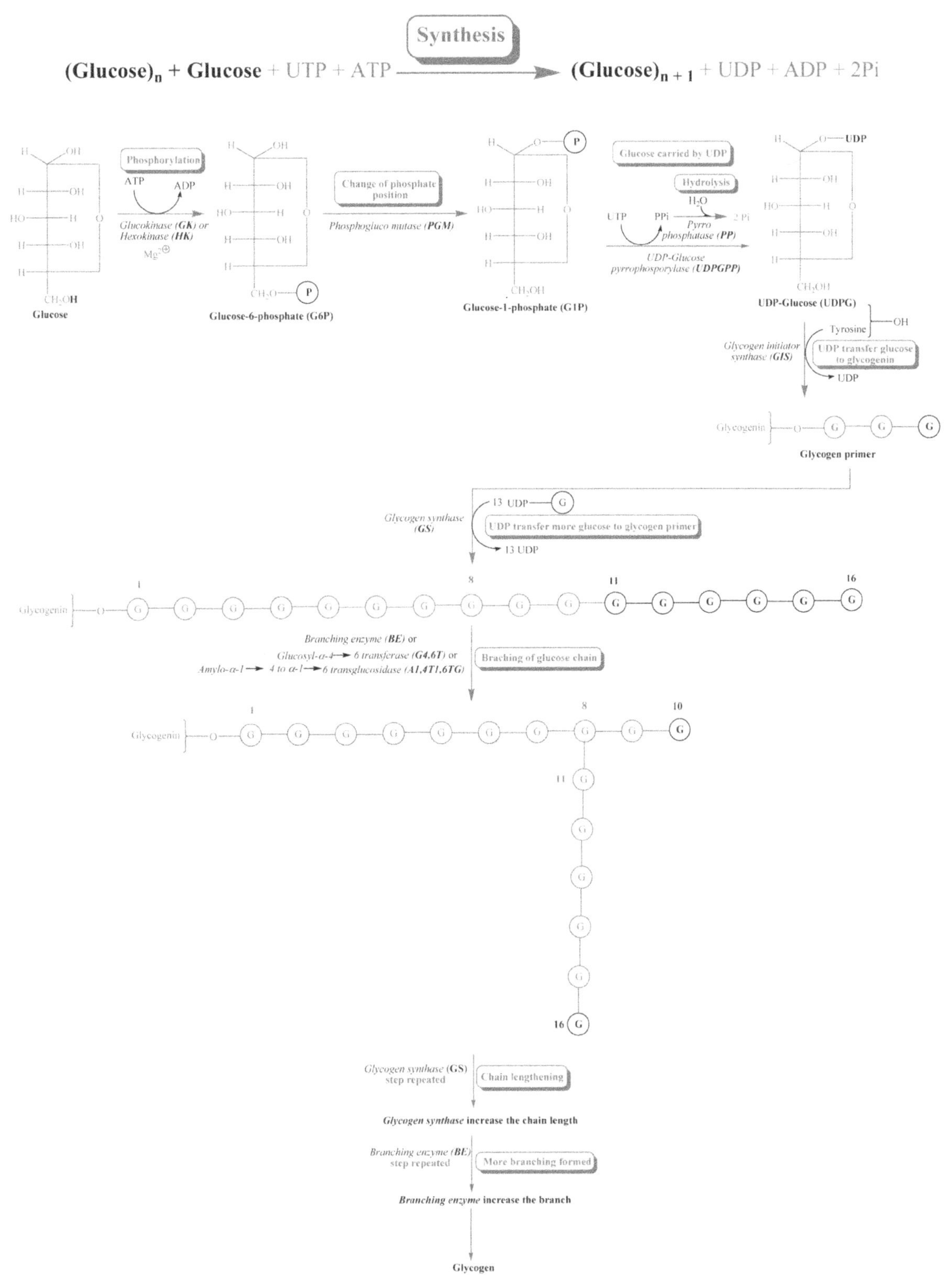

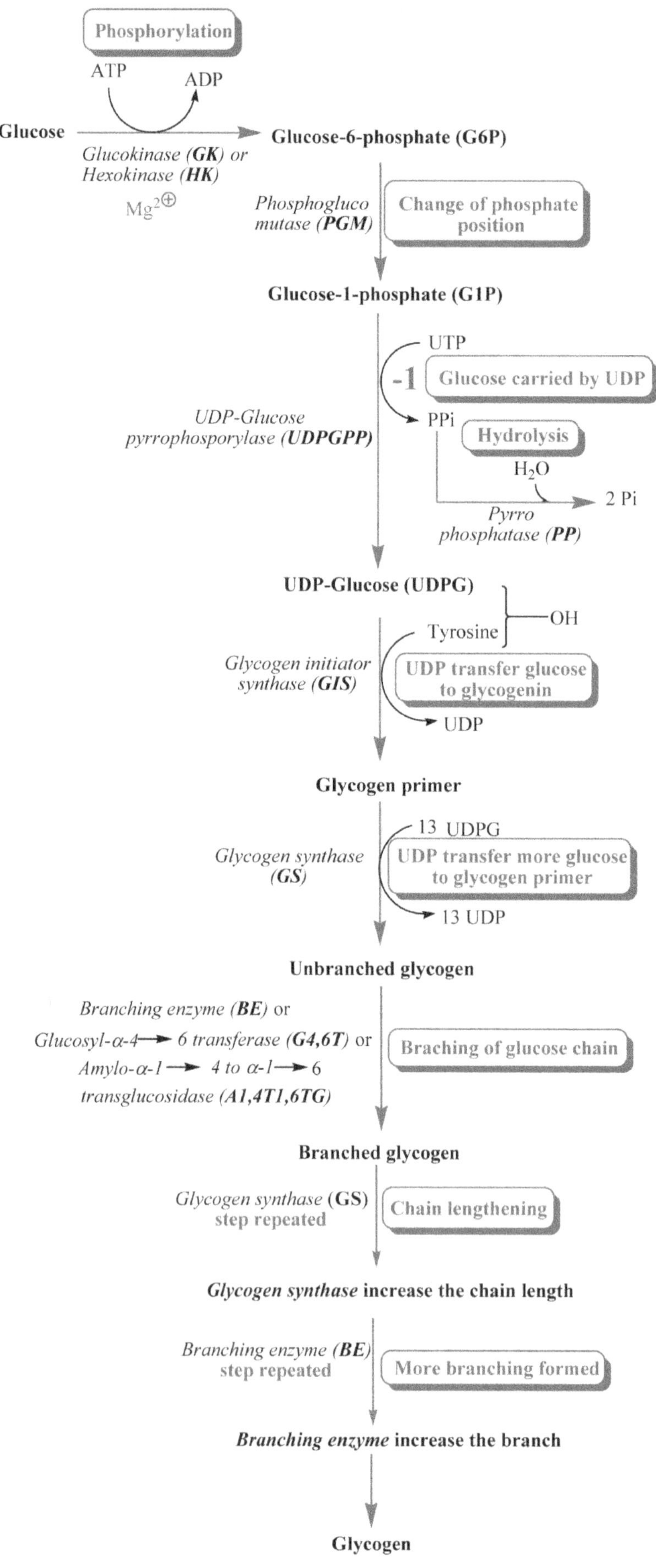
Phosphorylation
ATP
ADP
Glucose
Glucose-6-phosphate (G6P)
Glucokinase (GK) or
Hexokinase (HK)
Mg2⊕
Phosphogluco
mutase (PGM)
Change of phosphate position
Glucose-1-phosphate (G1P)
UTP
-1
Glucose carried by UDP
UDP-Glucose
pyrrophosporylase (UDPGPP)
PPi
Hydrolysis
H2O
2 Pi
Pyrro
phosphatase (PP)
UDP-Glucose (UDPG)
Tyrosine
OH
Glycogen initiator
synthase (GIS)
UDP transfer glucose to glycogenin
UDP
Glycogen primer
13 UDPG
Glycogen synthase
(GS)
UDP transfer more glucose to glycogen primer
13 UDP
Unbranched glycogen
Branching enzyme (BE) or
Glucosyl-α-4→6 transferase (G4,6T) or
Amylo-α-1→4 to α-1→6
transglucosidase (A1,4T1,6TG)
Braching of glucose chain
Branched glycogen
Glycogen synthase (GS)
step repeated
Chain lengthening
Glycogen synthase increase the chain length
Branching enzyme (BE)
step repeated
More branching formed
Branching enzyme increase the branch
Glycogen

Glycogenolysis

Definition: Glycogeno indicates "glycogen" and in Greek lysis means "breakdown / dissolution". **It is defined as breakdown of stored glycogen in liver and muscle into glucose.**

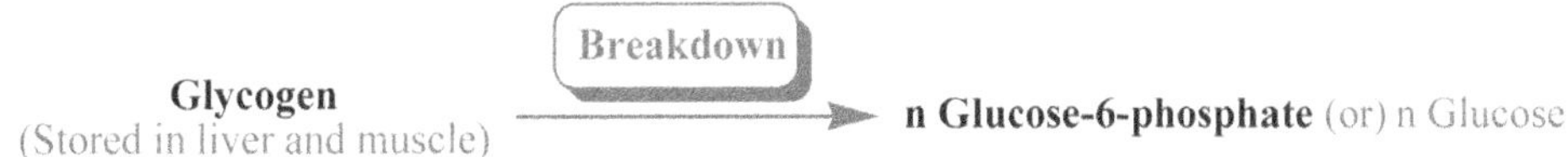

Pathway:

1. In the first step of glycogenolysis, glycogen undergoes phosphorylation reaction by reacting with inorganic phosphate in presence of *glycogen phosphorylase* (*GP*) (Substrate is "glycogen" and the type of reaction is "phosphorolysis") and liberates glucose-1-phosphate (G1P). This process of phosphorolysis continues until four glucose residues remains on either side of branching point. The molecule which contains four glucose residues on either side of branching point is called as "limit dextrin" which cannot be further degraded by *glycogen phosphorylase* (*GP*).
2. In the next step, *glucosyl-4,4-transferase* (*G4,4T*) (Glucose is transferred from α-1,4 linkage to α-1,4 linkage) removes 3 to 4 residues of glucose and transfer them to other chain. The linkage in both the breaking point and attaching point is α-1,4 linkage. ***Glucosyl-4,4-transferase* (*G4,4T*) is the first *debranching enzyme* (*DB*) of glycogenolysis.**
3. **The second *debranching enzyme* (*DB*) i.e., "*amylo-α-1,6-glucosidase*" (*A1,6G*)** (Break of α-1.6 glycosidic linkage) debranches the branching point glucose and removes as free glucose not as glucose phosphate. It only breaks the α-1,6 linkage and not transfers unlike *glucosyl-4,4-transferase* (*G4,4T*).
4. The resulted intermediate is again attacked by *glycogen phosphorylase* (*GP*) and produces glucose-1-phosphate (G1P).
5. Further, phosphate group present in 1st position of glucose-1-phosphate (G1P) is shifted to 6th position and produces glucose-6-phosphate (G6P). The enzyme responsible is *phospho gluco mutase* (*PGM*) (In change of position of phosphate group involved reactions, the enzymes acted are "*mutase*" and the substrate is "glucose-1-phosphate (G1P)").
6. Glucose-6-phosphate (G6P) can either undergo glycolysis or converted to glucose. *Glucose-6-phosphatase* (*G6Pase*) is present in liver, kidney and intestine thereby leads to glucose. Liver is the major glycogen storage organ to provide glucose into circulation to be utilized by various other tissues. In case of muscle and brain *glucose-6-phosphatase* (*G6Pase*) is absent thereby leads to glycolysis. Even though some free glucose is produced in these organs by *amylo-α-1,6-glucosidase* (*A1,6Gase*) enzyme.
7. The ratio of glucose-1-phosphate (G1P) and free glucose produced in glycogenolysis by combined effects of *glycogen phosphorylase* (*GP*) and *debranching enzyme* (*DB*) is 8:1. *Debranching enzyme* (*DB*) cleaves the glycogen branches by two enzyme activities present on a single polypeptide; hence it is a bifunctional enzyme.
8. *Lysosomal acid maltase* (*LAM*) or *acid maltase* (*AM*) or *α-1,4-glucosidase* (*α1,4G*) (Breaking of α-1.6 glycosidic linkage) is a lysosomal enzyme which continuously degrades a small quantity of glycogen. Significance of this pathway is not clear. However, deficiency of this enzyme cause glycogen accumulation and leads to serious glycogen storage disease type - II or Pompe's disease.

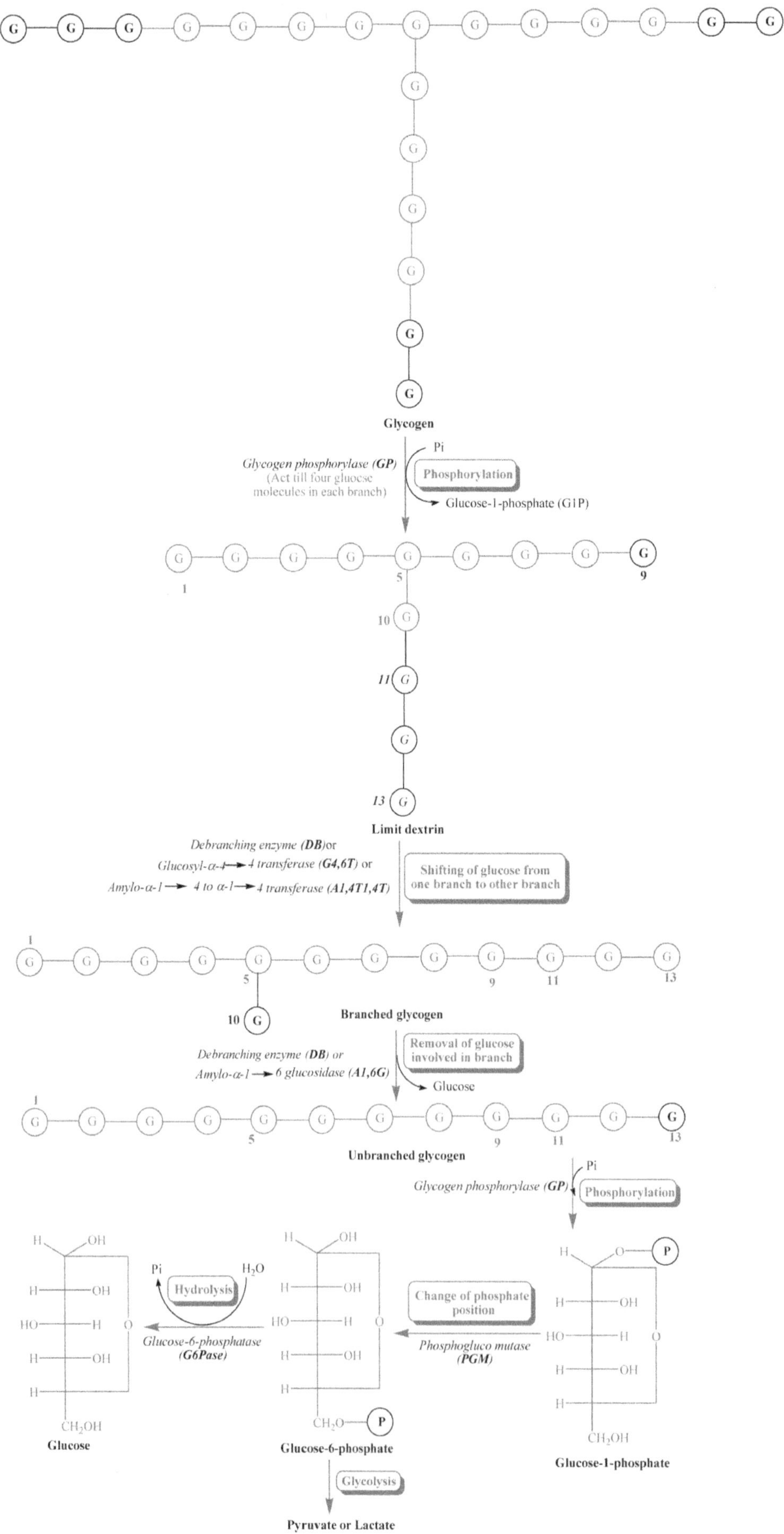

Glycogen
Glycogen phosphorylase (GP)
(Act till four gluocse molecules in each branch)
Pi
Phosphorylation
Glucose-1-phosphate (G1P)
Limit dextrin
Debranching enzyme (DB) or
Glucosyl-α-4 → 4 transferase (G4,6T) or
Amylo-α-1 → 4 to α-1 → 4 transferase (A1,4T1,4T)
Shifting of glucose from one branch to other branch
Branched glycogen
Debranching enzyme (DB) or
Amylo-α-1 → 6 glucosidase (A1,6G)
Removal of glucose involved in branch
Glucose
Unbranched glycogen
Glycogen phosphorylase (GP)
Phosphorylation
Glucose-1-phosphate
Change of phosphate position
Phosphogluco mutase (PGM)
Glucose-6-phosphate
Hydrolysis
H_2O
Glucose-6-phosphatase (G6Pase)
Glucose
Glycolysis
Pyruvate or Lactate

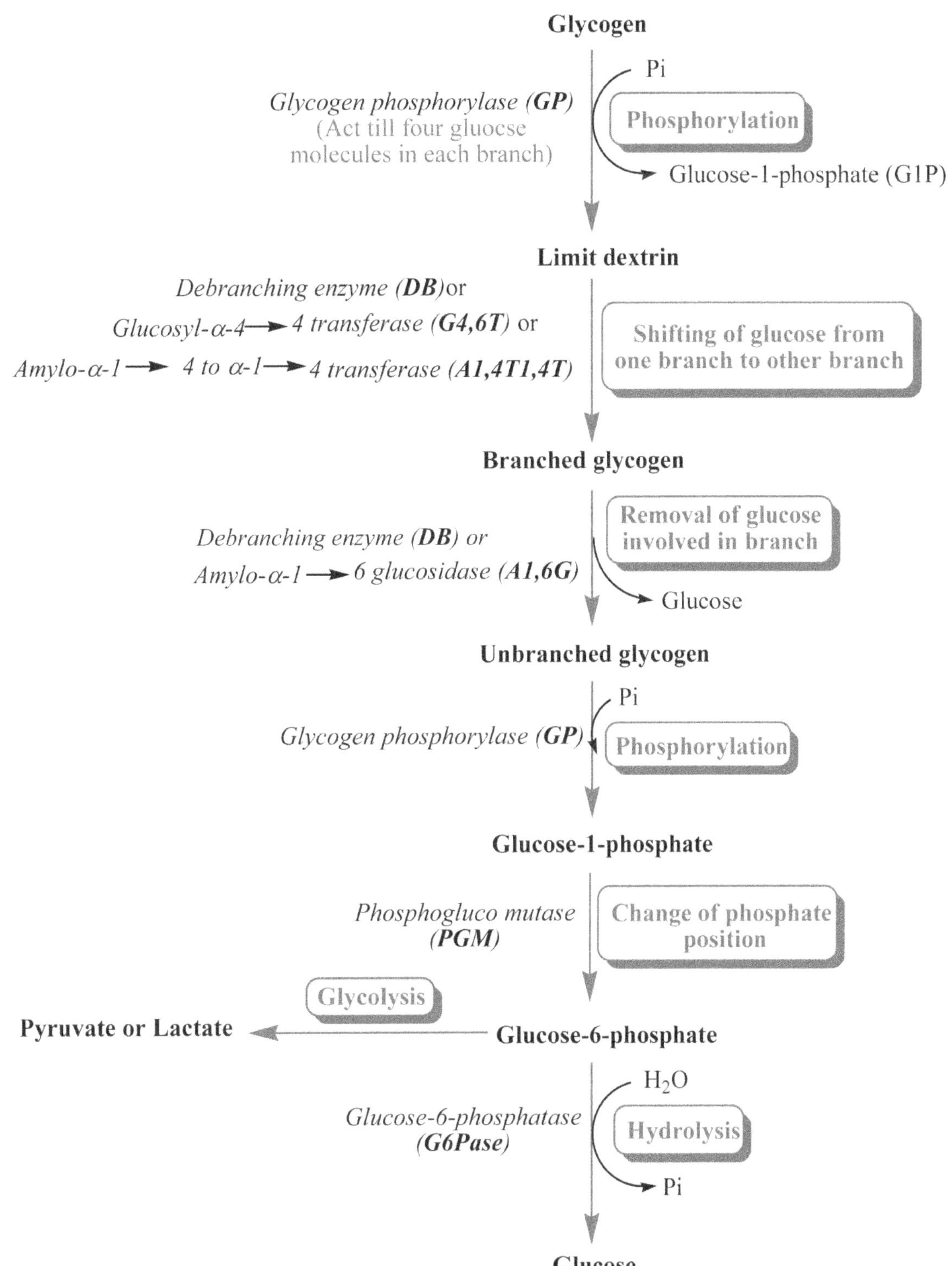

Glycogen Storage Diseases

The diseases which are related to glycogenesis and glycogenolysis are commonly known as glycogen storage diseases. The various glycogen storage diseases are summarized in Table 2.6 along with its responsible enzyme.

Table 2.6 Glycogen storage diseases & their characteristic features.

S. No.	Type of glycogen storage diseases	Disease name	Enzyme responsible	Characteristic features
1	Type – I	Von-Gierke's disease or Type – I glycogenosis	*Glucose-6-phosphatase* (*G6Pase*)	Glycogen accumulates in liver and kidney leads to fasting hypoglycemia, lactic acidemia, hyperlipidemia and hyperuricemia.
2	Type – II	Pompe's disease	*Lysosomal α-1,4-glucosidase* (*α1,4G*) or *acid maltase* (*AM*)	Increased glycogenesis leads to accumulation of glycogen in all tissues particularly heart
3	Type – III	Cori's disease or Forbe's disease or Limit dextrinosis	*Debranching enzyme* (*DE*) or *Amylo-α-1,6-glucosidase* (*A1,6G*)	Decreased debranching of limit dextrin leads to accumulation of branched chain glycogen (Similar to Type – I but mild).
4	Type – IV	Anderson's disease or Amylopectinosis	*Glucosyl-α-4,6-transferase* (*G4,6T*) or *Amylo-α-1,4 to α-1,6-transglucosidase* (*α1,4T1,6TG*)	Increased concentration of un branched glycogen and accumulates in liver.
5	Type – V	Mc Ardle's disease or Type – V glycogenosis	*Glycogen phosphorylase* (*GP*) (In muscle)	Decreased muscle contraction leads to muscle cramps. Storage of glycogen in muscle increases.
6	Type – VI	Her's disease	*Glycogen phosphorylase* (*GP*) (In liver)	Blood glucose level decreased leads to liver enlargement. Mild hypoglycemia and ketosis also seen.
7	Type – VII	Taruis disease	*Phospho fructo kinase* (*PFK*)	Increased glucose-6-phosphate (G6P) and muscle cramps due to exercise.
8	Type – VIII, Type –IX, Type – X, Type – XI	---------	Enzymes involved in activating and deactivating liver phosphorylase	Rare.

Von-Gierke's disease:

It is due to lack of *glucose-6-phosphatase* (**G6Pase**) enzyme hence glucose-6-phosphate (G6P) is not converted into glucose. It leads to the following clinical conditions.

1. **Fasting hypoglycemia:** During fasting period, biological system depends on non-carbohydrate sources for its glucose demand. Due to lack of *glucose-6-phosphatase* (*G6Pase*), non-carbohydrate sources are not converted into glucose and thereby not enough glucose is released from liver into blood. Hence blood glucose level is decreased.
2. **Lactic acidemia:** Due to lack of *glucose-6-phosphatase* (*G6Pase*), glucose is not synthesized from lactate. Hence, concentration of lactate in blood is increased and pH is lowered.
3. **Hyperlipidemia:** Due to blockage of gluconeogenesis, more fats are mobilized to meet the energy requirements which results in increased plasma free fatty acids and ketone bodies.
4. **Hyperuricemia:** In other way, accumulated glucose-6-phosphate (G6P) is diverted to HMP pathway leads to production of ribose-5-phosphate (R5P) which increases the cellular level of phospho ribosyl pyrophosphate (PRPP) and increases the purine metabolism to uric acid. Elevated level of uric acid is associated with deposition of uric acid crystals in soft tissues that leads to a disease called gouty arthritis.

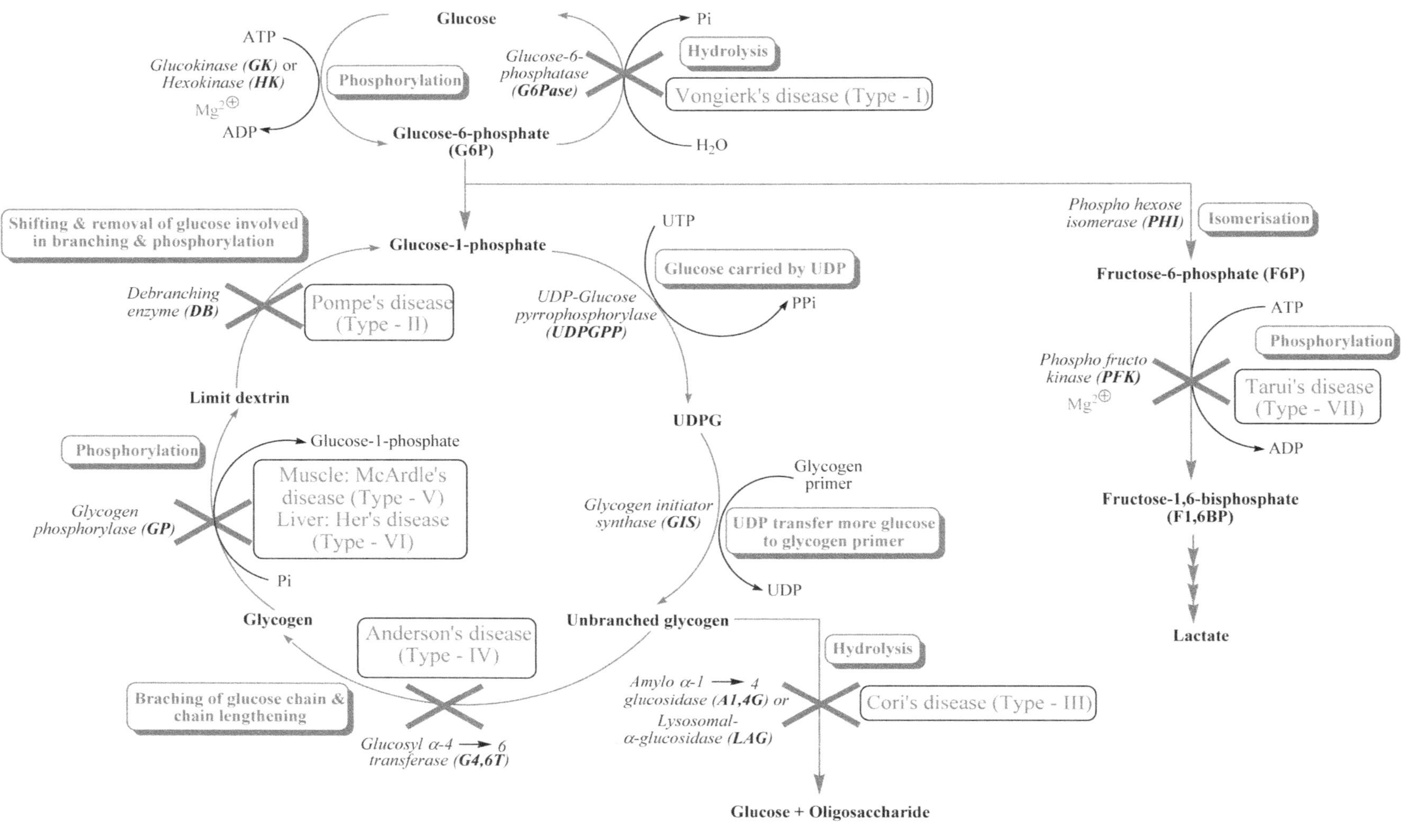
Glucose
ATP
Glucokinase (GK) or Hexokinase (HK)
Mg^{2+}
ADP
Phosphorylation
Glucose-6-phosphate (G6P)
Glucose-6-phosphatase (G6Pase)
Hydrolysis
Vongierk's disease (Type - I)
Pi
H_2O
Shifting & removal of glucose involved in branching & phosphorylation
Glucose-1-phosphate
Debranching enzyme (DB)
Pompe's disease (Type - II)
UDP-Glucose pyrrophosphorylase (UDPGPP)
UTP
Glucose carried by UDP
PPi
UDPG
Limit dextrin
Phosphorylation
Glucose-1-phosphate
Glycogen phosphorylase (GP)
Muscle: McArdle's disease (Type - V)
Liver: Her's disease (Type - VI)
Pi
Glycogen initiator synthase (GIS)
Glycogen primer
UDP transfer more glucose to glycogen primer
UDP
Glycogen
Unbranched glycogen
Anderson's disease (Type - IV)
Braching of glucose chain & chain lengthening
Glucosyl α-4 → 6 transferase (G4,6T)
Hydrolysis
Amylo α-1 → 4 glucosidase (A1,4G) or Lysosomal-α-glucosidase (LAG)
Cori's disease (Type - III)
Glucose + Oligosaccharide
Phospho hexose isomerase (PHI)
Isomerisation
Fructose-6-phosphate (F6P)
ATP
Phosphorylation
Phospho fructo kinase (PFK)
Mg^{2+}
Tarui's disease (Type - VII)
ADP
Fructose-1,6-bisphosphate (F1,6BP)
Lactate

Diabetes Mellitus

Diabetes mellitus also called as diabetes, is a carbohydrate metabolic disorder in which blood glucose levels are elevated due to decreased circulating insulin level. The following are the symptoms of diabetes mellitus such as a) Polyuria (frequent urination), b) Polydipsia (excessive thirst), c) Polyphagia (excessive hunger), d) Excess sweating, e) Hyperlipidemia, f) Dry mouth and itching skin, g) Blurred vision, h) Yeast infections, i) Slow healing sores or cuts, j) Pain or numbness in feet or legs and k) Weight loss.

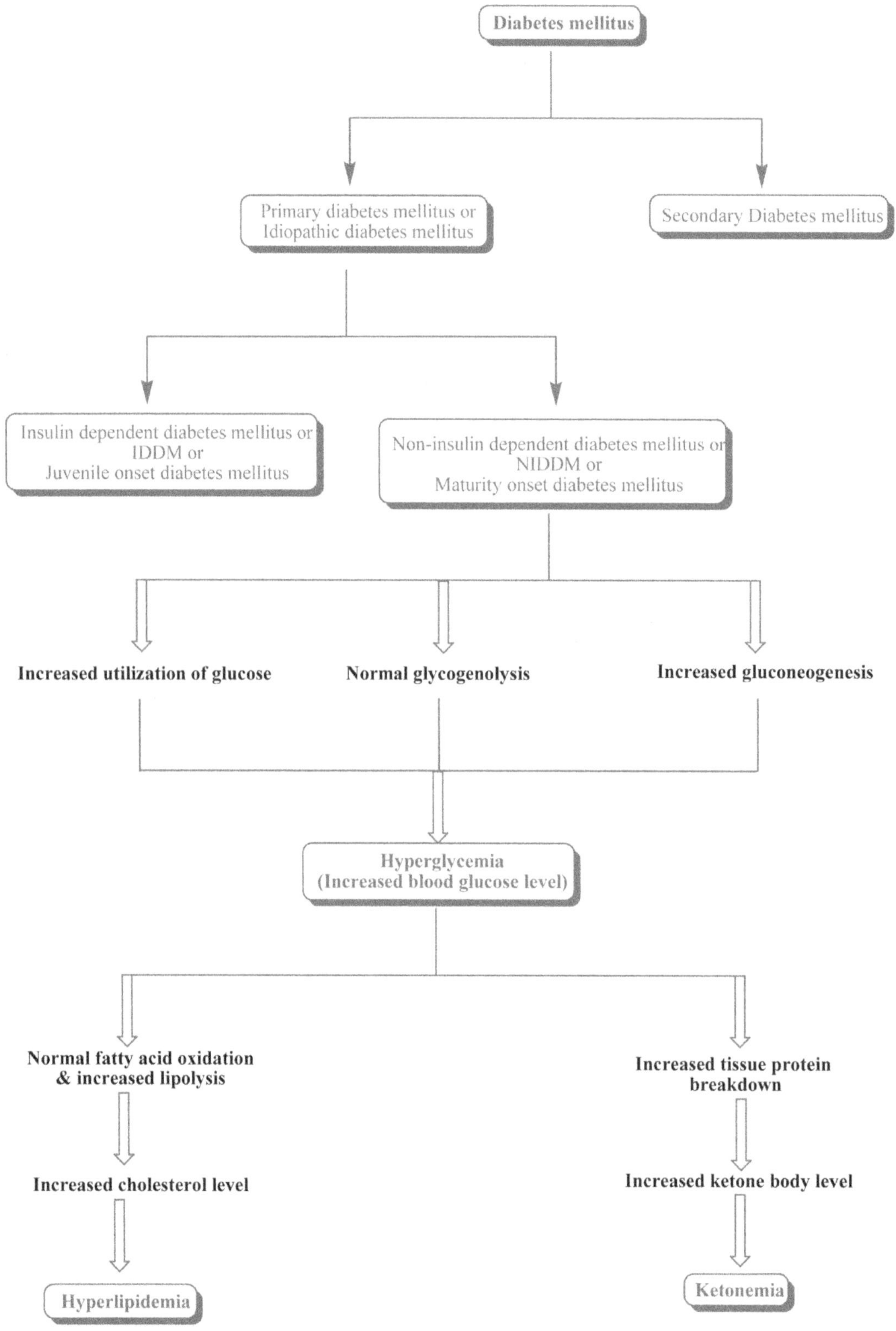

Classification

Diabetes mellitus are broadly classified into two major types namely 1) Primary diabetes mellitus, 2) Secondary diabetes mellitus. Clinically primary diabetes mellitus also known as idiopathic diabetes mellitus is more important than secondary diabetes mellitus. It is due to defect in insulin secretion. It is further classified into 1) Type - I diabetes mellitus and 2) Type–II diabetes mellitus.

Type - I diabetes mellitus: Also known as insulin dependent diabetes mellitus or IDDM or Juvenile onset diabetes mellitus. This diabetes mellitus is dependent on insulin. It is more common in younger people between 10-15 years. In this type of diabetes, there is a complete destruction of β-cells of islets of langerhans. Hence, circulating insulin level is low to very low. This leads to increased blood glucose level. Treatment for IDDM is administration of insulin.

Type - II diabetes mellitus: Also known as non-insulin dependent diabetes mellitus or NIDDM or maturity onset diabetes mellitus. This diabetes mellitus is not dependent on insulin. This type of diabetes mellitus is most common. It is common in elder people (more than 40 years). In this type of diabetes, there is no complete destruction of β-cells of islets of langerhans. Hence circulating insulin level is low. This leads to increased blood glucose level. Treatment for NIDDM is administration of oral hypoglycemic agents.

Regulation of Carbohydrate Metabolism or Regulation of Blood Glucose Level

The rate limiting enzyme of glycogenesis is *glycogen synthase* (*GS*) and the rate limiting enzyme of glycogenolysis is *glycogen phosphorylase* (*GP*). Hence *glycogen synthase* (*GS*) and *glycogen phosphorylase* (*GP*) regulate the carbohydrate metabolism. These enzymes are regulated by the three different mechanisms.

1. Allosteric regulation.
2. Hormonal regulation (Insulin stimulates glycogenesis and inhibits glycogenolysis whereas glucagon and nor-epinephrine inhibit glycogenesis and stimulates glycogenolysis)
3. Effect of calcium (Calcium stimulates glycogenolysis)

1. **Allosteric Regulation:**

   The process of regulating carbohydrate metabolism by the availability of substrate and energy level is known as allosteric regulation. When glucose and energy levels are available in high amount, *glycogen synthase* (*GS*) (glycogenesis) is activated and *glycogen phosphorylase* (*GP*) (glycogenolysis) is inhibited. On the other hand, when glucose and energy levels are available in low amount *glycogen synthase* (*GS*) (glycogenesis) is inhibited and *glycogen phosphorylase* (*GP*) (glycogenolysis) is activated. Allosteric regulation of blood glucose level is depicted in Figure 2.3.

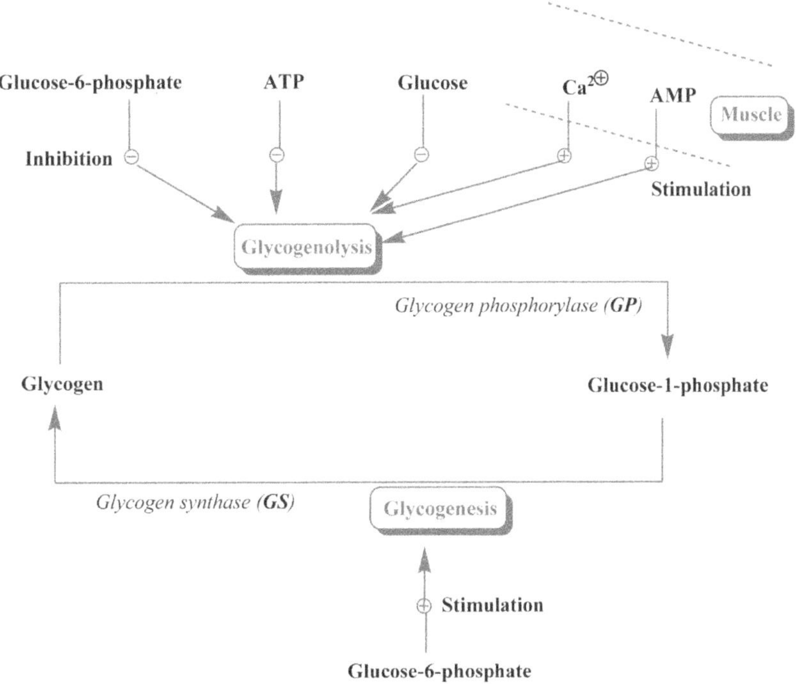

Figure 2.3 Allosteric regulation of blood glucose level.

2. **Hormonal Regulation:**

Enzyme proteins are covalently modified by hormones by either phosphorylation or dephosphorylation which results in glycogenesis or glycogenolysis. In general, phosphorylation leads to degradation of glycogen and dephosphorylation leads to synthesis of glycogen. Overall effects of hormones in carbohydrate metabolism are summarized into two major categories.

1. **Insulin:** Increased level of insulin stimulates glycogenesis and inhibits glycogenolysis because insulin inhibits the conversion of active form of *adenylate cyclase* from inactive form of *adenylate cyclase* in plasma membrane.
2. **Glucagon and epinephrine:** Increased level of glucagon, nor-epinephrine and epinephrine inhibits glycogenesis and stimulates glycogenolysis because in plasma membrane it promotes the conversion of active form of *adenylate cyclase* from its inactive form. Effect of glucagon and epinephrine on glycogenesis and glycogenolysis is presented in Figure 2.4 and Figure 2.5, respectively. In addition, effect of insulin on glycogenesis and glycogenolysis is presented in Figure 2.6.

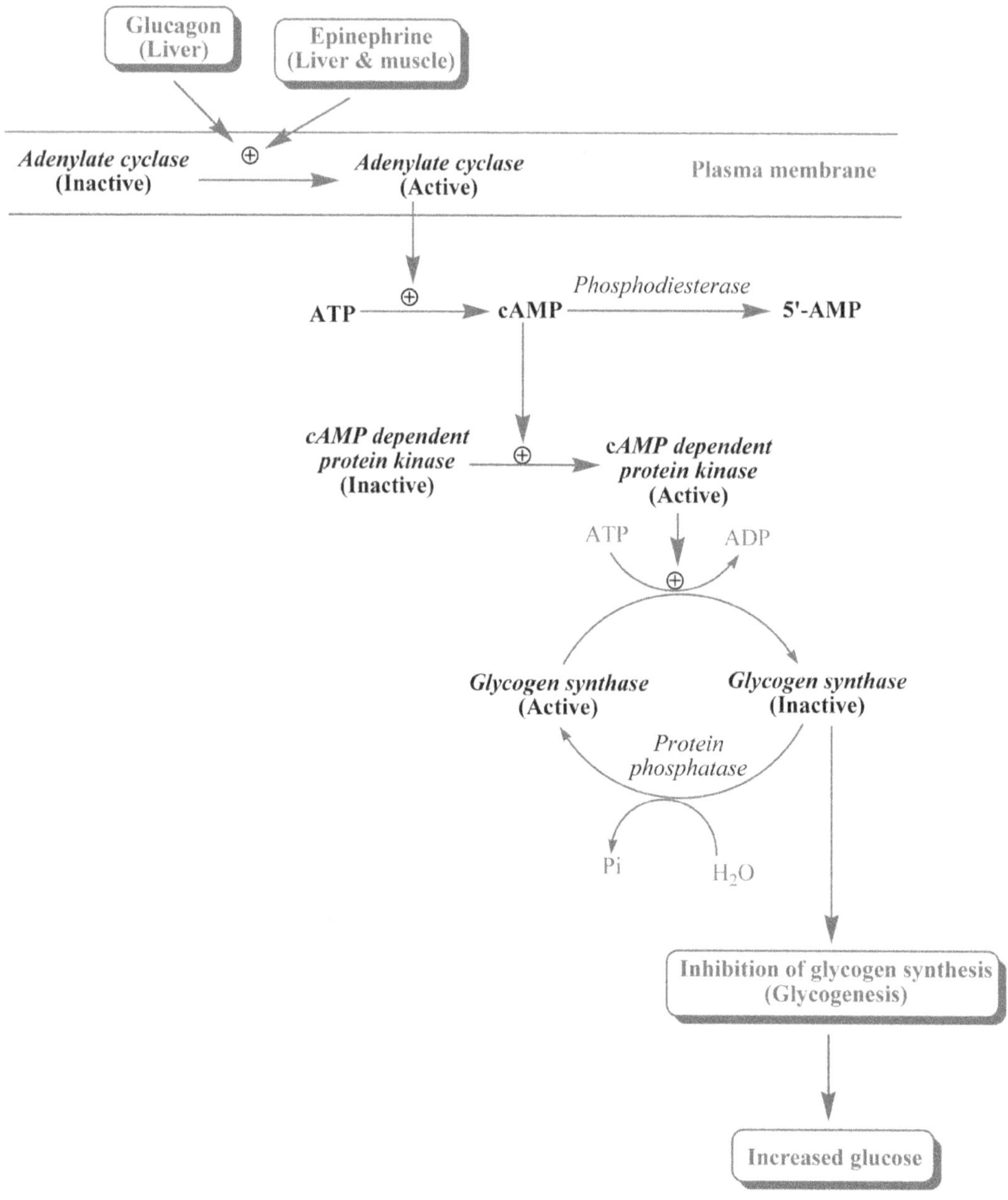

Figure 2.4 Effect of glucagon and epinephrine on glycogenesis.

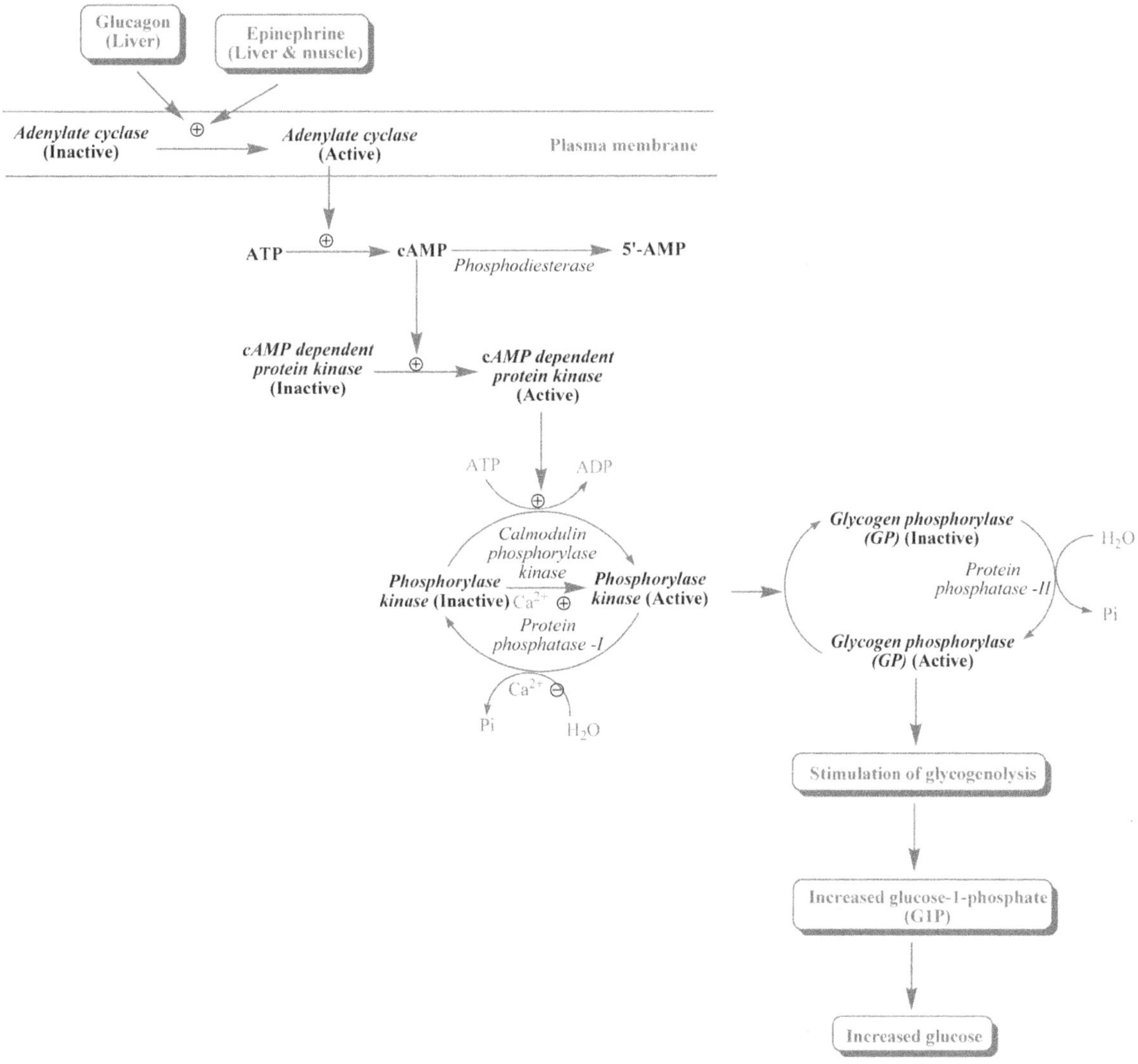

Glucagon (Liver)
Epinephrine (Liver & muscle)
Adenylate cyclase (Inactive) ⊕ → *Adenylate cyclase* (Active)
Plasma membrane
ATP ⊕ → cAMP → 5'-AMP
Phosphodiesterase
cAMP dependent protein kinase (Inactive) ⊕ → *cAMP dependent protein kinase* (Active)
ATP ADP ⊕
Calmodulin phosphorylase kinase
Phosphorylase kinase (Inactive) Ca^{2+} ⊕ → *Phosphorylase kinase* (Active)
Protein phosphatase -I
Ca^{2+} ⊖
Pi H_2O
Glycogen phosphorylase (GP) (Inactive)
Protein phosphatase -II
H_2O Pi
Glycogen phosphorylase (GP) (Active)
Stimulation of glycogenolysis
Increased glucose-1-phosphate (G1P)
Increased glucose

Figure 2.5 Effect of glucagon and epinephrine on glycogenolysis.

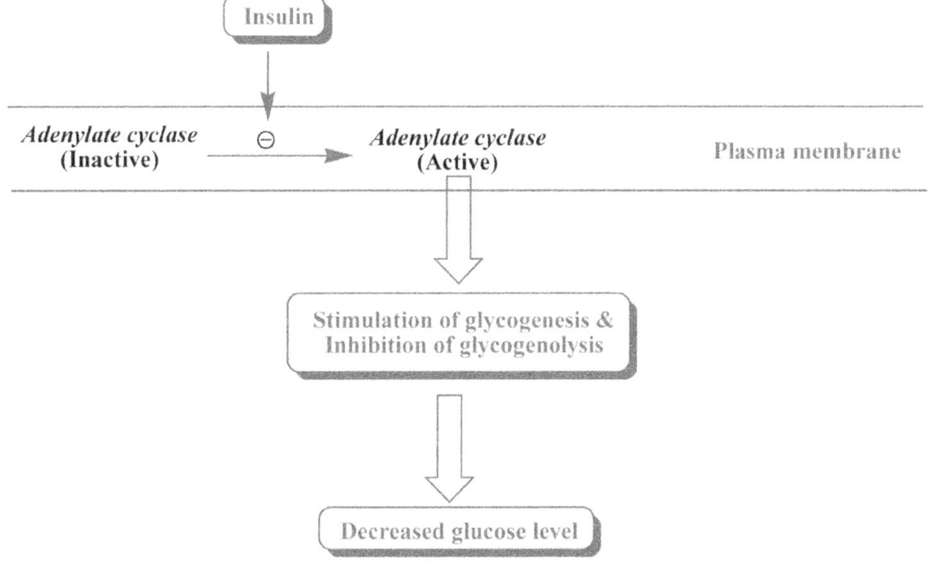

Figure 2.6 Effect of insulin on glycogenesis and glycogenolysis.

3. **Effect of Calcium:**

   Generally, release of calcium from sarcoplasmic reticulum leads to reaction with a protein called calmodulin and produces calcium-calmodulin complex. This formed complex activates *glycogen phosphorylase* (*GP*) which leads to stimulation of glycogenolysis ultimately glucose level increased.

Biological Oxidation

Oxidation is defined as addition of oxygen (or) loss of hydrogen (or) loss of electrons and reduction is defined as loss of oxygen (or) gain of hydrogen (or) gain of electron. The electron lost in the oxidation is accepted by acceptor which is said to be reduced. Both oxidation and reduction are coupled with each other. Hence oxidation-reduction reactions are commonly known as redox reaction (If one compound is getting oxidized the other one must reduce). **Example:** Inter conversion of Fe^{2+} (ferrous ion) to Fe^{3+} (ferric ion).

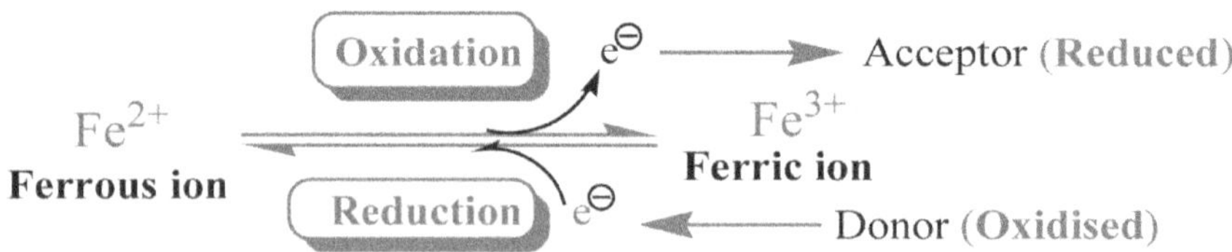

If the oxidation reduction reaction takes place in biological system then it is known as biological redox reaction (or) simply biological oxidation. The general oxidation-reduction principle is applicable to biological systems also. **Example:** The oxidation of NADH + H^+ to NAD^+ is coupled with simultaneous reduction of FMN to $FMNH_2$. In this example NADH + H^+ / NAD^+ and FMN / $FMNH_2$ are called as redox pair which differ in their tendency to lose or gain electrons.

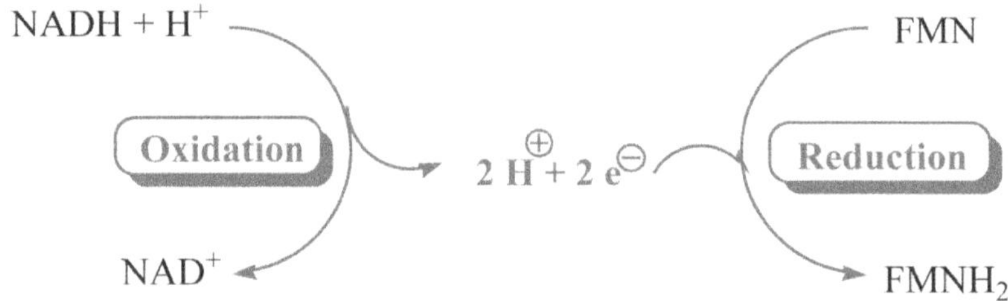

Co-Enzyme System Involved in Biological Oxidation

Co-enzymes are defined as the non-protein, organic, low molecular weight and easily dialyzable substances associated with the functions of enzymes.

Holoenzyme (Active enzyme) ⟶ Apoenzyme (Protein part) + Co-enzyme (Non protein part)

The followings are the various co-enzymes which are involved in biological oxidation. They are,

1. Flavin mononucleotide (FMN)
2. Flavin adenine dinucleotide (FAD)
3. Nicotinamide adenine dinucleotide (NAD^+)
4. Nicotinamide adenine dinucleotide phosphate ($NADP^+$)
5. Lipoic acid

Details of these co-enzymes along with its chemical structure is explained in enzyme topic (Unit-5).

Synthesis of ATP

ATP is generally synthesized by phosphorylation reaction from ADP and inorganic phosphate. Generally, the phosphorylation reaction used to synthesize ATP is broadly classified into two different types.

1. Substrate level phosphorylation
2. Oxidative phosphorylation

Substrate Level Phosphorylation

In this type of phosphorylation, ATP is directly synthesized in the metabolism during oxidation of substrate without involvement of ETC (Electron Transport Chain). To produce ATP, high energy phosphates are transferred usually from high energy compounds such as 1,3-bisphosphoglycerate, phosphoenol pyruvate (intermediates of glycolysis) and succinyl CoA (intermediates of citric acid cycle).

Example 1: 1,3-Bisphospho glycerate (1,3-BPG) produced 3-phospho glycerate (3-PG) by dephosphorylation reaction in presence of *phospho glycero kinase* (PGK) (In ATP / GTP involved reactions the enzymes acted are "*kinase*" and the substrate is "1,3-bisphospho glycerate").

COO—P, H—C—OH, CH_2O—P **1,3-Bisphospho glycerate (1,3-BPG)** → (Dephosphorylation; ADP → ATP, +1; *1,3-Bisphospho glycerokinase* ***(1,3-BPGK)***; Mg^{2+}) → COO^{-}, H—C—OH, CH_2O—P **3-Phospho glycerate (3-PG)**

Example 2: Phosphoenolpyruvate undergoes dephosphorylation and produce pyruvate in enol form in presence of *pyruvate kinase* (PK) (PEP) (In ATP / GTP involved reactions, the enzymes acted are "*kinase*" and the product formed is "pyruvate").

COO^{-}, C—O—P, $=CH_2$ **Phosphoenol pyruvate (PEP)** → (Dephosphorylation; ADP → ATP, +1; *Pyruvate kinase* ***(PK)***; Mg^{2+} (or) Mn^{2+}) → COO^{-}, C—**OH**, $=CH_2$ **Pyruvate (Enol form)**

Example 3: Succinyl CoA is hydrolyzed into succinate with loss of co-enzyme A. The reaction is catalyzed by *succinate thiokinase* (STK) enzyme (In ATP / GTP involved reactions, the enzymes acted are "*kinase*", sulphur atom of CoA is involved and the product formed is "succinate"). One GDP is converted into GTP in this step by reacting with inorganic phosphate.

$CH_2—COO^{-}$, $CH_2—C(=O)—$**SCoA** **Succinyl CoA** → (Hydrolysis; GDP, Pi → GTP; H_2O → CoASH; *Succinate thiokinase* ***(STK)***) → $CH_2—COO^{-}$, $CH_2—COO^{-}$ **Succinate**

Oxidative Phosphorylation

In aerobic organism, oxidative phosphorylation is the major source of ATP. Oxidative phosphorylation is defined as the process of synthesizing ATP from ADP and Pi (inorganic phosphate) with the involvement ETC (electron transport chain). In general, the transport of electrons through the ETC is linked with the release of free energy. Oxidative phosphorylation is taking place in complex-V of inner mitochondrial membrane.

Phosphorous oxygen ratio (P:O): The phosphorous oxygen ratio i.e., P:O is defined as the number of inorganic phosphate molecules utilized for ATP generation for every atom of oxygen consumed. Otherwise it represents the number of molecules of ATP synthesized per pair of electrons carried through ETC. In general, the phosphorous oxygen ratio (P:O) for mitochondrial oxidation of NADH is three.

$$NADH + H^+ + \frac{1}{2}O_2 + 3\ ADP + 3\ Pi \longrightarrow NAD^+ + 3\ ATP + H_2O$$

The phosphorous oxygen ratio (P:O) for mitochondrial oxidation of $FADH_2$ is two.

$$FADH_2 + \frac{1}{2}O_2 + 2\ ADP + 2\ Pi \longrightarrow FAD + 2\ ATP + H_2O$$

Ten and six protons are pumped across the mitochondrial membrane by NADH + H^+ and $FADH_2$, respectively. Four protons are required for the synthesis of one ATP. Hence, there is a strong evidence that the phosphorous oxygen ratio (P:O) for mitochondrial oxidation of NADH + H^+ and $FADH_2$, is 2.5 and 1.5, respectively.

Site of oxidative phosphorylation in ETC: In ETC, there are three exergonic site which results in the synthesis of 3 ATP molecules.

1. Oxidation of $FMNH_2$ by Co-enzyme Q
2. Oxidation of cytochrome b by cytochrome c_1.
3. *Cytochrome oxidase* reaction.

Each one of the above sites represents the coupling site for the synthesis of one ATP. NADH + H^+ pass through all three coupling sites that results in production of three ATP. Whereas, $FADH_2$ by passing the first coupling site and pass through only last two coupling sites results in production of two ATP.

Energetic of oxidative phosphorylation: The simplified reactions involved in the transport of electrons to redox pair $\frac{1}{2}O_2$ / H_2O (E_0: + 0.82 V) from redox pair NAD^+ / NADH + H^+ (E_0: - 0.32 V) is represented as follows,

$$\frac{1}{2}O_2 + NADH + H^+ \longrightarrow H_2O + NAD^+$$

Between these two redox pairs the redox potential difference is 1.14 V [$\Delta E_0 = E_0$ of accepted redox pair - E_0 of donated redox pair i.e., 0.82 - (-0.32) which is 0.82 + 0.32)]. This 1.14 V redox potential equals to 52 Cal/mol of energy. In ETC, from the above electron transfers three ATPs are generated. Hence, the total energy of these three ATPs is 21.9 Cal/mol (One ATP energy is 7.3 Cal/mol. Hence, for three ATPs it is 7.3 X 3 = 21.9). From this, the energy conservation efficiency is calculated as follows,

$$\text{Energy Conservation Efficiency} = \frac{\text{Energy of 3 ATPs}}{\text{Total energy}} \times 100 = \frac{21.9}{52} \times 100 = 42\%$$

Thus, only 42 % of energy is trapped in the form of three ATPs when NADH + H^+ are oxidized and the remaining energy is lost as heat. This lost heat is not a waste one because it is necessary to maintain body temperature and it allows continuous generation of ATP in ETC.

Mechanism of Oxidative Phosphorylation:

The mechanism involved in oxidative phosphorylation is tried to explain by several hypothesis. Out of several mechanisms proposed for oxidative phosphorylation the following three are most important.

1. Chemical coupling mechanism
2. Chemiosmotic mechanism
3. Conformational coupling mechanism

1. **Chemical coupling mechanism:** In the year 1953, Edward Slater proposed this hypothesis. According to this mechanism, in ETC during the course of electron transfer, ADP reacts with inorganic phosphate and produces a series of phosphorylated high energy intermediates which are utilized for synthesis of ATP. This reaction is believed to be analogous to the substrate level phosphorylation reactions occurring in glycolysis and TCA cycle. In addition, till date no evidence could prove this hypothesis since all attempts made to isolate any one of the phosphorylated high energy intermediates are not successful.

ADP + Pi ⟶ Several phosphorylated high energy intermediates ⟶ ATP

2. **Chemiosmotic mechanism:** This mechanism is widely accepted and it was proposed in the year 1961 by Peter Mitchell. This mechanism clearly explains the utilization of electrons transport in ETC for the production of ATP from ADP and inorganic phosphate. The energy stored in battery separated by positive and negative charges is generally used for comparison of chemiosmotic mechanism and is represented in Figure 2.7.

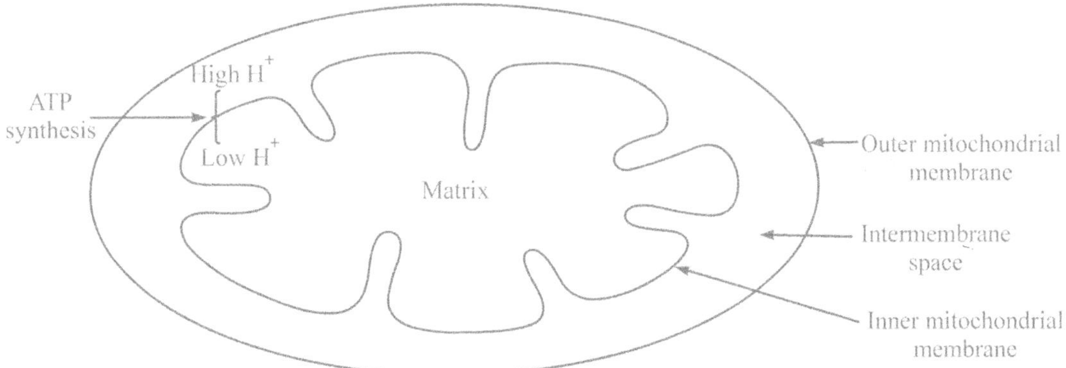

Figure 2.7 Outline of chemiosmotic mechanism for oxidative phosphorylation.

The inner mitochondrial membrane is impermeable to ions such as protons (H^+) and hydroxyl ions (OH^-). In ETC, across the coupling membrane (i.e., inner mitochondrial membrane) protons are translocated along with the transport of electrons to the inter membrane space from mitochondrial matrix. Electrochemical gradient or proton gradient takes place as a result of pumping of protons. The reason behind is accumulation of more protons (H^+) on the outer side of the inner mitochondrial membrane than the inner side. This formed electrochemical gradient or proton gradient due to flow of electrons in ETC is sufficient enough for the synthesis of ATP from ADP and inorganic phosphate. The electrochemical gradient or proton gradient is utilized by the enzyme known as *ATP synthase* present in complex–V of inner mitochondrial membrane and produces ATP. The enzyme is also known as *ATPase* as it hydrolyzes ATP into ADP and inorganic phosphate. *ATP synthase* is a complex enzyme and are made up of two functional subunits namely F_1 and F_0. The structure of *ATP synthase* is comparable with the structure of lollipops. ATP is synthesized when the protons accumulated on the inter membrane space re-enter into the mitochondrial matrix. Chemiosmotic mechanism for oxidative phosphorylation is schematically represented in Figure 2.8.

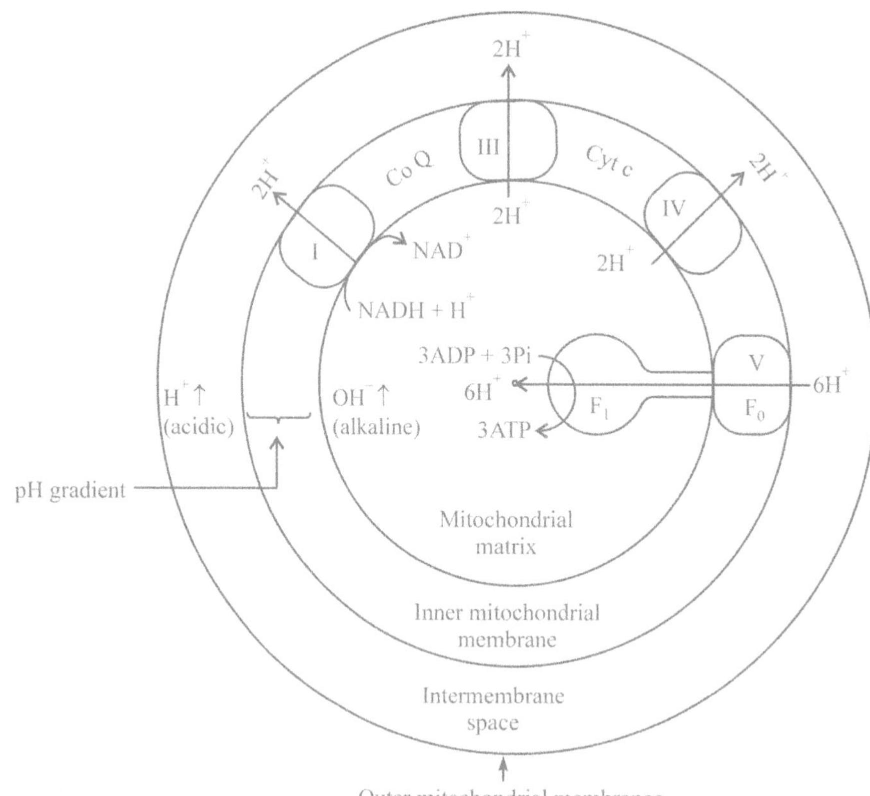

Figure 2.8 Schematic representation of chemiosmotic mechanism for oxidative phosphorylation.

Evidence for chemiosmotic mechanisms: There are several evidences available for supporting chemiosmotic mechanisms.

1. ATP synthesis takes place in inner mitochondrial membrane only.
2. Inner mitochondrial membrane is impermeable to various ions such as H^+, K^+ etc.
3. Additions of proton in inter membrane space of mitochondria results in increased ATP synthesis.
4. Any substances which increases the membrane permeability leads to decreased ATP synthesis. **Example:** 2, 4-Dinitrophenol (2,4-DNP).

3. **Conformational coupling mechanism:** According to this mechanism, inner mitochondrial membrane undergoes some conformational changes therefore ADP and Pi (inorganic phosphate) come close to each other during electron transfer in ETC which results in formation of ATP. There is an evidence for this mechanism as inner mitochondrial membrane undergoes conformational changes and it is explained by rotary motor model for ATP generation.

   Rotary motor model for ATP generation: In 1964 Paul Boyer proposed that ATP is synthesized due to a conformational change in the mitochondrial membrane proteins. Now this hypothesis of Paul Boyer is considered as rotary motor or engine driving model or binding change model which is widely accepted. The enzyme *ATP synthase* is a complex one present in complex–V of inner mitochondrial membrane and it contains two major sub complexes namely F_0 and F_1. To the sub complex F_0 composed of channel protein C subunits, *F_1-ATP synthase* is attached. *F_1-ATP synthase* consist of three subunits namely α, β and γ. Generally, γ subunit is present centrally and is surrounded by alternative α and β subunits. Three α, three β and one γ subunit is present in *F_1-ATP synthase*.

   The γ subunit is rotated physically in response to proton flux leads to induction of conformational changes in β_3 subunit results in release of ATP. Different conformations were adapted by the three β subunits of *F_1-ATP synthase* according to the binding change mechanism. One subunit has O (open) conformation; the second one has L (loose) conformation; and the third one has T (tight) conformation. γ subunit rotation is induced by protons through unknown mechanism. This leads to conformational changes in β subunits. In L-conformation, ADP and inorganic phosphate binds to β subunits. When this L-site of β subunits changed to T-conformation, ATP is synthesized. The O-site is changed to L-conformation which binds to ADP and inorganic phosphate. The T-site is changed to O-conformation and releases ATP. This conformational change of β subunits is repeated and three ATPs are generated for each rotation. The release of ATP from O-conformation is energy dependent whereas synthesis of ATP is not dependent on energy. This is very crucial in synthesis of ATP by rotary motor model. This enzyme *ATP synthase* acting as a proton driving motor is a good example for rotary catalysis. Hence, in the world the smallest molecular motor is *ATP synthase*. Rotary motor model for ATP generation is represented in Figure 2.9.

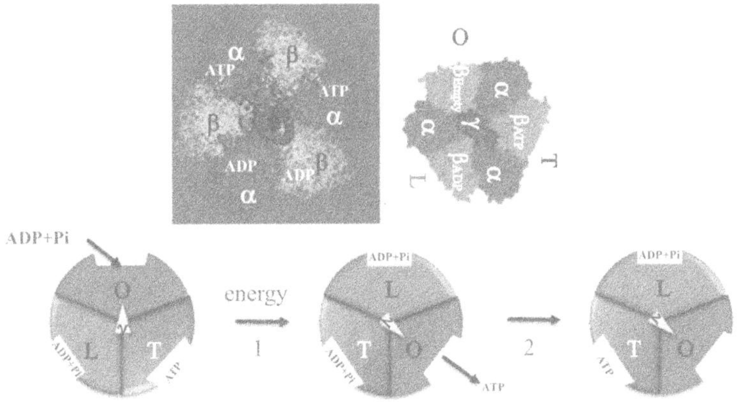

Figure 2.9 Rotary motor model for ATP generation.

INHIBITORS OF OXIDATIVE PHOSPHORYLATION

Oxidative phosphorylation can be inhibited by the following components.

1. Uncouplers
2. Ionophores
3. Inhibitors of *ATP synthase*
4. Inhibitors of adenine nucleotide carrier.

1. **Uncouplers:** These are the substances which uncouple or delink the transport of electrons in ETC during oxidative phosphorylation. Uncoupler oxidizes the reducing equivalents such as NADH + H^+ and $FADH_2$ without production of ATP. **Example:** 2,4-Dinitrophenol (2,4-DNP) and physiological uncouplers such as thyroxine, thermogenin and long chain fatty acids.
2. **Ionophores:** Ionophores is defined as lipophilic substances which increases the membrane permeability of various ions such as H^+, K^+, Cl^-, HCO_3^-, Na^+ etc. across the biological membrane. Even uncouplers are proton ionophores (uncouplers increase the membrane permeability of H^+ ions). **Example:** Valinomycin, gramicidin-A and nigericin are K^+ ionophores; 2,4-dinitophenol (2,4-DNP) is H^+ ionophores.
3. **Inhibitors of *ATP synthase*:** *ATP synthase* is an enzyme responsible for the synthesis of ATP. Hence, inhibition of *ATP synthase* may lead to decreased ATP synthesis. **Example:** Oligomycin
4. **Inhibitors of adenine nucleotide carrier:** ADP is an important component for the synthesis of ATP. Hence decreased supply of ADP may lead to decreased synthesis of ATP. This type of inhibitors inhibits adenine nucleotide carrier which leads to block of adequate supply of ATP. **Example:** Atractyloside

Electron Transport Chain (ETC) or Respiratory Chain or Electron Transport System (ETS)

Through a series of biochemical reactions, energy rich biomolecules such as carbohydrates (specifically glucose), amino acids and fatty acids are oxidized in body into carbon dioxide and water. During these metabolic reactions from various metabolic intermediates the reducing equivalents are transferred into co-enzyme NAD^+ and FAD to produce NADH + H^+ and $FADH_2$ respectively. Through electron transport chain (ETC) these two reduced coenzymes finally reduce oxygen to water. Free energy loss is usually associated with ETC. From ADP and inorganic phosphate, ATP is synthesized by utilizing the part of this free energy . ETC is important for regeneration of oxidized form of reducing equivalent NAD^+ and FAD. Overview of biological oxidation and ETC are represented in Figure 2.10 and 2.11, respectively.

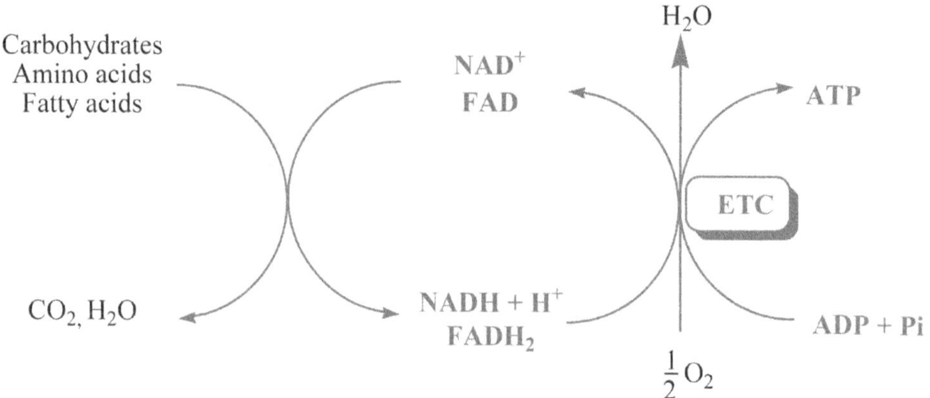

Figure 2.10 Overview of biological oxidation.

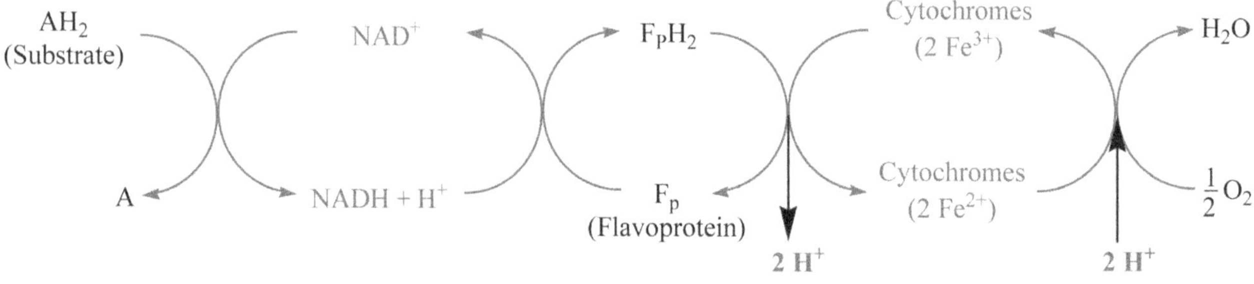

Figure 2.11 Overview of electron transport chain (ETC).

Mitochondria: Mitochondria are considered as the power house of the cell because mitochondria are the centre for metabolic oxidation reactions. The reduced coenzymes like NADH + H^+ and $FADH_2$ are oxidized to NAD^+ and FAD respectively in ETC of mitochondrion with energy liberation in the form of ATP. Five distinct parts are present in mitochondria. They are,

1. Outer mitochondrial membrane
2. Inner mitochondrial membrane
3. Inter membrane space
4. The cristae and
5. The mitochondrial matrix

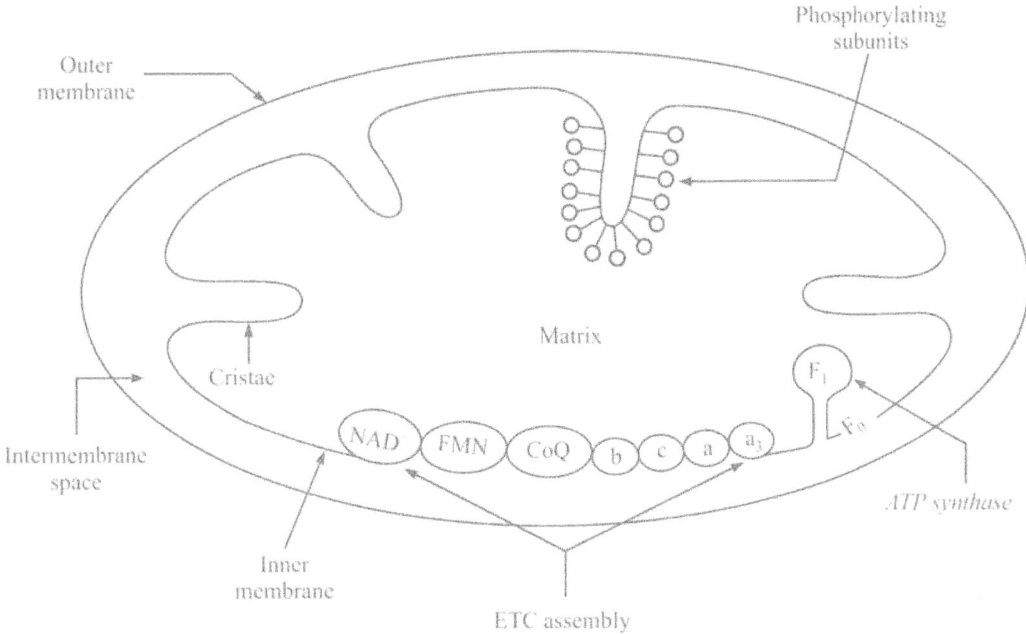

Figure 2.12 Structure of mitochondria depicting ETC.

In the inner mitochondrial membrane of the mitochondria, ETC and ATP synthesizing systems are located which is a specialized structure and rich in proteins. Inner mitochondrial membrane is impermeable to ions like sodium (Na^+), potassium (K^+), proton (H^+), etc. and small molecule like ADP, ATP, etc. The surface area of the inner mitochondrial membrane is greatly increased by forming cristae (highly folded membrane). The centre of ATP production i.e., a specialized particle phosphorylating subunits which look likes lollipops are present in the inner surface of the inner mitochondrial membrane. The mitochondrial matrix is the interior ground substance of the mitochondria. The enzymes involved in TCA cycle, oxidation of amino acids and β-oxidation of fatty acids are rich in the mitochondrial matrix. Structure of mitochondria depicting ETC is presented in Figure 2.12.

Mechanism of ETC

Five distinct enzyme or respiratory complexes are present in the inner mitochondrial membrane of the mitochondria. They are complex–I, complex–II, complex–III, complex–IV and complex–V. Electrons are carried by the first four complexes i.e., complex–I to complex–IV and the ATP is synthesized in complex–V. Certain mobile electron carriers such as, NADH, co-enzyme Q, cytochrome C and oxygen are present in ETC besides these five enzyme complexes. The electrons are transported collectively by the complex–I to complex–IV and the mobile electron carriers. Finally, the electrons react with oxygen and produced water. ETC of mitochondria utilizes the largest portion of oxygen consumed by the body. Mechanism of ETC with multiprotein complexes involved in ETC is represented schematically in Figure 2.13.

Components of ETC: There are the five major components which are distinct carriers that participate in the electron transport chain. These carriers are sequentially arranged and carry electrons from the substrate and finally combine with oxygen to produce water. The five major components of ETC are, 1) Nicotinamide nucleotides, 2) Flavoproteins, 3) Iron-sulphur proteins, 4) Co-enzyme Q and 5) Cytochromes.

1. **Nicotinamide nucleotide:** NAD^+ and $NADP^+$ are the two coenzymes of vitamin B_3 i.e., niacin. Out of these two, NAD^+ is actively involved in ETC. Generally, from the substrates (AH_2) such as glyceraldehyde-3-phosphate, pyruvate, isocitrate, α-ketoglutarate and malate, NAD^+ removes two hydrogen and reduced to $NADH + H^+$ in presence of *dehydrogenase* enzyme.

Redox reaction

$$\underset{\textbf{Substrate}}{AH_2} + NAD^+ \underset{\textit{Dehydrogenase}}{\rightleftharpoons} \underset{\textbf{Product}}{A} + NADH + H^+$$

Whereas $NADP^+$ is reduced to $NADPH + H^+$ in presence of $NADP^+$ dependent *dehydrogenase* enzyme which is not a substrate for ETC. $NADPH + H^+$ is mainly involved in fatty acid synthesis and cholesterol synthesis

2. **Flavoproteins:** *NADH-coenzyme Q reductase* or *NADH dehydrogenase* and *succinate-coenzyme Q reductase* or *succinate dehydrogenase* are the two important flavoproteins of the ETC. Prosthetic group present in flavoprotein *NADH dehydrogenase* is FMN. The co-enzyme FMN is converted to $FMNH_2$ by accepting two electrons and protons from $NADH + H^+$. *NADH dehydrogenase* is closely associated with iron-sulphur (Fe-S) proteins or non-heme iron (NHI) proteins.

$$FMN + NADH + H^+ \xrightarrow[\text{NADH-coenzyme Q reductase or NADH dehydrogenase}]{\text{Reduction}} FMNH_2 + NAD^+$$

Prosthetic group present in flavoprotein *succinate dehydrogenase* is FAD. The coenzyme FAD is converted to $FADH_2$ by accepting two electrons and protons from succinate. *Succinate dehydrogenase* is also closely associated with iron-sulphur (Fe-S) proteins or non-heme iron (NHI) proteins.

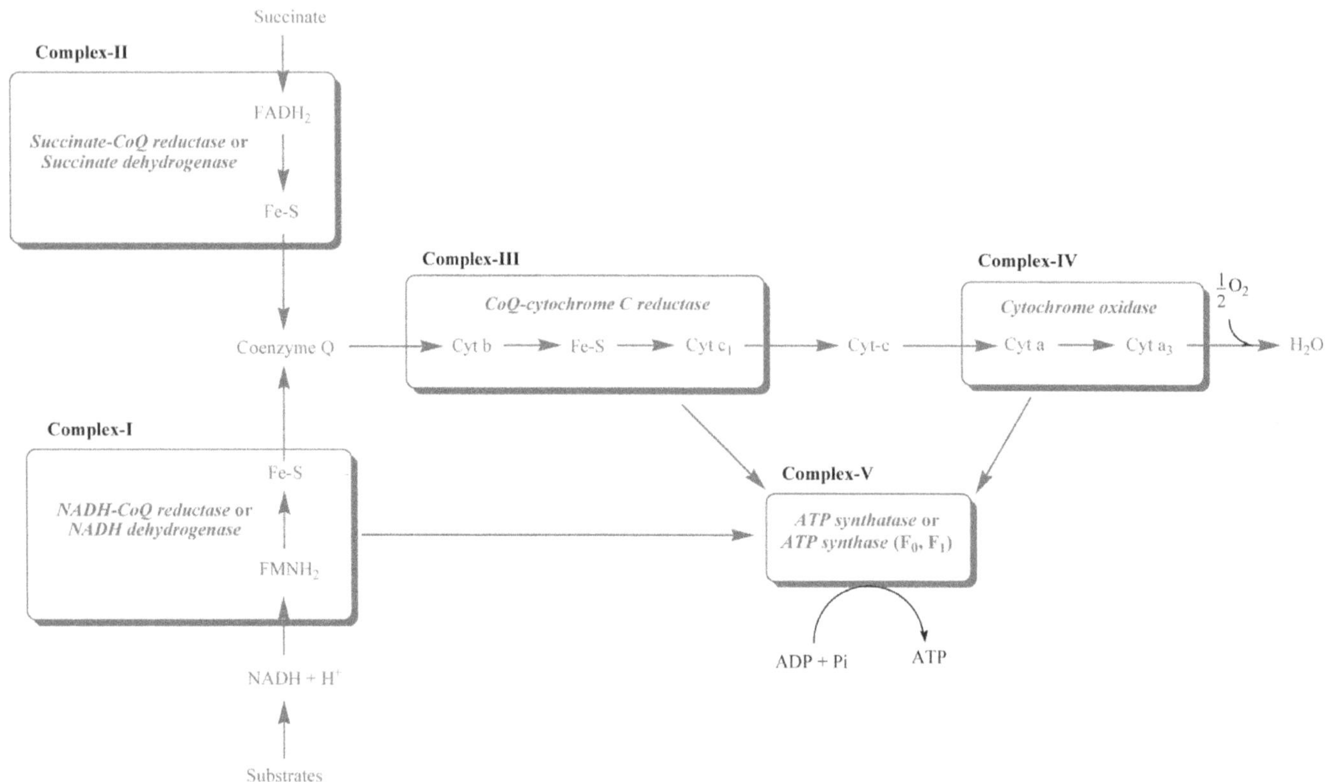

Figure 2.13 Mechanism of ETC with multiprotein complexes involved in ETC.

$$FAD + Succinate \xrightarrow[\text{Succinate-coenzyme Q reductase or Succinate dehydrogenase}]{\text{Reduction}} FADH_2 + Fumarate$$

3. **Iron-sulphur (FeS) proteins:** There are about six iron-sulphur proteins which are involved in ETC and the exact mechanism involved in iron-sulphur protein is not clearly understood. In generals iron-sulphur proteins exist in two forms such as ferric i.e., Fe^{3+} (oxidized) and ferrous i.e., Fe^{2+} (reduced) which are inter convertible. Out of several iron-sulphur proteins, one is involved in the transfer of electron form $FMNH_2$ to coenzyme Q; the other one is involved in the transfer of electron form $FADH_2$ to coenzyme Q; the next one is the transfer of electron form cytochrome b to cytochrome c_1.
4. **Co-enzyme Q:** It is ubiquitous in living system; hence, it is also known as ubiquinone. Co-enzyme Q is a quinone derivative with a variable isoprenoid side chain. Quinone ring with ten isoprenoid unit side chain is present in mammalian tissues, hence it is commonly known as co-enzyme Q_{10} or CoQ_{10}. Co-enzyme Q is a lipophilic electron carrier. It accepts electron from both $FMNH_2$ produced in ETC and $FADH_2$ produced outside ETC (**Example:** *Succinate dehydrogenase, acyl CoA dehydrogenase*, etc.) In some organism like mycobacteria, co-enzyme Q is not present, hence, in these organism vitamin K performs the similar functions of co-enzyme Q. In body co-enzyme Q is directly synthesized because in animal there is no known vitamin precursors for co-enzyme Q .

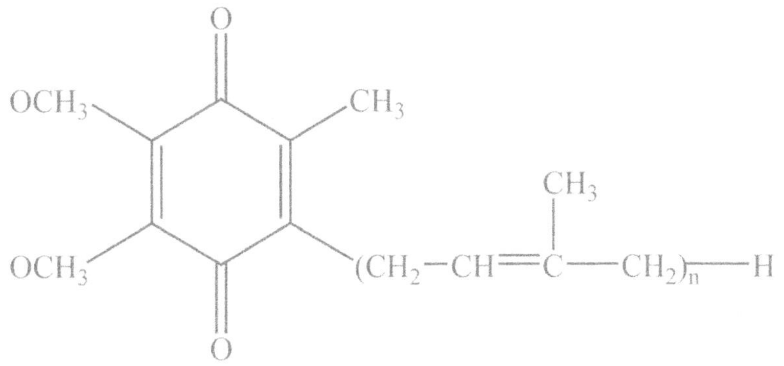

O
OCH_3 CH_3
CH_3
OCH_3 $(CH_2-CH=C-CH_2)_n-H$
O

5. **Cytochromes:** In general, cytochromes are hemoprotein containing heme as prosthetic group. Porphyrin ring with iron atom is present in heme. Compared to other hemoproteins such as hemoglobin, methemoglobin, heme present in cytochromes is different. In cytochromes, the iron is present in both reduced (ferrous i.e., Fe^{2+}) and oxidized (ferric i.e., Fe^{3+}) form alternatively which is essential for the transport of electrons in ETC. In case of other hemoproteins such as hemoglobin, methemoglobin, heme is present only in ferrous (Fe^{2+}) state.

   Depending upon the types of heme present and the respective absorption spectrum, initially three cytochromes are designated as cytochrome a, cytochrome b and cytochrome c. Latter, several additional cytochromes are discovered which are designated as cytochrome c_1, cytochrome b_1 and cytochrome a_3.

   Electrons are transported from co-enzyme Q into cytochromes in the following orders b, c_1, c, a and a_3. These cytochromes act as an effective electron carrier due to the presence of reversible oxidation–reduction property of heme iron present in it.

   Heme group and 104 amino acid containing small protein is cytochrome c (Molecular weight: 13,000). With an intermediate redox potential, cytochrome c acts as a central molecule in ETC. Cytochrome c can be easily extracted because it is loosely bounded in the inner mitochondrial membrane.

   In ETC, the terminal component is *cytochrome oxidase*. Cytochromes a and a_3 are collectively known as *cytochrome oxidase*. This is the only cytochrome which can directly react with molecular oxygen atom. Additionally, *cytochrome oxidase* also contains copper besides iron. Like iron, this copper also undergoes oxidation –reduction (cupric i.e., Cu^{2+} - curprous i.e., Cu^{+}) during the transport of electrons. Finally, water is produced in ETC from the transported electrons, free protons and the molecular oxygen atom.

Inhibitors of ETC:

There are many site specific ETC inhibitors. Generally, inhibitors block the electron transport by binding with one component of ETC. This may lead to the accumulation of reduced components before the inhibitor

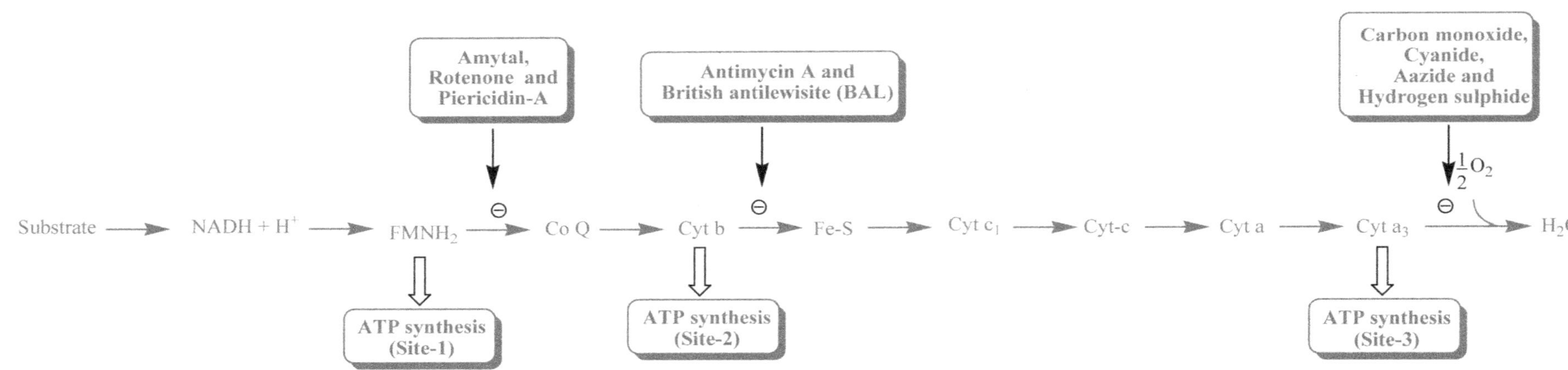

Figure 2.14 ETC with sites of ATP synthesis and inhibitors.

blockade step and oxidized components after the inhibitor blockade step. ATP synthesis i.e., phosphorylation mainly depends on ETC. Hence, ATP synthesis is also inhibited by the site specific ETC inhibitors. The inhibitors may act on three different sites of ATP synthesis as follows.

1. **Inhibitors at site-1:** The following chemical agents inhibits the synthesis of ATP in site-1 of ETC i.e., NADH and co-enzyme Q. **Example:** Amytal (barbiturate drug), rotenone (fish poison) and piericidin-A (antibiotic).
2. **Inhibitors at site-2:** The compounds inhibit the synthesis of ATP in site-2 of ETC i.e., cytochrome b and cytochrome c. **Example:** Antimycin-A (antibiotic) and British antilewisite i.e., BAL (Antidote used for war gas).
3. **Inhibition at site-3:** The compounds inhibit the synthesis of ATP in site-3 of ETC i.e., *cytochrome oxidase*. **Example:** Carbon monoxide (reacts with reduced form of cytochrome), cyanide and azide (reacts with oxidized form of cytochrome) and hydrogen sulphide (reacts with both oxidized and reduced form of cytochrome).

The most potent inhibitor of ETC is cyanide. It blocks the ETC by binding with the ferric ion of *cytochrome oxidase* which leads to death. Tissue asphyxia (mostly in CNS) is the reason behind the cyanide death. ETC with sites of ATP synthesis and inhibitors are presented in Figure 2.14.

PROBABLE QUESTIONS

PART – A: Multiple Choice Questions

1. Out of the following pathways which one is not an oxidative pathway?
   (a) Glycolysis (b) HMP shunt pathway
   (c) Glycogenesis (d) Uronic acid pathway
2. In which of the following category the degradative process will come.
   (P) Anabolism (Q) Catabolism
   (R) Metabolism (S) Excretion.
   Choose the correct option.
   (a) P and Q is correct (b) R and S is correct
   (c) P is correct (d) Q is correct
3. Which one of the following statement is false for glycolysis?
   (a) It is an oxidative pathway (b) ATPs are generated
   (c) Operative only in presence of oxygen (d) It is very essential for brain
4. In which of the following organs insulin dependent glucose transport is occurring?
   (P) Skeletal muscle (Q) Adipose tissue
   (R) Erythrocyte (S) Brain.
   Choose the correct one.
   (a) P and Q (b) P and S
   (c) Q and R (d) R and S
5. Which of the following substance inhibits phosphotriose isomerase enzyme?
   (a) Iodoacetate (b) Arsenite
   (c) Fluoride (d) Bromohydroxy acetone phosphate
6. For optimum activity of *pyruvate dehydrogenase* & *α-ketoglutarate dehydrogenase* which one is correct?
   (P) THF (Q) NAD^+
   (R) Lipoamide (S) TPP

Choose the correct option.

(a) P is not required and Q, R & S are required
(b) Q is not required and P, R & S are required
(c) R is not required and P, Q & S are required
(d) S is not required and P, Q & R are required

7. How many ATPs are generated in TCA cycle?
(a) 24 (b) 30
(c) 12 (d) 8

8. Citric acid cycle is regulated by which enzyme?
(P) *Citrate synthase* (Q) *Aconitase*
(R) *α-Ketoglutarate dehydrogenase* (S) *Isocitrate dehydrogenase.*
Choose the correct option.
(a) P, Q & R (b) Q, R & S
(c) P, R & S (d) P, Q & S

9. Which intermediate of TCA cycle is involved in lipid metabolism?
(a) Oxaloacetate (b) Citrate
(c) α-Ketoglutarate (d) Succinate

10. Which of the following takes place in glyoxylate cycle?
(a) Glucose to pyruvate (b) Glucose to glycogen
(c) Fat to glucose (d) Glucose to fat

11. One of the following enzyme(s) in glycolysis catalyzes an irreversible reaction.
(P) *Hexokinase* (Q) *Phosphofructokinase*
(R) *Pyruvate kinase* (S) *Aldolase.*
Choose the correct option.
(a) P, Q & R (b) Q, R & S
(c) P, R & S (d) P, Q & S

12. Muscle can't be utilize pyruvate / lactate for the synthesis of glucose. What is the reason behind this?
(P) *Glucose-6-phosphatase* (Q) *Frutose-1,6-bisphosphatase*
(R) *Glucose-1,6-bisphosphatase* (S) *Fructose-6-phosphatase.*
Choose the correct option.
(a) Absence of Q & R (b) Absence of R & S
(c) Absence of P & S (d) Absence of P & Q

13. Synthesis of 2,3-bisphosphoglycerate occurs in which of the following tissue?
(a) Liver (b) Kidney
(c) Erythrocyte (d) Brain

14. How many ATPs are generated when one glucose molecule is completely oxidized in anaerobic condition?
(a) 38 (b) 24
(c) 2 (d) 8 27.

15. Why TCA cycle is the central pathway of metabolism of the cell?
    (a) It occurs in the center of the cell
    (b) Its intermediates are commonly used by other metabolic reactions
    (c) All other metabolic pathways depend upon it
    (d) None of the above
16. In what form does the product of glycolysis enter the TCA cycle?
    (a) Acetyl CoA (b) Pyruvate
    (c) NADH (d) Glucose
17. Why does the glycolytic pathway continue in the direction of glucose catabolism?
    (a) There are essentially three irreversible reactions that act as the driving force for the pathway
    (b) High levels of ATP keep the pathway going in a forward direction
    (c) The enzymes of glycolysis only function in one direction
    (d) Glycolysis occurs in either direction
18. What is the role of *kinase* enzyme?
    (P) Removes phosphate groups of substrates
    (Q) Uses ATP to add a phosphate group to the substrate
    (R) Uses NADH to change the oxidation state of the substrate
    (S) Removes water from a double bond.
    Choose the correct option.
    (a) P & Q (b) R & S
    (c) P & R (d) Q & S
19. Which of the following is not a good source for carbohydrate synthesis?
    (P) Pyruvate (Q) Glycerol
    (R) Odd chain fatty acid (S) Even chain fatty acid.
    Choose the correct option.
    (a) Only R (b) Only S
    (c) Both R & S (d) Both P & Q
20. How many ATPs are needed for the addition of each glucose residue in glycogenesis?
    (a) 1 (b) 2
    (c) 3 (d) 4
21. How many ATPs are generated & utilized in conversion of phosphoenol pyruvate to pyruvate & vice versa, respectively?
    (P) One generated (Q) Two generated
    (R) One utilized (S) Two utilized.
    Choose the correct option.
    (a) P & S (b) Q & R
    (c) P & R (d) Q & S
22. Which of the following enzyme regulates glycogenesis?
    (a) *Glycogen synthase* (b) *Glycogen phosphorylase*
    (c) *Hexokinase* (d) *Phosphogluco mutase*

23. Deficiency of *glucose-6-phosphatase* causes which disease?
   (a) Pompe's disease
   (b) Cori's disease
   (c) Anderson's disease
   (d) Von-Gierke's disease
24. Which of the following one is correct?
   (P) Glucagon stimulates gluconeogenesis
   (Q) Glucogenic amino acids stimulates gluconeogenesis
   (R) Glucose stimulates gluconeogenesis
   (S) Acetyl CoA stimulates gluconeogenesis.

   Choose the correct option.
   (a) P, Q & R is correct; S is wrong
   (b) Q, R & S is correct; P is wrong
   (c) P, Q & S is correct; R is wrong
   (d) P, R & S is correct; Q is wrong
25. Her's disease is due to deficiency of which of the following enzyme?
   (a) *Glycogen phosphorylase*
   (b) *Phosphofructo kinase*
   (c) *Lysosomal-α-glucosidase*
   (d) *Glucosyl-(4,6)-transferase*
26. Which of the following linkages are present in glycogen?
   (P) α-1,4-Glycosidic linkage
   (Q) β-1,4-Glycosidic linkage
   (R) α-1,6-Glycosidic linkage
   (S) β-1,6-Glycosidic linkage.

   Choose the correct option.
   (a) Both P & Q
   (b) Both P & R
   (c) Both P & S
   (d) Both Q & S
27. In which of the following metabolic pathways ATPs are not directly utilized or produced?
   (a) Glycolysis
   (b) Uronic acid pathway
   (c) HMP shunt
   (d) Glycogenolysis
28. Which is the connecting link between HMP shunt & lipid synthesis?
   (a) Ribose
   (b) NADPH
   (c) Sedoheptulose-7-phosphate
   (d) NADH
29. Wernicke-Korsakoff syndrome is due to the alteration of which of the following?
   (a) *Transketolase*
   (b) *Transaldolase*
   (c) *Glucose-6-phosphate dehydrogenase*
   (d) *Gluconolactone hydrolase*
30. Which of the following enzyme is a lysosomal enzyme?
   (P) *Amylo-α-1,6-glucosidase*
   (Q) *Amylo-α-1,4-glucosidase*
   (R) *Glucosyl-(α-4-6)-transferase*
   (S) *Glucosyl-(α-4-4)-transferase.*

   Choose the correct option.
   (a) Only P
   (b) Both P & Q
   (c) Both R & S
   (d) Only Q
31. In which of the following metabolic pathways free sugar / sugar acids are involved?
   (a) Glycolysis
   (b) Uronic acid pathway
   (c) HMP shunt
   (d) Glycogenolysis
32. Deficiency of which of the following causes essential pentoseuria?
   (a) *Glucuronidase*
   (b) *L-Gulonolactone oxidase*
   (c) *Xylitol dehydrogenase*
   (d) *Phosphogluco mutase*

33. Which of the following non-vitamin co-enzyme is a carrier of monosaccharide in glycogen synthesis?
    (P) UDP (Q) CDP
    (R) ATP (S) SAM.
    Choose the correct option.
    (a) Only P (b) Only Q
    (c) Both R & S (d) Both P & Q
34. Which of the following enzyme is absent in primates which is responsible for the synthesis of ascorbic acid?
    (a) *Glucuronidase* (b) *L-Gulonolactone oxidase*
    (c) *Xylitol dehydrogenase* (d) *Phosphogluco mutase*
35. Which is a good precursor for glucosamine?
    (a) Galactose-1-phosphate (b) Galactose-6-phosphate
    (c) Fructose-1-phosphate (d) Fructose-6-phosphate
36. Which of the following are characteristic features of Von Gierke's disease?
    (P) Fasting hypoglycemia (Q) Hypolipidemia
    (R) Lactic acidemia (S) Gouty arthritis.
    Choose the correct option.
    (a) P, Q & R (b) Q, R & S
    (c) P, R & S (d) P, Q & S
37. Dietary xylulose can participate in other metabolisms by entering through which of the following pathway?
    (a) HMP shunt pathway (b) Sorbitol pathway
    (c) Uronic acid pathway (d) Glycolysis
38. Essential fructosuria is due to deficiency of which of the following enzyme?
    (a) *Aldose reductase* (b) *Sorbitol dehydrogenase*
    (c) *Aldolase B* (d) *Fructokinase*
39. The FMNH2 is oxidized by ____________
    (a) Cytochrome-c (b) - 0.22
    (c) Cytochrome-a (d) - 0.32
40. Which complex of inner mitochondrial membrane is the site of oxidative phosporylation?
    (a) III (b) IV
    (c) V (d) VI
41. Inner mitochondrial membrane is impermeable to which of the following ions?
    (a) H^+ (b) K^+
    (c) OH^- (d) All
42. Which of the following antibiotics act as ionophores for potassium ions.
    (a) Antimycin & Valinomycin (b) Piercidin-A & Valinomycin
    (c) Nigercin & Valinomycin (d) Antimycin & Piercidin-A
43. Protein that contains a nucleic acid derivative of riboflavin is called ________
    (a) Nucleic acid (b) Amino acid
    (c) Flavoprotein (d) None

44. NADP-linked *dehydrogenase* catalyzes ________

(a) Glucose 6-phosphate+$NADP^+$ ↔ 6-phosphogluconate + NADPH + H^+

(b) Lactate + NAD^+ pyruvate + NADH + H^+

(c) Pyruvate + CoA + NAD^+ acetyl-CoA + CO_2 + NADH + H^+

(d) L-Malate + NAD^+ oxaloacetate + NADH + H^+

45. A lipid-soluble benzoquinone with a long isoprenoid side chain is?

(a) Ubiquinone (b) Cytochrome-b

(c) Cytochrome-c (d) Cytochrome-a

46. The only membrane bound enzyme in the citric acid cycle is ________

(a) *Succinate dehydrogenase* (b) *NADH dehydrogenase*

(c) *ATP synthase* (d) *Acyl CoA dehydrogenase*

47. In ETC, complex-I is also called ________

(a) *NADH dehydrogenase* (b) *Succinate dehydrogenase*

(c) Cytochrome bc1 complex (d) *Cytochrome oxidase*

48. In ETC, complex-II is also called ________

(a) *NADH dehydrogenase* (b) *Succinate dehydrogenase*

(c) Cytochrome bc1 complex (d) *Cytochrome oxidase*

49. In ETC, complex-III is also called ________

(a) *NADH dehydrogenase* (b) *Succinate dehydrogenase*

(c) Cytochrome bc1 complex (d) *Cytochrome oxidase*

50. In ETC, complex-IV is also called ________

(a) *NADH dehydrogenase* (b) *Succinate dehydrogenase*

(c) Cytochrome bc1 complex (d) *Cytochrome oxidase*

51. In mitochondria, hydride ions are removed from substrates by ________

(a) NAD-linked *dehydrogenases* (b) NADP-linked *dehydrogenases*

(c) *ATP synthase* (d) *Succinate dehydrogenases*

52. Which of the following is the prosthetic group of *NADH dehydrogenase*?

(a) NADH (b) FAD

(c) NADPH (d) FMN

53. If mitochondria were blocked at the site of NADH oxidation and were treated with succinate as substrate, what would the P : O ratio is?

(a) Same as that normally produced by succinate

(b) One more than normally produced by succinate

(c) One less than normally produced by succinate

(d) Zero

54. ATP synthesis by chemiosmosis is by __________

(a) *ATP dehydrogenase* (b) *Gyrase*

(c) *ATP synthase* (d) *Dehydrogenase*

Key for Multiple Choice Questions

1. (c)	2. (d)	3. (c)	4. (a)	5. (d)
6. (a)	7. (c)	8. (c)	9. (b)	10. (c)
11. (a)	12. (d)	13. (c)	14. (c)	15. (b)
16. (a)	17. (a)	18. (a)	19. (b)	20. (b)
21. (a)	22. (a)	23. (d)	24. (c)	25. (a)
26. (b)	27. (c)	28. (b)	29. (a)	30. (d)
31. (b)	32. (c)	33. (a)	34. (b)	35. (d)
36. (c)	37. (c)	38. (d)	39. (b)	40. (c)
41. (d)	42. (c)	43. (c)	44. (a)	45. (a)
46. (a)	47. (a)	48. (b)	49. (c)	50. (d)
51. (a)	52. (d)	53. (a)	54. (c)	

PART – B: Short Answers

1. Write briefly about the metabolic derangements in diabetes mellitus.
2. Write a note on glycogen storage diseases.
3. Write the reactions of Kreb's cycle.
4. What are the glycogen storage diseases?
5. Explain the terms: a) Hypoglycemia; b) Gluconeogenesis.
6. Write short notes on diabetes mellitus.
7. Write short notes on glycogen storage diseases.
8. Write a short note on hormonal regulation of blood glucose levels & diabetes mellitus.
9. Write about glycolysis pathway, energetic & significance.
10. Write the sequence of glycolysis reactions.
11. Explain pentose phosphate pathway.
12. Describe the process of gluconeogenesis in carbohydrate metabolism.
13. Define gluconeogenesis & glycogenolysis.
14. Give the significance of pentose phosphate pathway.
15. Explain the salient features of gluconeogenesis & its regulation.
16. Write a detailed note on inhibitors of ETC.

PART – C: Long Answers

1. Explain HMP pathway and its significance.
2. Explain the steps involved in gluconeogenesis and explain its significance.
3. Explain Kreb's cycle with its regulation.
4. Explain the steps involved in glycolytic pathway and mention the energetic under aerobic and anaerobic conditions.
5. How does insulin and epinephrine regulate glycogen metabolism?
6. Outline the steps involved in glycolysis. The role of HMP shunts in the carbohydrate metabolism.
7. Write in detail about the difference between the gluconeogenesis and glycogenesis.
8. Explain how does hormones regulate glycogenesis.

9. Outline the hormonal regulations of carbohydrate metabolism.
10. Write about citric acid cycle pathway, energetic & significance.
11. Explain pentose phosphate pathway & its significance.
12. Explain any two of the following: a) Glycogenolysis, b) HMP shunt, c) Glycogenesis.
13. Explain the following: a) TCA cycle, b) Glycolysis
14. Explain the citric acid cycle.
15. Write a brief account of glycolysis.
16. Write a detailed note on gluconeogenesis.
17. Describe about TCA cycle and add a note on effect of inhibitors and regulation of TCA cycle.
18. Describe the TCA cycle, its regulation & energy yield in it.
19. Sketch the pentose phosphate pathway & explain its physiological significance.
20. How does blood glucose levels are regulated? Explain the different methods of regulation in detail.
21. Explain about ETC & its mechanism.
22. Explain substrate level phosphorylation with suitable example.
23. Write an essay on electron transport chain & oxidative phosphorylation.
24. Write the biosynthesis of ATP.
25. Explain the different mechanism or hypothesis proposed for oxidative phosphorylation.
26. Explain rotary motor model for ATP generation. Add a note on inhibitors of oxidative phosphorylation.

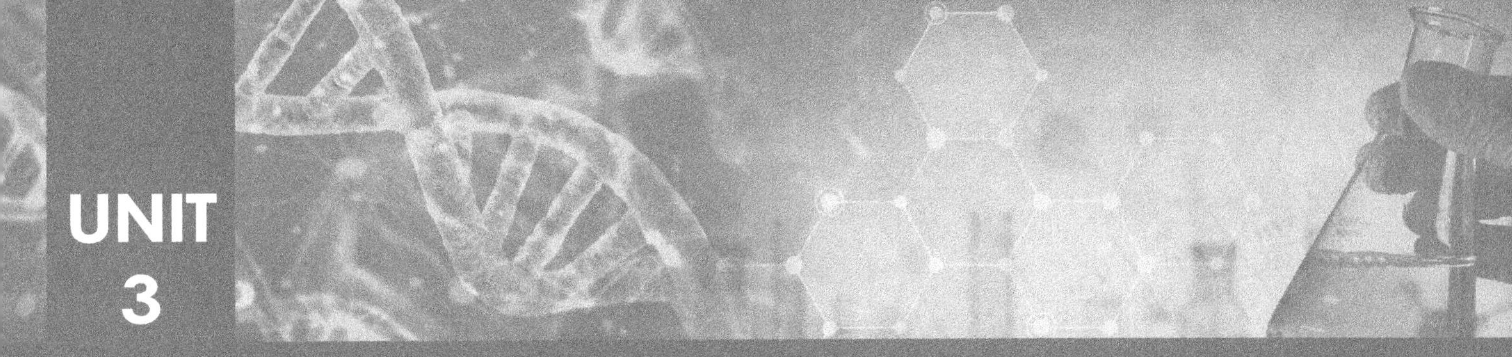

Lipid Metabolism and Amino Acid Metabolism

Lipid Metabolism

Lipid metabolism includes fatty acid oxidation, fatty acid synthesis, lipogenesis, ketogenesis, ketolysis, and cholesterol metabolism, etc.

Fatty Acid Oxidation

Fatty acid undergoes oxidation and produces small metabolites such as acetyl CoA (mostly). Fatty acid oxidation is broadly classified into four major types based on the position where the oxidation takes place as follows,

1. α-Oxidation
2. β-Oxidation
3. γ-Oxidation
4. ω-Oxidation

Out of these different types, the most predominant one occurring in the body is β-oxidation. The other types of fatty acid oxidations such as α-oxidation, γ-oxidation and ω-oxidation are minor pathways.

β-Oxidation of Fatty Acids

Definition:

In the body, fatty acids are mainly oxidized by β-oxidation. **It is defined as the oxidation that takes place on the β-carbon atom of the fatty acids with the sequential removal of two carbon fragments as acetyl CoA.** In the body, fatty acid oxidation takes place in most of the tissues but for energy requirements, some tissues such as the brain, erythrocytes and adrenal medulla cannot utilize fatty acids.

Stages involved:

There are three important steps involved in β-oxidation of fatty acids. They are,

1. Fatty acid activation in cytosol.
2. Transport of acyl CoA from cytosol to mitochondria.
3. Proper β-oxidation in mitochondrial matrix.

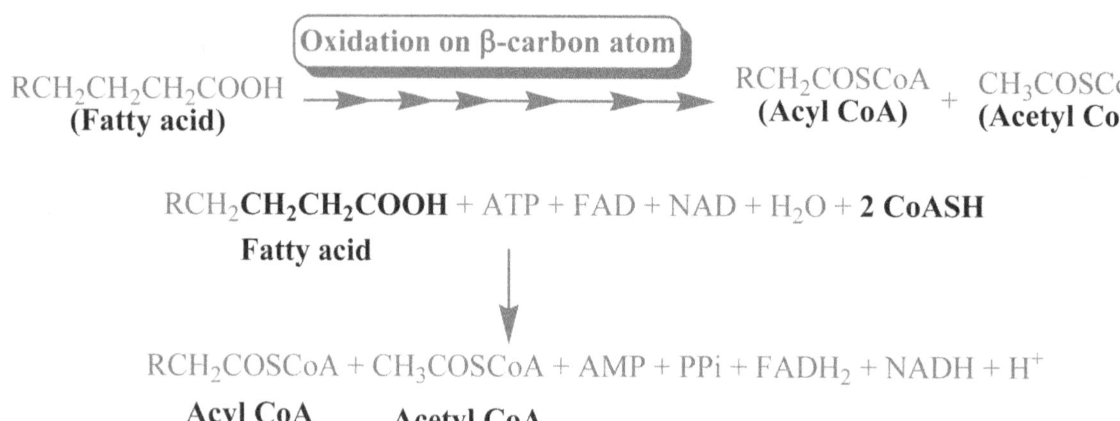

Stage 1 (Fatty acid activation in cytosol):

The active form of fatty acids is known as acyl CoA. In this stage, fatty acids are converted into acyl CoA in cytosol by the enzyme called "*acyl CoA synthetase* (*ACS*) or *thiokinase* (*TK*)". It involves two steps.

1. In the first step, fatty acid reacts with ATP in the presence of *acyl CoA synthetase* (*ACS*) or *thiokinase* (*TK*) that produces acyladenylate with the liberation of pyrophosphate (PPi). The total reaction is made irreversible by an immediate elimination of pyrophosphate into inorganic phosphate (Pi) through hydrolysis in the presence of *pyrophosphatase* (Substrate is "pyrophosphate" and the type of reaction is "hydrolysis").
2. In the next step, acyladenylate reacts with co-enzyme A to produce acyl CoA and AMP. This step is also catalyzed by the same enzyme involved in first step i.e., *acyl CoA synthetase* (*ACS*) (The product formed is "acyl CoA" and the type of reaction is "synthetic") or *thiokinase* (*TK*) (In ATP / GTP involved reactions, the enzymes acted are "*kinase*" and "sulphur" atom of co-enzyme A is also involved in reaction). *Kinase* enzyme needs magnesium ion as co-factors for its activity. In this step, one ATP is converted into AMP (2 ATP is utilized i.e., 1 ATP for ATP to ADP and other 1 ATP for ADP to AMP).

There are 3 different types of fatty acids based on length of the carbon chain. Hence, three different thiokinases are available to activate these fatty acids. They are,

(a) *Long chain thiokinase* (Activates fatty acid containing 9 to 20 carbon atoms)
(b) *Medium chain thiokinase* (Activates fatty acid containing 4 to 9 carbon atoms)
(c) *Short chain thiokinase* (Activates fatty acid containing less than 4 carbon atoms)

Stage 2 (Transport of acyl CoA from cytosol to mitochondria):

Acyl CoA is impermeable to the inner mitochondrial membrane. Therefore, the transport of acyl CoA will not occur by a simple diffusion. Hence, a special transport system known as a **carnitine carrier system or carnitine shuttle** performs this one. Carnitine carrier system transfers acyl CoA from cytosol to mitochondria. This carrier system is a very good example for facilitated diffusion and the carnitine carrier system is presented in Figure 3.1. This stage involves four steps.

1. **Formation of acyl carnitine:** Carnitine is chemically β-hydroxy-γ-trimethyl aminobutyrate. In the first step, acyl group of acyl CoA is transferred to carnitine to produce acyl carnitine in the presence of *carnitine acyl transferase – I* or *CAT – I* (Substrate is "carnitine" and the group transferred is "acyl group"). *CAT– I,* is present in the outer surface of the inner mitochondrial membrane.
2. **Transport of acyl carnitine from cytosol to mitochondrial matrix:** Acyl carnitine is transported from cytosol to mitochondrial matrix by a specific carrier protein.

$$R-CH_2-CH_2-\overset{\overset{O}{\|}}{C}-OH$$

Fatty acid
(Inactive form)

Acyl CoA synthetase or *Thiokinase*

ATP

- 2 Esterification or Transfer of AMP

PPi → 2 Pi (*Pyrophosphatase*, H_2O)

$$R-CH_2-CH_2-\overset{\overset{O}{\|}}{C}-AMP$$

Acyladenylate

Acyl CoA synthetase or *Thiokinase*

CoASH

Substitution

AMP

$$R-CH_2-CH_2-\overset{\overset{O}{\|}}{C}-SCoA$$

Acyl CoA
(Active form of fatty acid)

3. **Release of acyl CoA in mitochondrial matrix:** In this step, the acyl carnitine entered in the mitochondrial matrix liberates acyl CoA and carnitine by reacting with co-enzyme A in the presence of *carnitine acyl transferase – II* or *CAT – II* (Substrate is "carnitine" and the group transferred is "acyl group"). *CAT – II* is present in the inner mitochondrial membrane.
4. **Carnitine returns to cytosol:** Finally, released carnitine is transported from mitochondrial matrix to cytosol for reuse.

The cells have two separate pools of co-enzyme A i.e., cytosolic and mitochondrial. Hence, the co-enzyme A used for activation in the first stage is different from the one that combines with the acyl carnitine in the mitochondria to form acyl CoA. Malonyl CoA inhibits *carnitine acyl transferase – I* or *CAT – I*. Malonyl CoA is a key metabolite involved in the fatty acid synthesis that takes place in cytosol. In other words, while the fatty acid synthesis is in progress (reflected in high concentration of malonyl CoA), their oxidation does not occur because the carnitine shuttle is impaired.

Stage 3 (Proper β-oxidation in mitochondrial matrix):

Two carbon fragment "acetyl CoA" is liberated in each cycle of the proper β-oxidation. This stage involves four steps and the following are the sequence of four chemical reactions that take place in the mitochondrial matrix during proper β-oxidation. They are 1) Oxidation, 2) Hydration, 3) Oxidation, 4) Cleavage.

1. **Oxidation:** At first, acyl CoA undergoes oxidation with FAD by losing two hydrogen atoms in the presence of *acyl CoA dehydrogenase* (*ACAD*) (In NAD^+ / FAD involved reactions. the enzymes acted are "*dehydrogenase*" and the substrate is "acyl CoA"). One hydrogen is lost from α-carbon and the other hydrogen is lost from β-carbon. Hence, a double bond is formed between α- and β-carbon atoms and the product formed is known as α, β-unsaturated acyl CoA or Δ^2-trans enoyl CoA. ***Acyl CoA dehydrogenase* is the rate limiting enzyme of β-oxidation and it regulates the β-oxidation of fatty acid.** In this step, one FAD is converted into $FADH_2$ **(2 ATP is generated).**

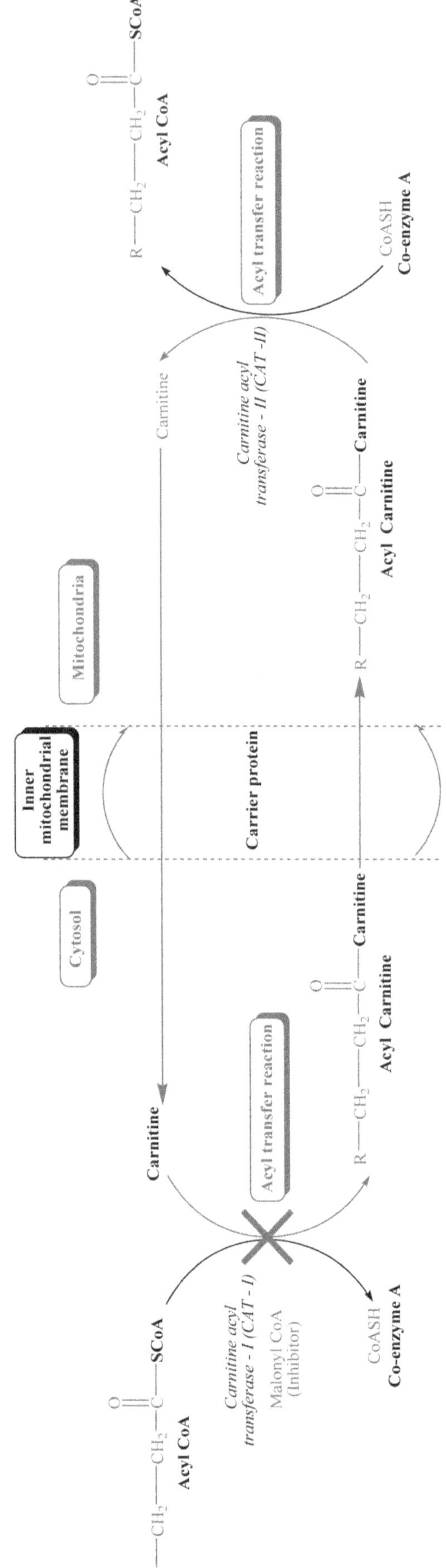

Figure 3.1 Carnitine shuttle or Carnitine carrier system.

2. **Hydration:** In this step, Δ^2-trans enoyl CoA is reacted with water molecules and produces β-hydroxy acyl CoA. Hydrogen is attached to α-carbon and the hydroxyl group is attached to β-carbon. This reaction is catalyzed by *enoyl CoA hydratase* (*ECAH*) (Substrate is "enoyl CoA" and the type of reaction is "hydration").
3. **Oxidation:** β-Hydroxy acyl CoA further oxidized by NAD^+ and produces β-keto acyl CoA in presence of β-*hydroxy acyl CoA dehydrogenase* (βHACAD) (In NAD^+ / FAD involved reactions, the enzymes acted are "*dehydrogenase*" and the substrate is "β-hydroxy acyl CoA"). In this oxidation, one hydrogen atom is lost from β-carbon and the other hydrogen is lost from the β-hydroxyl group. Hence, a double bond is formed between β-carbon and β-oxygen atoms. In other words, secondary alcohol is oxidized to keto group. In this step, one NAD^+ is converted into NADH + H^+ (3 ATP is generated).

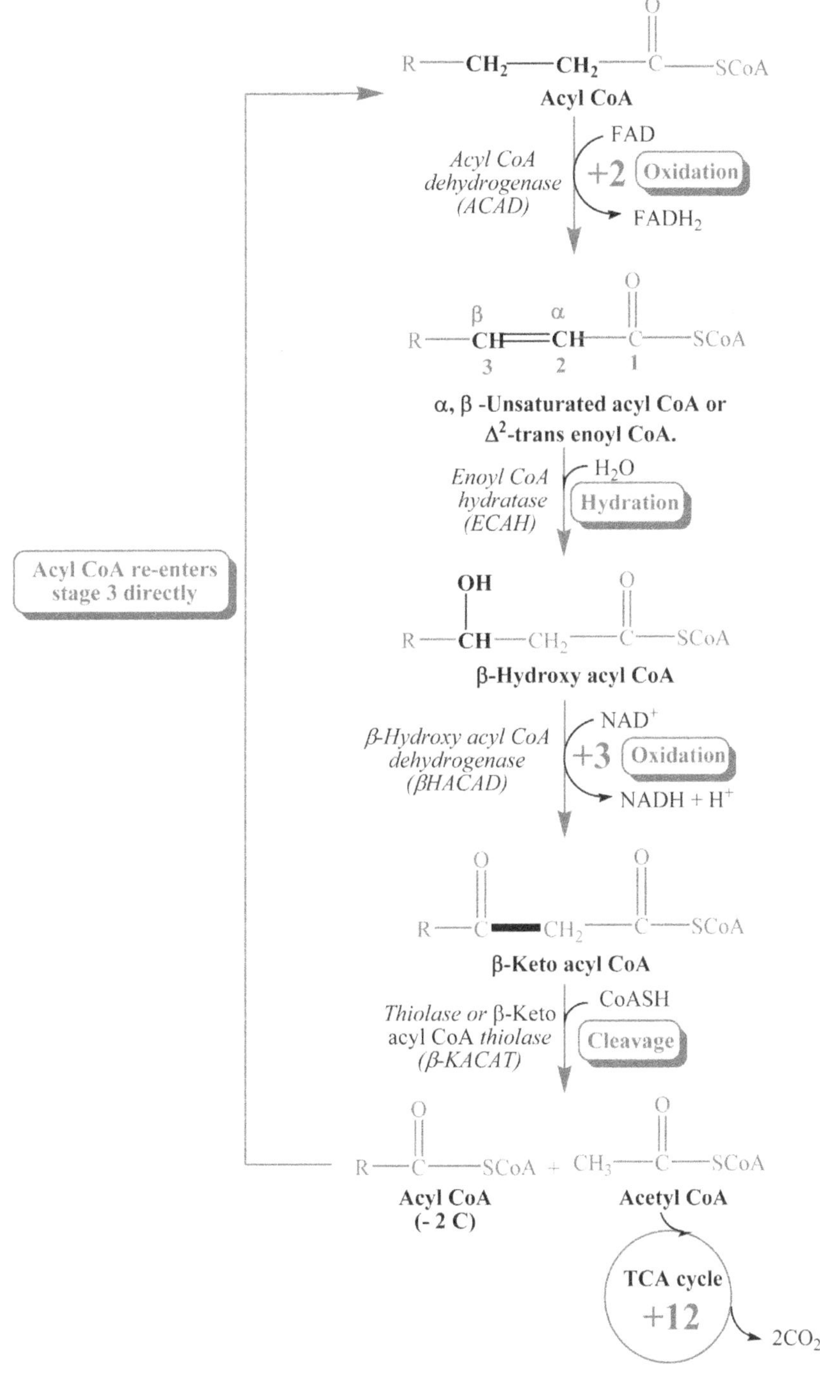

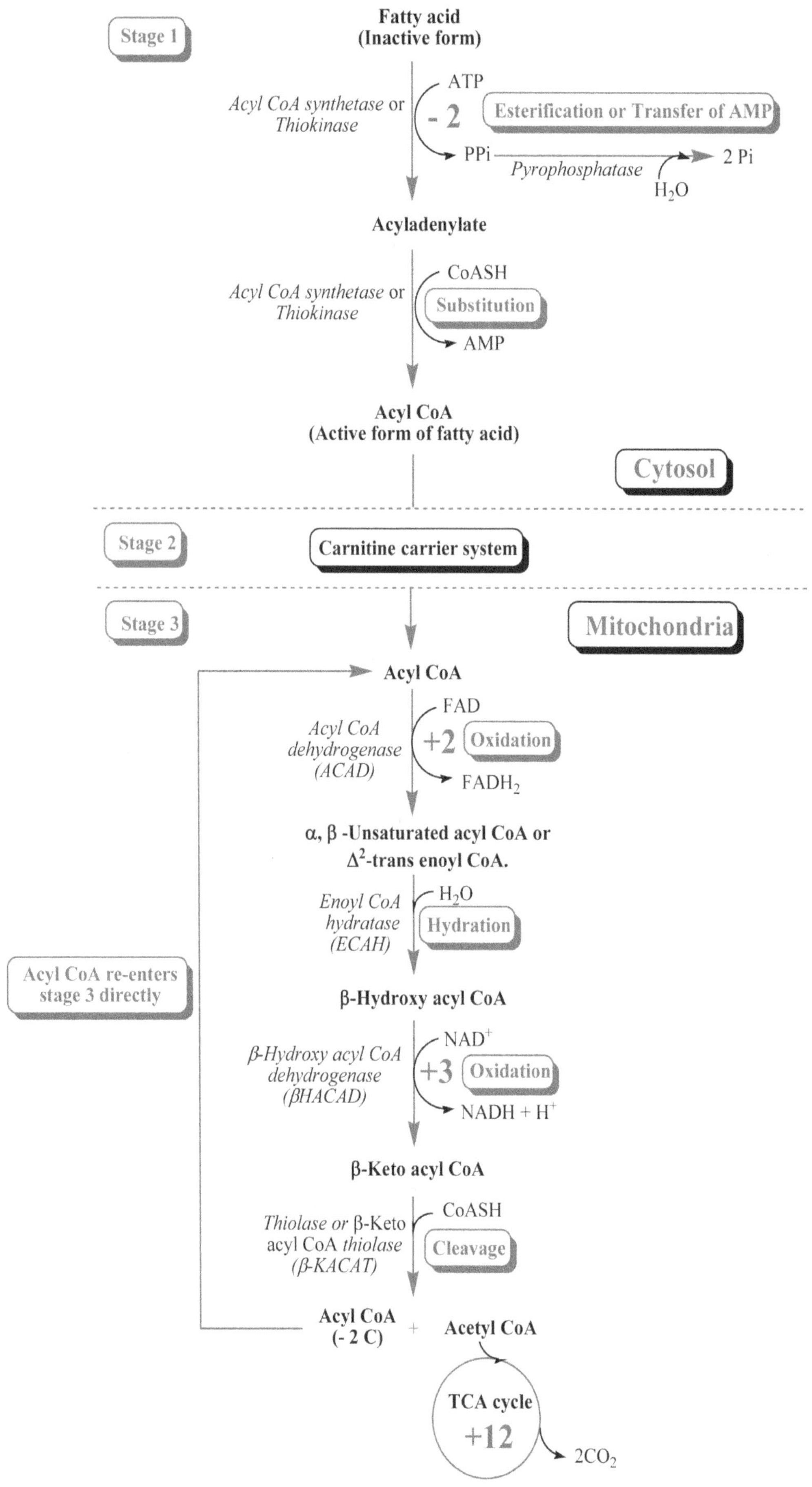

Stage 1
Fatty acid
(Inactive form)
Acyl CoA synthetase or Thiokinase
ATP
- 2
Esterification or Transfer of AMP
PPi
Pyrophosphatase
2 Pi
H_2O
Acyladenylate
Acyl CoA synthetase or Thiokinase
CoASH
Substitution
AMP
Acyl CoA
(Active form of fatty acid)
Cytosol
Stage 2
Carnitine carrier system
Stage 3
Mitochondria
Acyl CoA
Acyl CoA dehydrogenase (ACAD)
FAD
+2
Oxidation
$FADH_2$
α, β -Unsaturated acyl CoA or
Δ^2-trans enoyl CoA.
Enoyl CoA hydratase (ECAH)
H_2O
Hydration
Acyl CoA re-enters stage 3 directly
β-Hydroxy acyl CoA
β-Hydroxy acyl CoA dehydrogenase (βHACAD)
NAD^+
+3
Oxidation
$NADH + H^+$
β-Keto acyl CoA
Thiolase or β-Keto acyl CoA thiolase (β-KACAT)
CoASH
Cleavage
Acyl CoA
(- 2 C)
+
Acetyl CoA
TCA cycle
+12
$2CO_2$

4. **Cleavage:** This is the final reaction in which β-keto acyl CoA reacts with co-enzyme A in the presence of *thiolase* or *β-keto acyl CoA thiolase* (The type of reaction is "thiolytic cleavage" and the substrate is "β-keto acyl CoA") and produces acyl CoA with two carbon less than the original and liberates two carbon fragment acetyl CoA. The new acyl CoA re-enters proper β-oxidation step and it continues till the fatty acid is completely oxidized.

   The overall reaction involved in each cycle of proper β-oxidation can be written as follows.

Acyl CoA (with "n" carbon) + FAD + NAD^+ + H_2O + CoASH

↓ Proper β-oxidation (Per cycle)

Acyl CoA (with "n-2" carbon) + Acetyl CoA + $FADH_2$ + NADH + H^+

In the biological system, the most predominantly occurring β-oxidation is β-oxidation of saturated even carbon fatty acid. Hence, the above discussion is with respect to that one.

Oxidation of palmitic acid:

Palmitic is a sixteen-carbon containing fatty acid. It undergoes β-oxidation by the above method and produces energy.

$$CH_3-(CH_2)_{14}-\overset{\displaystyle O}{\overset{\|}{C}}-OH$$

Palmitic acid

In the first stage, palmitic acid is activated to its active form palmitoyl CoA with utilization of 2 ATP in cytosol by *thiokinase*. Later, palmitoyl CoA is transported from cytosol to mitochondrial matrix by facilitated diffusion through special carrier protein using a carnitine carrier system. The second stage is catalyzed by *carnitine acyl transferase* or *CAT*. In the final stage, the palmitoyl CoA undergoes proper β-oxidation in the mitochondrial matrix by a four-step process and liberates 2 carbon fragment acetyl CoA and acyl CoA with 2 carbon less than the original. This obtained acyl CoA (2 carbon less) further undergoes four-step proper β-oxidation again and produce corresponding acyl CoA (2 carbon less than substrate acyl CoA) and acetyl CoA. As palmitoyl CoA contains 16 carbons, the proper β-oxidation cycles are repeated for 7 times and produces 8 acetyl CoA totally. The produced acetyl CoA is oxidized to carbon dioxide by entering into TCA cycle and produce 12 ATP. The overall reaction involved in the oxidation of one mole of palmitic acid is summarized in the below equation.

$CH_3(CH_2)_{14}COOH$ + ATP + 7 FAD + 7 NAD + 7 H_2O + 8 CoASH

Palmitic acid

↓ β–Oxidation

8 $CH_3COSCoA$ + AMP + PPi + 7 $FADH_2$ + 7 NADH + 7 H^+

Palmitoyl CoA

Energetic of palmitic acid β-oxidation:

Energy generation is the ultimate aim in fatty acid metabolism. The energy obtained in complete β-oxidation of palmitic acid is summarized in Table 3.1 and Figure 3.2.

Table 3.1 Energetic of palmitic acid β-oxidation.

S. No	Mechanism or molecule involved	No. of ATP generated or utilized per cycle or mole	No. of cycles or moles involved	Total ATP generated or utilized
Proper β-oxidation cycle in mitochondrial matrix				
1	One FAD is reduced to $FADH_2$ (One $FADH_2$ is equals to 2 ATP)	+ 2	7	+ 14
2	One NAD^+ is reduced to NADH + H^+ (One NADH + H^+ is equals to 3 ATP)	+ 3	7	+ 21
TCA cycle				
3	One acetyl CoA is oxidized to carbondioxide	+ 12	8	+ 96
Total ATP generated by one mole of palmitic acid (+14 + 21 + 96)				**+ 131**
Activation of palmitic acid in cytosol				
4	One ATP is converted into AMP	- 2	1	- **2**
Net ATP generated by one mole of palmitic acid through complete **β-oxidation** (131 - 2)				**129**

The standard free energy of palmitic acid (one mole) = 2340 Cal

The energy yielded by β–oxidation of palmitic acid (one mole) = 129 ATP = 129 × 7.3 Cal = 941.7 Cal [1 ATP = 7.3 Cal]

The energey conversion efficiency of palmitic acid β-oxidation $= \frac{941.7}{2340} \times 100 = 40.24\ \%$

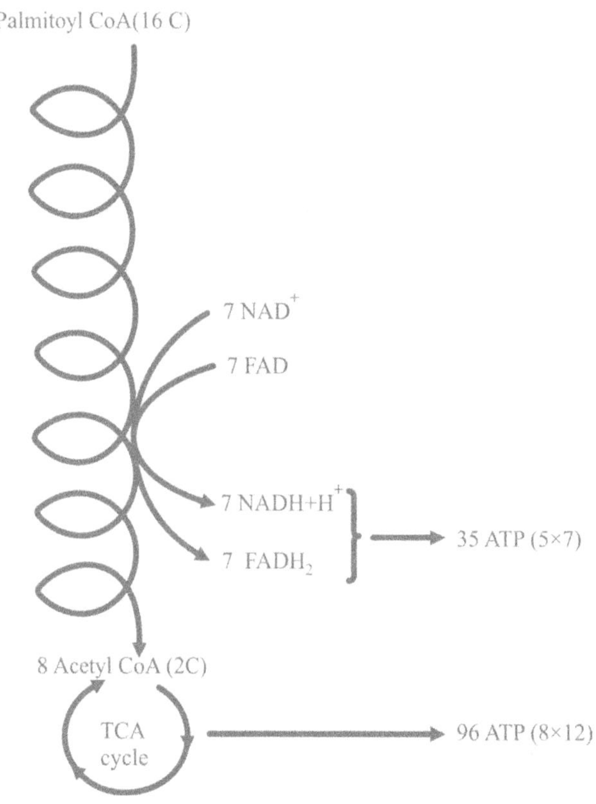

Figure 3.2 Energetic of palmitic acid β-oxidation - Overview.

Metabolic disorder:

1. **Sudden infant death syndrome (SIDS):** In general, an overnight unexpected death of healthy infants is known as SIDS and the real cause for this syndrome is not known. Now, it was identified that at least 10 % of SIDS is due to the deficiency of *medium chain acyl CoA dehydrogenase* (*MCACAD*). The frequency of this enzyme defect is 1 in 10,000 births and the prevalent is more than phenylketonuria. Soon after eating or feeding babies, glucose is the principle source of energy. The glucose utilization and its level are decreased after a few hours. Hence, simultaneously, the fatty acid oxidation must increase to meet the energy requirements. Hence, in infants blocking of β-oxidation due to the deficiency of *medium chain acyl CoA dehydrogenase* (*MCACAD*) leads to sudden death.
2. **Jamaican vomiting sickness:** This metabolic disorder is caused by eating unripe ackee fruit which contains an unusual toxic amino acid known as hypoglycin-A. *Acyl CoA dehydrogenase* (ACAD) is inhibited by this hypoglycin-A. Hence, fatty acid β-oxidation is blocked leads to several complications. Jamaican vomiting sickness is characterized by severe hypoglycemia, vomiting, and convulsion. In severe conditions, it produces coma and death, if untreated.

Ketone Bodies Metabolism

Ketone bodies are defined as a water-soluble chemical substance present in biological systems possessing carbonyl groups and yielding energy. Following are three important ketone bodies present in biological systems 1) Acetone, 2) Acetoacetate, 3) β-Hydroxybutyrate or 3-Hydroxybutyrate. Out of these three, acetone and acetoacetate are called as "true ketone bodies" because it contains carbonyl group; whereas β-hydroxybutyrate is not a true ketone body due to the lack of carbonyl keto group in structure. However, it is considered a ketone body due to its structural similarities or relationship with acetoacetate. Except acetone, other two ketone bodies undergoe metabolism and produce energy. Acetone is not metabolized in the body.

$CH_3-C(=O)-CH_3$

Acetone
(True ketone body;
Not metabolized)

$CH_3-C(=O)-CH_2-COOH$

Acetoacetate
(True ketone body;
Metabolized and yield energy)

$CH_3-\underset{\beta}{C}H(OH)-\underset{\alpha}{C}H_2-COOH$

β-Hydroxy butyrate
(Not true ketone body;
Metabolized and yield energy)

Ketone bodies metabolism is generally divided into 2 major pathways such as,

1. Ketogenesis
2. Ketolysis

Ketogenesis

Definition: It is defined as a series of chemical reactions occurring in the biological system to produce ketone bodies from acetyl CoA.

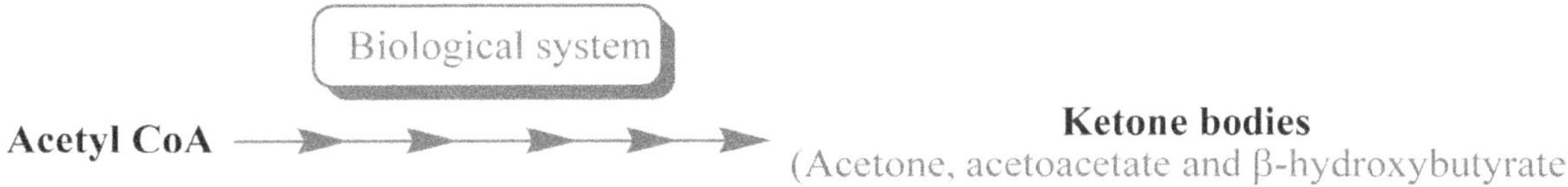

Pathway: Mainly ketogenesis occurs in the liver and the enzymes involved in ketogenesis are present in the mitochondrial matrix. Acetyl CoA, needed for the synthesis of ketone bodies is generally obtained from the oxidation of fatty acids, pyruvate or some amino acids particularly ketogenic amino acids like leucine, lysine, phenylalanine, etc. (because they are degraded to acetoacetate and acetyl CoA). The following are the various reactions involved in ketogenesis.

1. Initially, two molecules of acetyl CoA are condensed together and produce acetoacetyl CoA with loss of co-enzyme A in presence of *β-ketoacyl CoA thiolase* (*βKACAT*) or *β-ketothiolase* (*βKT*) or simply *thiolase* (The type of reaction is "thiolytic cleavage" and the product is "acetoacetyl CoA" which is "β-keto acyl CoA"). This is the enzyme involved in the final step of proper β-oxidation of fatty acids. Hence, this reaction is considered as reverse reactions of *thiolase* catalyzed reaction in β-oxidation.

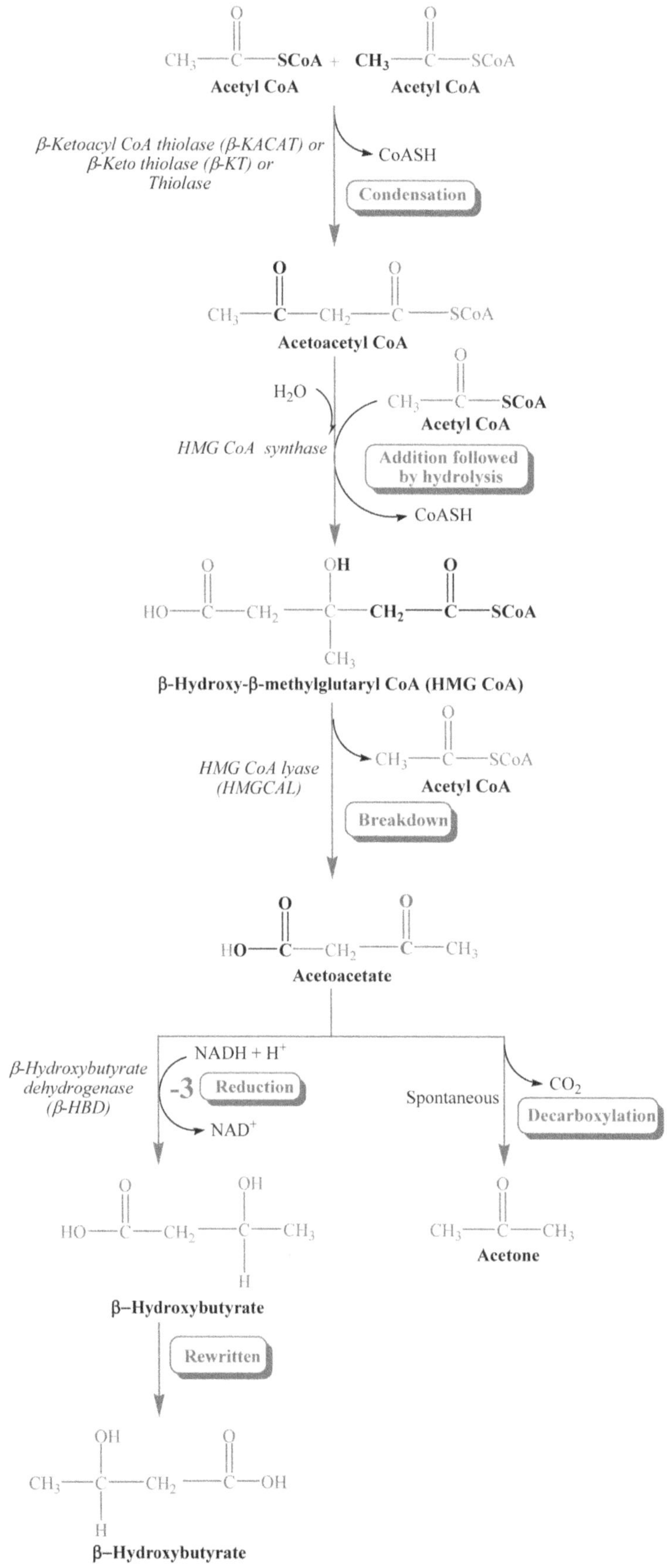

$CH_3-C(=O)-SCoA + CH_3-C(=O)-SCoA$
Acetyl CoA **Acetyl CoA**

β-Ketoacyl CoA thiolase (β-KACAT) or β-Keto thiolase (β-KT) or Thiolase
→ CoASH
Condensation

$CH_3-C(=O)-CH_2-C(=O)-SCoA$
Acetoacetyl CoA

H_2O
HMG CoA synthase
$CH_3-C(=O)-SCoA$ **Acetyl CoA**
Addition followed by hydrolysis
→ CoASH

$HO-C(=O)-CH_2-C(OH)(CH_3)-CH_2-C(=O)-SCoA$
β-Hydroxy-β-methylglutaryl CoA (HMG CoA)

HMG CoA lyase (HMGCAL)
→ $CH_3-C(=O)-SCoA$ **Acetyl CoA**
Breakdown

$HO-C(=O)-CH_2-C(=O)-CH_3$
Acetoacetate

β-Hydroxybutyrate dehydrogenase (β-HBD)
$NADH + H^+$
-3 Reduction
→ NAD^+

Spontaneous
→ CO_2
Decarboxylation

$HO-C(=O)-CH_2-C(OH)(H)-CH_3$
β–Hydroxybutyrate

$CH_3-C(=O)-CH_3$
Acetone

Rewritten

$CH_3-C(OH)(H)-CH_2-C(=O)-OH$
β–Hydroxybutyrate

2. Another molecule of acetyl CoA reacts with acetoacetyl CoA and one molecule of water in the presence of *HMG CoA synthase* (*HMGCAS*) (Product is "HMG CoA" and the type of reaction is "synthesis") and produce β-hydroxy-β-methylglutaryl CoA (HMG CoA) and co-enzyme A. The basic reaction involved in this step is addition followed by hydrolysis. This step is the rate limiting step of ketogenesis. Hence, ***HMG CoA synthase* (*HMGCAS*) regulates ketogenesis.**
3. In the succeeding step, HMG CoA undergoes breakdown reaction and produced one of the ketone body acetoacetate with liberation of one molecule of acetyl CoA. This reaction is catalyzed by *HMG CoA lyase* (*HMGCAL*) (Substrate is "HMG CoA" and the type of reaction is "lysis or breakdown").
4. From the ketone body acetoacetate, the remaining two ketone bodies are synthesized. Acetoacetate spontaneously undergoes decarboxylation with the removal of carbon dioxide from carboxylic group and produces the other ketone body "acetone".
5. In another way, acetoacetate is reduced using NADH + H^+ results in the formation of β-hydroxybutyrate and NAD^+ in presence of *β-hydroxybutyrate dehydrogenase* (*βHBD*) (In NAD^+ / $NADP^+$ involved reaction, the enzymes acted are "*dehydrogenase*" and the product is "β-hydroxybutyrate"). In this reaction, one mole of NADH + H^+ is converted to NAD^+ **(3 ATPs are utilized).**

From the liver, ketone bodies are easily transported to other tissues because they are water soluble. For peripheral tissues like skeletal muscle, cardiac muscle, renal cortex, etc., two ketone bodies namely acetoacetate and β-hydroxybutyrate serve as important sources of energy. Ketone bodies cannot be utilized by tissues that lack mitochondria such as erythrocytes. During starvation and diabetes mellitus, the supply of glucose to the tissues is short; hence in such situations ketone bodies production and utilization becomes more significant. For the brain and the other parts of CNS, ketone bodies are the major fuel source during prolonged starvation. Utilization of fatty acids by the brain for energy is very limited. 50 to 70 % of the brain's energy demands are rectified by ketone bodies only. During the period of food deprivation, this is an adaptation for the survival of the organism.

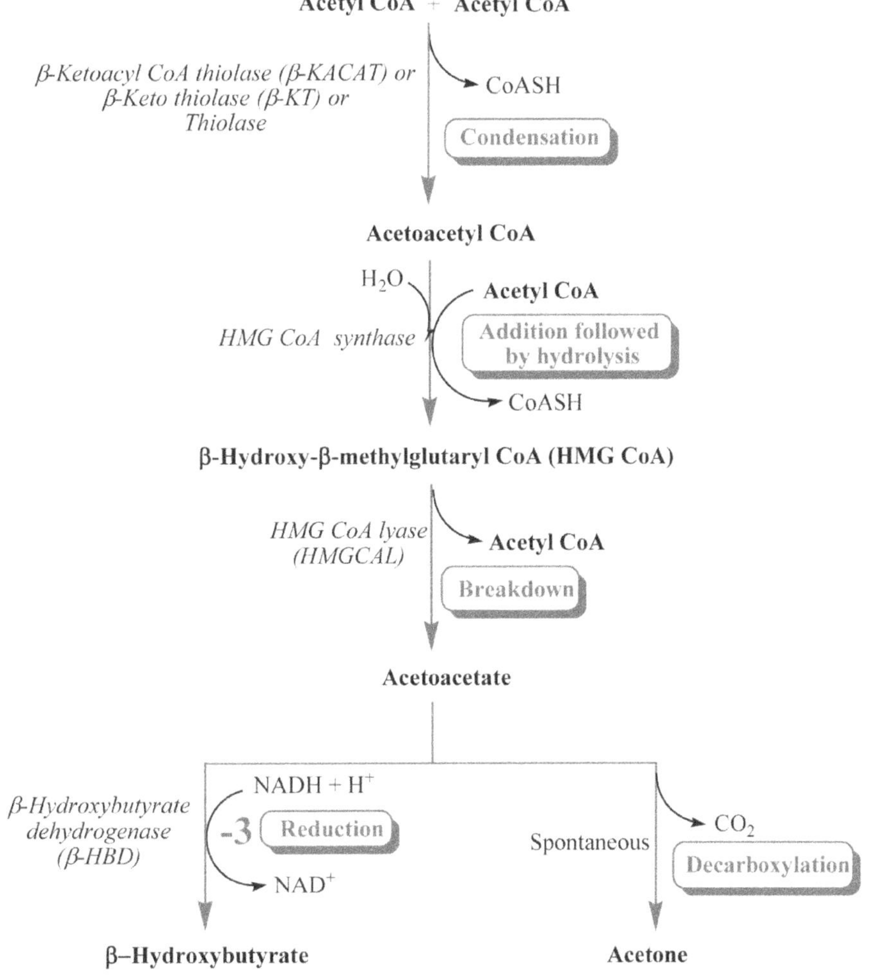

Regulation of ketogenesis:

Overproduction of ketonebodies take place when carbohydrates are not available to the tissues. This is due to excessive utilization of fatty acid to meet the energy requirements of the cells. Ketogenesis is stimulated by the hormone glucagon and inhibited by insulin. In diabetes mellitus, increased ratio of glucagon / insulin promotes ketogenesis due to disturbances in carbohydrate and lipid metabolism.

In general, ketogenic substances such as fatty acid and ketogenic amino acids like leucine, lysine, tyrosine, etc. promote ketogenesis. Conversely, anti-ketogenic substances such as glucose, glycerol and glucogenic amino acids like glycine, alanine, serine, glutamate, etc. inhibits ketogenesis.

Ketolysis

Definition: It is defined as a series of chemical reactions occurring in the biological system to break ketone bodies acetoacetate and β-hydroxybutyrate into acetyl CoA.

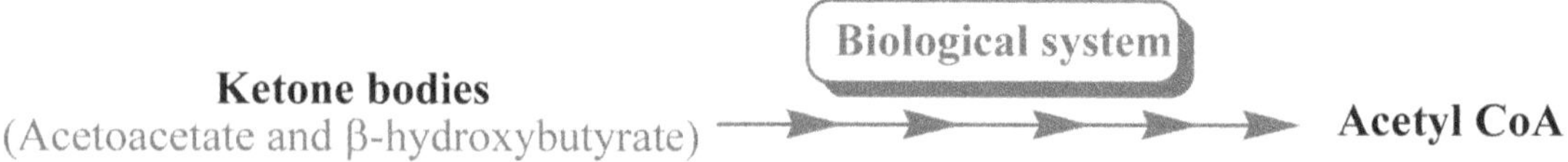

Pathway: Ketolysis is the reverse of ketogenesis with a slight modification. The following are the various reactions taking place in conversion of ketone bodies like acetoacetate and β-hydroxybutyrate into acetyl CoA.

1. The first step is the reversal of the last step of ketogenesis. In this step, β-hydroxybutyrate is oxidized to acetoacetate using NAD^+ in presence of *β-hydroxybutyrate dehydrogenase* (*βHBD*) (In NAD^+ / $NADP^+$ involved reactions, the enzymes acted are "*dehydrogenase*" and the substrate is "β-hydroxybutyrate"). In this reaction, one mole of NAD^+ is converted to NADH + H^+ (**3 ATPs are generated**).
2. Later, acetoacetate is activated to its active form acetoacetyl CoA by succinyl CoA in the presence of mitochondrial enzyme *thiophorase* (TP) which is otherwise known *succinyl CoA acetoacetate CoA transferase* (*SCACT*) (Substrate is "acetoacetate and succinyl CoA" and the type of reaction is "transfer of co-enzyme A"). In this reaction, co-enzyme A is simply transferred from TCA cycle intermediate succinyl CoA to acetoacetate. After donating co-enzyme A, succinyl CoA is converted to succinate. Liver cannot utilize ketone bodies due to lack of *thiophorase* (*TP*).
3. Finally, acetoacetyl CoA reacts with co-enzyme A in presence of *β-ketoacyl CoA thiolase* (*βKACAT*) or *β-ketothiolase* (*βKT*) or simply *thiolase* (The type of reaction is "thiolytic cleavage" and the substrate is "β-keto acyl CoA") and produces 2 moles of acetyl CoA. This reaction is similar to *thiolase* catalyzed reaction in β-oxidation of fatty acid or reversal of the first step of ketogenesis.

Metabolic disorders of ketone bodies metabolism

In healthy individuals, there is a constant synthesis of ketone bodies by the liver and their utilization by extrahepatic tissues. The normal level of ketone bodies in the blood is 1 mg/dl. Only very low quantities of ketone bodies are excreted in urine and cannot be detected by routine Rothera's test. When there is an imbalance between ketogenesis and ketolysis the following metabolic disorder may occur.

1. **Ketonemia:** It is defined as an increased level of ketone bodies in the blood due to their overproduction rather than the deficiency of their utilization (Rate of ketogenesis exceeds the rate of ketolysis).
2. **Ketonuria:** It is a clinical condition in which more quantities of ketone bodies are excreted in the urine. Generally, active fat metabolism is indicated by the appearance of ketone bodies in urine. Some body weight programs are designed to encourage a reduction in carbohydrate and total calorie intake until ketone bodies appear in the urine.
3. **Ketosis:** The combined effect of ketonemia and ketonuria is known as ketosis. The common feature of ketosis is the smell of acetone in breath. Usually, it is associated with starvation and uncontrolled diabetes mellitus.

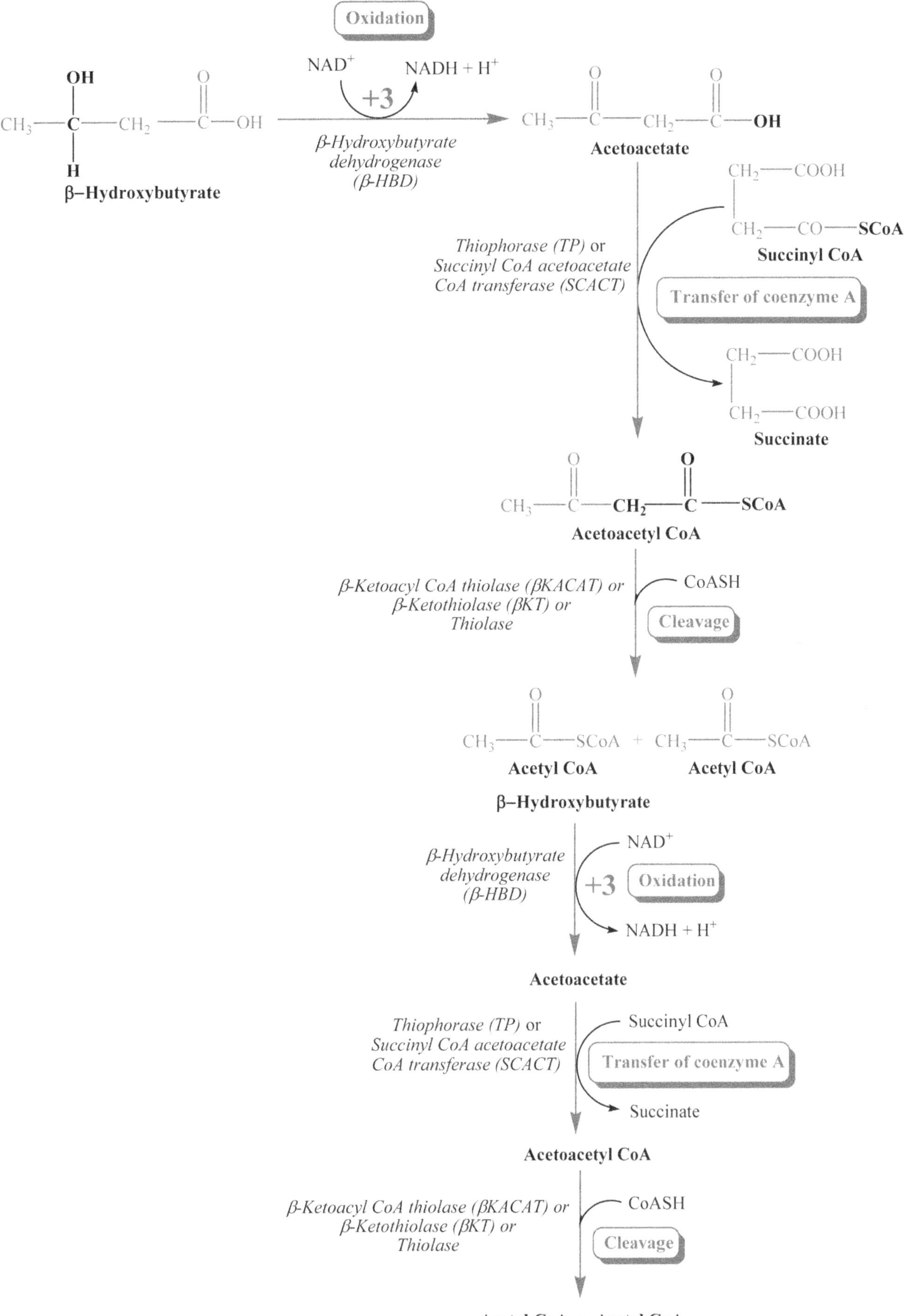
Oxidation
NAD+
NADH + H+
+3
OH
CH3—C—CH2—C—OH
H
β–Hydroxybutyrate
β-Hydroxybutyrate dehydrogenase (β-HBD)
CH3—C—CH2—C—OH
Acetoacetate
CH2—COOH
CH2—CO—SCoA
Succinyl CoA
Thiophorase (TP) or Succinyl CoA acetoacetate CoA transferase (SCACT)
Transfer of coenzyme A
CH2—COOH
CH2—COOH
Succinate
CH3—C—CH2—C—SCoA
Acetoacetyl CoA
β-Ketoacyl CoA thiolase (βKACAT) or β-Ketothiolase (βKT) or Thiolase
CoASH
Cleavage
CH3—C—SCoA + CH3—C—SCoA
Acetyl CoA
Acetyl CoA
β–Hydroxybutyrate
β-Hydroxybutyrate dehydrogenase (β-HBD)
NAD+
+3
Oxidation
NADH + H+
Acetoacetate
Thiophorase (TP) or Succinyl CoA acetoacetate CoA transferase (SCACT)
Succinyl CoA
Transfer of coenzyme A
Succinate
Acetoacetyl CoA
β-Ketoacyl CoA thiolase (βKACAT) or β-Ketothiolase (βKT) or Thiolase
CoASH
Cleavage
Acetyl CoA + Acetyl CoA

Fatty acid degradation is increased during starvation to meet the energy demands of the body. Hence, acetyl CoA is overproduced which cannot be fully handled by the TCA cycle. In addition, oxaloacetate deficiency (most of the oxaloacetate is diverted for the synthesis of glucose to meet essential requirements for tissues like the brain) also impairs the TCA cycle. Hence acetyl CoA is accumulated and it is diverted for the over synthesis of ketone bodies.

Diabetes mellitus is associated with insulin deficiency. In this condition, lipolysis is increased and carbohydrate metabolism is impaired which leads to the accumulation of acetyl CoA and increased ketogenesis. The ketone body concentration in blood and urine may reach 100 mg/dl and 500 mg/day, respectively in severe diabetes mellitus.

4. **Ketoacidosis:** Both acetoacetate and β-hydroxybutyrate are strong acids. Hence, increased concentration of ketone bodies decreases the pH and produce acidic condition known as ketoacidosis. Ketoacidosis combined with diabetes mellitus is commonly called **diabetic ketoacidosis** which is a dangerous disease. If untreated it may result in coma and death also. Ketosis due to starvation is not accompanied by ketoacidosis. Ketoacidosis is generally treated by using insulin which increases the glucose uptake by tissues and inhibits ketogenesis.

Denovo Synthesis of Fatty Acids

Fatty acids are synthesized and stored as triacylglycerols when excess dietary carbohydrates and amino acids are consumed. Cytosol fraction of the cell contains enzymes machinery for fatty acid synthesis and it is mainly takeing place in the liver, adipose tissue, kidney, and lactating mammary glands.

Components required: For the synthesis of fatty acids, the three important components needed are, a) Acetyl CoA (provides carbon skeleton), b) ATP (provides energy), c) NADPH (provides reducing equivalent).

Stages involved: Like β-oxidation of fatty acid, three stages are involved in the synthesis of fatty acid also. They are,

1. Synthesis of acetyl CoA and NADPH in cytosol.
2. Synthesis of malonyl CoA from acetyl CoA.
3. Reactions of *fatty acid synthase* (*FAS*) complex.

Stage 1 (Synthesis of acetyl CoA and NADPH in cytosol):

Synthesis of fatty acids needs acetyl CoA and NADPH as precursors. In mitochondria, oxidation of fatty acid and pyruvate, degradation of some amino acids carbon skeleton and catabolism of ketone bodies produces acetyl CoA. But mitochondrial membrane is impermeable to acetyl CoA. Hence, in mitochondria acetyl CoA reacts with oxaloacetate in presence of *citrate synthase* (*CS*) (Product is "citrate" and type of reaction is "synthesis") to produce citrate which is permeable to the mitochondrial membrane and transferred to the cytosol.

In cytosol, citrate undergoes breakdown to liberate acetyl CoA and oxaloacetate in presence of *citrate lyase* (*CL*) (Substrate is "citrate" and type of reaction is "lysis or breakdown"). The liberated oxaloacetate is converted into malate in presence of *malate dehydrogenase* (*MDH*) (In NAD^+ / $NADP^+$ involved reactions, the enzymes acted are "*dehydrogenase*" and the product is "malate"). Later, malate is converted to pyruvate in presence of *malic enzyme* (*ME*) or *malate dehydrogenase* (*MDH*) (In NAD^+ / $NADP^+$ involved reactions, the enzymes acted are "*dehydrogenase*" and the substrate is "malate") by oxidative decarboxylation. In this reaction, one mole of carbondioxide and NDPH + H^+ is synthesized which is utilized for the synthesis of fatty acid. The coupled transport of acetyl CoA with the production of carbon dioxide and NDPH + H^+ is highly advantageous to the cell for the biosynthesis of fatty acids.

Stage 2 (Synthesis of malonyl CoA from acetyl CoA):

This step is the rate-limiting step of the fatty acid synthesis. In this step, acetyl CoA undergoes carboxylation and produced malonyl CoA in presence of *acetyl CoA carboxylase* (*ACAC*) (Substrate is "acetyl

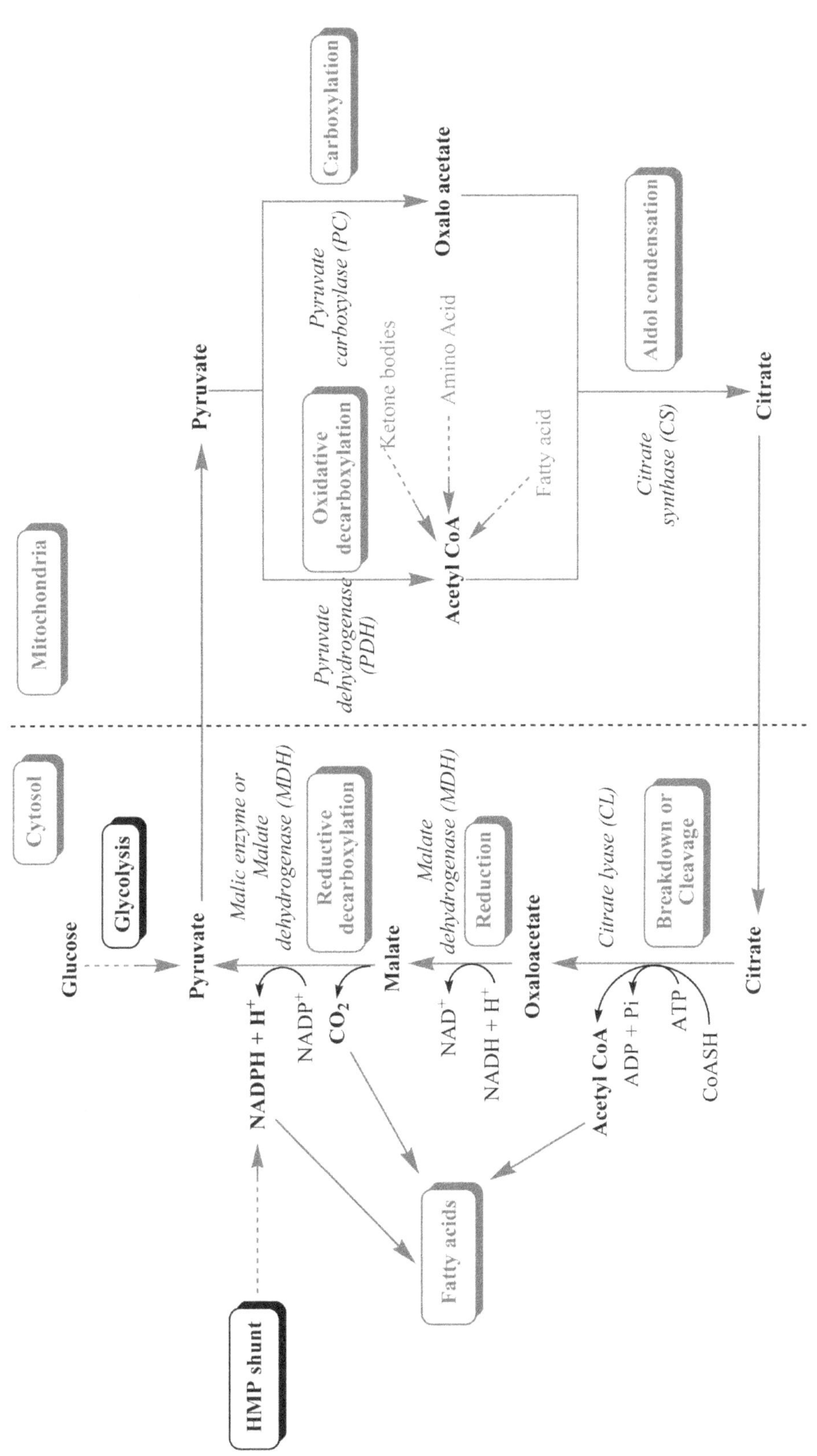
Cytosol
Mitochondria
Glucose
Glycolysis
Pyruvate
Pyruvate
Pyruvate dehydrogenase (PDH)
Oxidative decarboxylation
Pyruvate carboxylase (PC)
Carboxylation
Ketone bodies
Amino Acid
Fatty acid
Acetyl CoA
Oxalo acetate
Aldol condensation
Citrate synthase (CS)
Citrate
Citrate
Citrate lyase (CL)
Breakdown or Cleavage
ATP
CoASH
ADP + Pi
Acetyl CoA
Oxaloacetate
Malate dehydrogenase (MDH)
Reduction
NAD+
NADH + H+
Malate
Malic enzyme or Malate dehydrogenase (MDH)
Reductive decarboxylation
CO_2
NADP+
NADPH + H+
HMP shunt
Fatty acids

CoA" and the type of reaction is "carboxylation"). *Acetyl CoA carboxylase* (*ACAC*) needs biotin as a co-enzyme. In a carboxylation reaction, biotin acts as a carrier molecule. Biotin-enzyme reacts with carbondioxide in the presence of ATP to form a carboxybiotin-enzyme complex. This high energy complex handed over the carbondioxide to acetyl CoA to produce succinyl CoA. In this step, one ATP is converted into ADP and inorganic phosphate to provide the energy needed for the reaction. The mechanism of action of *acetyl CoA carboxylase* (*ACAC*) is similar to *pyruvate carboxylase*(*PC*).

$$CH_3-\overset{O}{\overset{\|}{C}}-SCoA \xrightarrow{\text{Rewritten}} H-CH_2-\overset{O}{\overset{\|}{C}}-SCoA$$

Acetyl CoA → Acetyl CoA

Acetyl CoA + CO_2 + ATP → (*Acetyl CoA carboxylase (ACAC)*, Biotin; Carboxylation) → Malonyl CoA + ADP + Pi

$$COOH-CH_2-\overset{O}{\overset{\|}{C}}-SCoA$$

Malonyl CoA

Stage 3 (Reactions of *fatty acid synthase* (*FAS*) complex):

Fatty acid synthase (*FAS*) complex is a multifunctional enzyme catalyzes the remaining reactions of fatty acid synthesis. *FAS* exists as a dimer with two identical units in eukaryotic cells including man. Seven different enzymes and a 4′-phosphopantetheine bound acyl carrier protein (ACP) is present in each monomer of the *FAS* complex. As a single unit this *FAS* complex catalyzes all seven reactions of stage 3 fatty acid synthesis; hence, dissociation of any one of *FAS* complex results in loss of enzyme activities. In eukaryotic cells (higher organism), an acyl carrier protein (ACP) is a part of the *FAS* complex; whereas in prokaryotic cells (lower organisms), ACP is not a part of the *FAS* complex and it is present separately. Seven reactions are catalyzed by seven different enzymes present in the *FAS* complex.

1. In the first step, ACP of *FAS* complex reacts with acetyl CoA and produces acetyl-S-ACP by transfer of acetyl group from acetyl CoA to ACP of the *FAS* complex. The reaction is catalyzed by *acetyl CoA-ACP transacylase* (Substrate is "acetyl CoA & ACP" of *FAS*, the type of reaction is "transfer" and the group transferred is "acetyl i.e., acyl"). Subsequently, the acetyl group is transferred to a cysteine residue of the enzyme from ACP to produce acetyl-S-enzyme. Hence, the ACP site becomes vacant.
2. Latter, malonyl CoA synthesized in stage 2 reacts with the above-formed acetyl-S-enzyme in presence of *malonyl CoA-ACP transacylase* (Substrate is "malonyl CoA & ACP" of *FAS*, the type of reaction is "transfer" and the group transferred is "malonyl") and produced acyl-S-ACP-malonyl-S-enzyme. In this step, the malonyl group is transferred from malonyl CoA to ACP of acetyl-S-enzyme.
3. In the next step, the acyl-S-ACP-malonyl-S-enzyme undergoes decarboxylation followed by addition to produce β-ketoacyl-S-ACP or simply β-ketoacyl-ACP. In this reaction initially, malonyl moiety attached to ACP loses the carboxyl group (added in stage 2 by *acetyl CoA carboxylase* (*ACAC*)) as carbondioxide and this carbondioxide is never incorporated into fatty acid carbon chain but the free energy lost by this decarboxylation is used for the addition takes place. Later, acetyl unit attached to cysteine is transferred to ACP and added to decarboxylated malonyl portion present in presence of

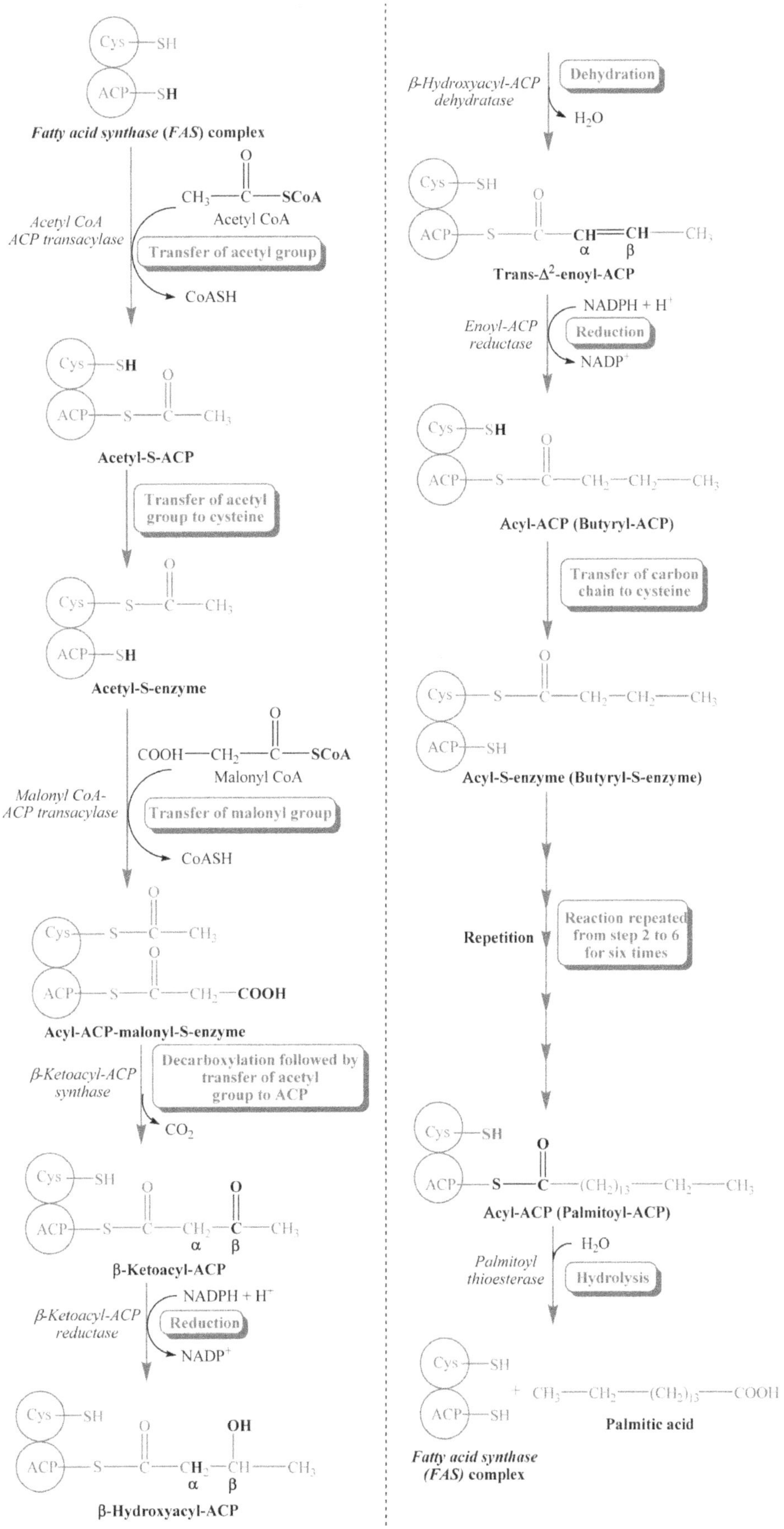

Cys—SH
ACP—SH
***Fatty acid synthase (FAS)* complex**

CH_3—C(=O)—SCoA
Acetyl CoA

Acetyl CoA ACP transacylase
Transfer of acetyl group
CoASH

Cys—SH
ACP—S—C(=O)—CH_3
Acetyl-S-ACP

Transfer of acetyl group to cysteine

Cys—S—C(=O)—CH_3
ACP—SH
Acetyl-S-enzyme

COOH—CH_2—C(=O)—SCoA
Malonyl CoA

Malonyl CoA-ACP transacylase
Transfer of malonyl group
CoASH

Cys—S—C(=O)—CH_3
ACP—S—C(=O)—CH_2—COOH
Acyl-ACP-malonyl-S-enzyme

β-Ketoacyl-ACP synthase
Decarboxylation followed by transfer of acetyl group to ACP
CO_2

Cys—SH
ACP—S—C(=O)—CH_2—C(=O)—CH_3
α β
β-Ketoacyl-ACP

β-Ketoacyl-ACP reductase
$NADPH + H^+$
Reduction
$NADP^+$

Cys—SH
ACP—S—C(=O)—CH_2—CH(OH)—CH_3
α β
β-Hydroxyacyl-ACP

β-Hydroxyacyl-ACP dehydratase
Dehydration
H_2O

Cys—SH
ACP—S—C(=O)—CH=CH—CH_3
α β
Trans-Δ^2-enoyl-ACP

Enoyl-ACP reductase
$NADPH + H^+$
Reduction
$NADP^+$

Cys—SH
ACP—S—C(=O)—CH_2—CH_2—CH_3
Acyl-ACP (Butyryl-ACP)

Transfer of carbon chain to cysteine

Cys—S—C(=O)—CH_2—CH_2—CH_3
ACP—SH
Acyl-S-enzyme (Butyryl-S-enzyme)

Repetition
Reaction repeated from step 2 to 6 for six times

Cys—SH
ACP—S—C(=O)—$(CH_2)_{13}$—CH_2—CH_3
Acyl-ACP (Palmitoyl-ACP)

Palmitoyl thioesterase
H_2O
Hydrolysis

Cys—SH
ACP—SH
***Fatty acid synthase (FAS)* complex**

+ CH_3—CH_2—$(CH_2)_{13}$—COOH
Palmitic acid

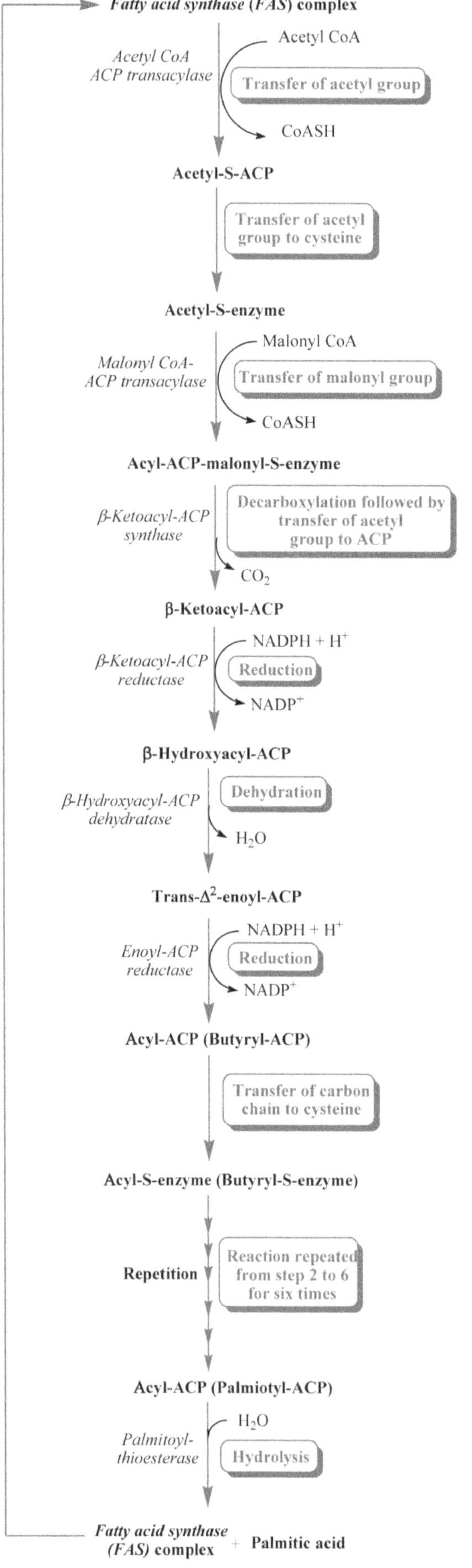
Fatty acid synthase (FAS) complex
Acetyl CoA
ACP transacylase
Acetyl CoA
Transfer of acetyl group
CoASH
Acetyl-S-ACP
Transfer of acetyl group to cysteine
Acetyl-S-enzyme
Malonyl CoA-ACP transacylase
Malonyl CoA
Transfer of malonyl group
CoASH
Acyl-ACP-malonyl-S-enzyme
β-Ketoacyl-ACP synthase
Decarboxylation followed by transfer of acetyl group to ACP
CO_2
β-Ketoacyl-ACP
β-Ketoacyl-ACP reductase
NADPH + H^+
Reduction
$NADP^+$
β-Hydroxyacyl-ACP
β-Hydroxyacyl-ACP dehydratase
Dehydration
H_2O
Trans-Δ^2-enoyl-ACP
Enoyl-ACP reductase
NADPH + H^+
Reduction
$NADP^+$
Acyl-ACP (Butyryl-ACP)
Transfer of carbon chain to cysteine
Acyl-S-enzyme (Butyryl-S-enzyme)
Repetition
Reaction repeated from step 2 to 6 for six times
Acyl-ACP (Palmiotyl-ACP)
Palmitoyl-thioesterase
H_2O
Hydrolysis
Fatty acid synthase (FAS) complex + Palmitic acid

β-ketoacyl-ACP synthase (The product formed is "β-ketoacyl-ACP" and the type of reaction is "synthesis").

4. The keto group of β-ketoacyl-ACP is reduced to secondary alcohol to produce β-hydroxyacyl-ACP in presence of *β-ketoacyl-ACP reductase* (The substrate is "β-ketoacyl-ACP" and the type of reaction is "reduction"). NADPH supplies the reducing equivalents for this reaction.

5. The produced β-hydroxyacyl-ACP undergoes dehydration in presence of *β-hydroxyacyl-ACP dehydratase* (The substrate is "β-hydroxyacyl-ACP" and the type of reaction is "dehydration") and produced α,β-unsaturated acyl-ACP or Δ^2-trans enoyl acyl-ACP. Hydrogen is removed from α-carbon and the hydroxyl group is removed from β-carbon atom of β-hydroxy acyl-ACP to loss water molecule. Hence, a double bond is formed between α- and β-carbon.

6. In the sixth step, Δ^2-trans enoyl acyl-ACP undergoes NADPH dependent reduction to produce acyl-ACP (butyryl-ACP) and the reaction is catalyzed by *enoylacyl-ACP reductase* (The substrate is "Δ^2-trans enoylacyl-ACP" and the type of reaction is "reduction").

   Now, the carbon chain attached to ACP of acyl-ACP (butyryl-ACP) is transferred to cysteine residue and the reactions of step 2 to step 6 are repeated for six more times. Each time the length of the fatty acid chain is increased to two carbon units which are obtained from malonyl CoA. Hence, at the end of the seventh cycle palmitate (a 16 carbon fully saturated fatty acid) bound ACP is produced, and in this step fatty acid synthesis is completed.

7. Finally, palmitate is separated from the *FAS* complex by simple hydrolysis reaction and the *FAS* complex is used again for the synthesis of fatty acids. This final step is catalyzed by *palmitoyl thioesterase* (The product formed is "palmitate", the substrate is "thioester" i.e., palmitoyl-ACP and the type of reaction is "hydrolysis").

Two carbon of palmitate is obtained from acetyl CoA directly and the remaining 14 carbon is also obtained from acetyl CoA only but indirectly through malonyl CoA. Hence, the overall reactions of palmitate synthesis can be summarized as follows,

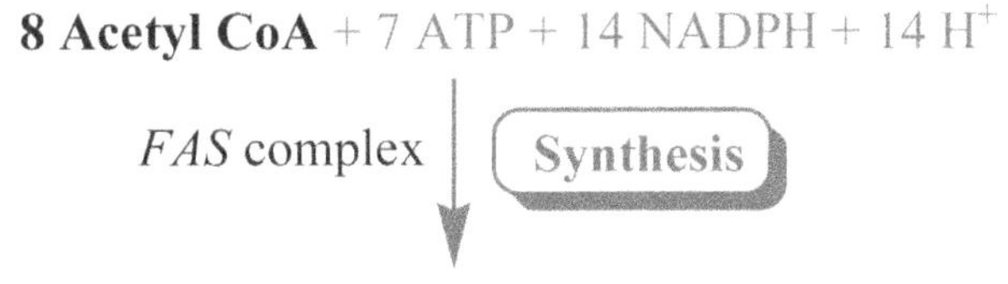

Cholesterol

Cholesterol is commonly known as animal sterol because it is found exclusively in animals and is chemically steroidal alcohol. Cholesterol contains both hydrophilic and hydrophobic regions in the structure; hence it is amphipathic in nature. In adults, 2 g of cholesterol is present per kg of body weight i.e., the total cholesterol present in 70 kg adult is 140 g (2 × 70). The chemical structure of cholesterol with the numbering of carbon atom is given below.

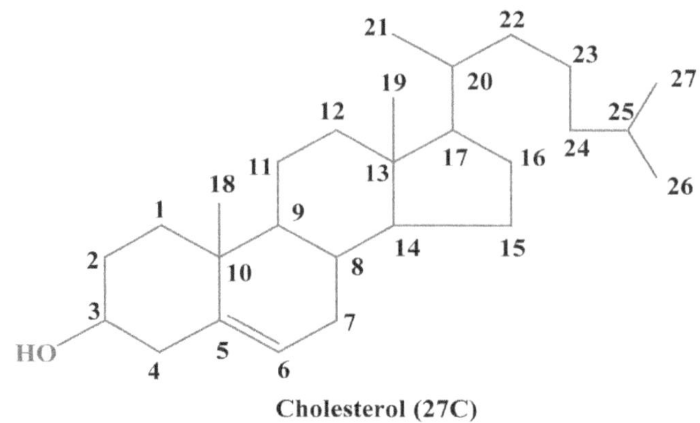

Cholesterol (27C)

Biological Significance of Cholesterol

Cholesterol performs many important biological functions. Hence, it is essential for life. Following are some important biological significance of cholesterol.

1. Cholesterol is the structural component of cell membrane.
2. All other steroidal compounds in the body are biosynthesized from cholesterol only.
3. Steroidal hormones are biosynthesized from cholesterol.
4. Cholesterol acts as a precursor for the synthesis of vitamin-D.
5. In addition, from cholesterol bile acids also biosynthesized in the body.
6. In general, lipids are biosynthesized in the form of lipoprotein only. Cholesterol is the essential component in the lipoproteins.
7. To liver, fatty acids are transported for oxidation as cholesteryl esters.

Degradation of Cholesterol

In humans, the ring structure (steroidal nucleus) of cholesterol cannot be metabolized. Unlike other compounds, cholesterol is not metabolized into carbondioxide and water. Instead of that cholesterol (about 50 %) is

1. Converted to bile acids (excreted in feces)
2. Act as a precursor for the synthesis of steroid hormones
3. Serves as a precursor for the synthesis of vitamin-D, coprostanol, and cholestanol.

Cholesterol, coprostanol, and cholestanol are called fecal sterol because these are steroidal alcohol excreted in feces also.

Conversion of Cholestrol into Bile Acids

Bile acids are 24 carbon-containing steroidal compounds with two to three hydroxyl (-OH) group in the steroidal ring and a side chain ending in the carboxyl (-COOH) group. Like cholesterol, bile acids are also amphipathic in nature because it contains both hydrophilic and hydrophobic regions in the structure. In the intestine, bile acids are actively participate in the digestion and absorption of lipids as emulsifying agents. Bile acids are biosynthesized in the liver by a series of a biochemical reaction. The following are some important steps involved in the biosynthesis of bile acids.

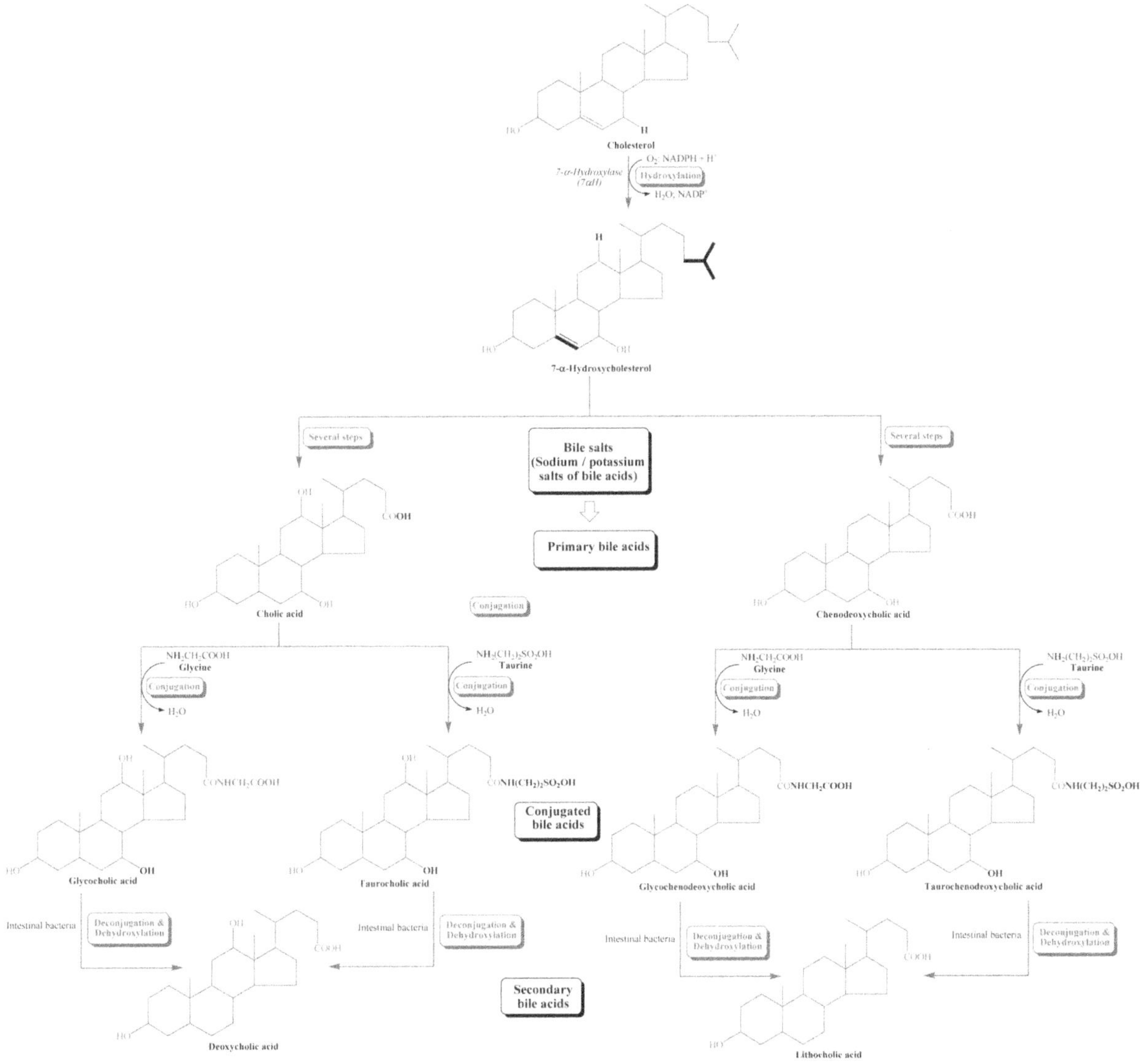

Cholesterol
7-α-Hydroxylase (7αH)
O_2; NADPH + H^+
Hydroxylation
H_2O; $NADP^+$
7-α-Hydroxycholesterol
Several steps
Bile salts (Sodium / potassium salts of bile acids)
Primary bile acids
Cholic acid
Conjugation
Chenodeoxycholic acid
NH_2CH_2COOH Glycine
$NH_2(CH_2)_2SO_2OH$ Taurine
H_2O
Conjugated bile acids
Glycocholic acid
Taurocholic acid
Glycochenodeoxycholic acid
Taurochenodeoxycholic acid
Intestinal bacteria
Deconjugation & Dehydroxylation
Secondary bile acids
Deoxycholic acid
Lithocholic acid

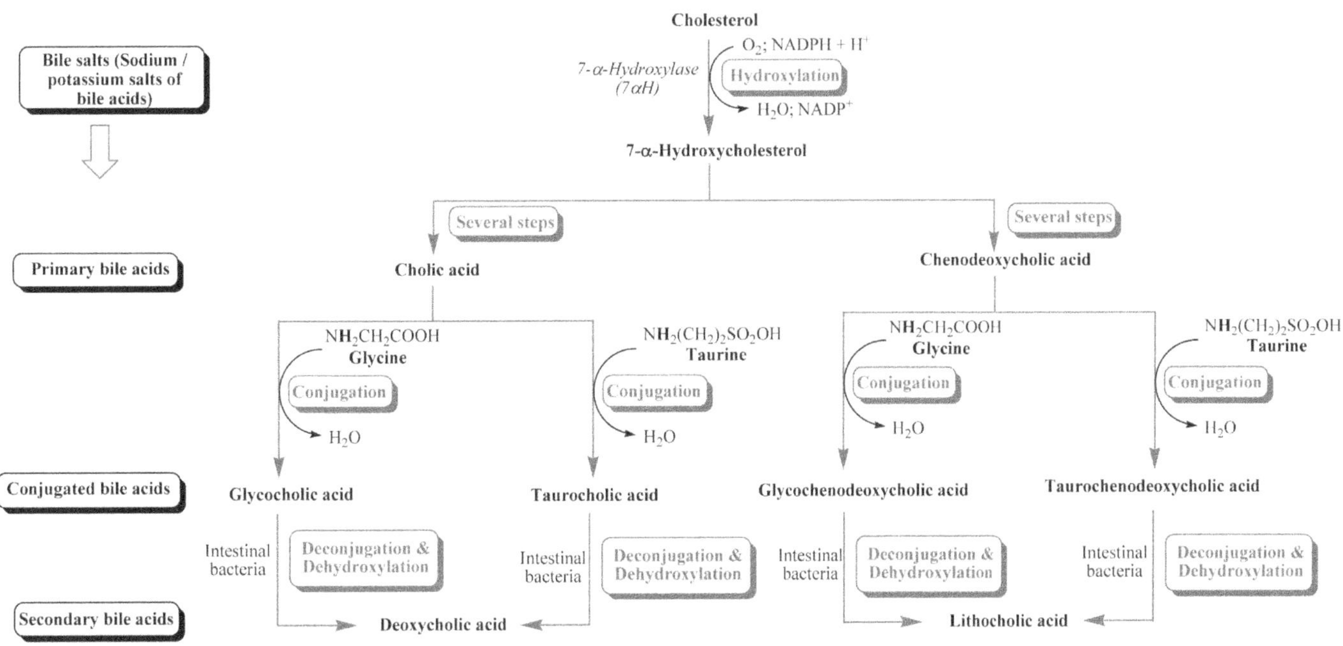

1. Initially, cholesterol undergoes hydroxylation at C-7 position to produce 7-α-hydroxy cholesterol in the presence of *7-α-hydroxylase* (7αH) (Type of reaction is "hydroxylation" and position of reaction is "7-α") with the involvement of NADPH and molecular oxygen. The NADPH is reduced to $NADP^+$ and one oxygen atom of molecular oxygen is removed as a water molecule and the other one is incorporated in C-7 position of cholesterol. **This step is a rate limiting step of bile acid production and the rate-limiting enzyme *7-α-hydroxylase* (7αH) is inhibited by bile acids.**
2. Later, through several biochemical reactions, primary bile acids such as cholic acid and chenodeoxycholic acid are synthesized from 7-α-hydroxy cholesterol. In bile, cholic acid is found in higher concentrations than chenodeoxycholic acid.
3. Conjugated bile acids such as glycocholic acid and taurocholic acid are synthesized when cholic acid is conjugated with amino acid glycine and taurine, respectively. Similarly, glycochenodeoxycholic acid and taurochenodeoxycholic acid are synthesized when chenodeoxycholic acid is conjugated with amino acid glycine and taurine, respectively. The conjugated bile acids are used as surfactants in the body. The sodium and potassium salts of conjugated bile acids are known as bile salts that are present in the bile.
4. In the intestine, secondary bile acids such as deoxycholic acid and lithocholic acid are produced by intestinal bacteria when a portion of conjugated bile acids undergoes deconjugation and dehydroxylation.

Conversion of Cholesterol into Steroid Hormones

Cholesterol serves as a precursor for the synthesis of steroid hormones. The following are five classes of steroid hormones that are synthesized from cholesterol in the body.

1. Glucocorticoids (**Example:** Cortisol)
2. Mineralocorticoids (**Example:** Aldosterone)
3. Progestins (**Example:** Progesterone)
4. Androgens (**Example:** Testosterone)
5. Estrogens (**Example:** Estradiol)

At first, from 27 carbons containing cholesterol, 21 carbons containing pregnenolone are synthesized. Pregnenolone is the common precursor for the synthesis of all steroid hormones. From pregnenolone, 21 carbons containing progesterone (progestin) are produced. From this progesterone-only cortisol, aldosterone, and estradiol are biosynthesized. Out of these three, cortisol and aldosterone contain 21 carbons; whereas estradiol contains only 18 carbons. For the convenience, the synthesis of hormones from cholesterol is divided into two pathways as follows, 1) Synthesis of adrenocorticoids, 2) Synthesis of steroid sex hormones.

1. **Synthesis of adrenocorticosteroids:**

   Adrenocorticosteroids or adrenocorticoids are produced by the adrenal cortex in adrenal glands. Based on their biological actions, adrenocorticoids are broadly classified into three different classes as follows.

   1. **Glucocorticoids:** Theses are 21 carbon steroids produced by zona fasciculate. They are opposite in action to insulin and affects the metabolism of glucose, amino acid, and fat. Cortisol or hydrocortisone is the most important glucocorticoid in humans. In rats, predominantly corticosterone is present.
   2. **Mineralocorticoids:** Theses are 21 carbon steroids produced by zona glomerulosa. It regulates electrolyte and water balance. The most important mineralocorticoid is aldosterone.
   3. **Androgens and estrogens:** Small quantities of androgens (19 carbon steroids) and estrogens (18 carbon steroids) are produced from the innermost adrenal cortex zona reticularis. Mostly gonads produce these hormones and it affects sexual development and functions. In the adrenal cortex, dehydroepiandrosterone is synthesized which is a precursor for the synthesis of androgens.

The various enzymes necessary for the synthesis of adrenocorticosteroids are present in mitochondria or endoplasmic reticulum and the reaction involved are explained below.

1. Initially, cholesterol lost 6 carbon fragments and produced pregnenolone in the presence *cytochrome P_{450} side chain cleavage* enzyme. Adrenocorticotropic hormone (ACTH) promotes this reaction.
2. Later, pregnenolone undergoes hydroxylation at C-17 position to produce 17-α-hydroxy pregnenolone in presence of *17-α-hydroxylase* (Type of reaction is "hydroxylation" and position of hydroxylation is "C-17α").
3. This formed 17-α-hydroxy pregnenolone undergoes two different reactions. In one way, it losses the side chain attached at C-17 by *lyase* enzyme followed by oxidation of alcohol group present in C-17 to ketone group results in the formation of dehydroepiandrosterone. In other way, it undergoes dehydrogenation at C-3 (secondary alcohol converted to ketone) in presence of *dehydrogenase* followed by isomerization (Position of double bond shifted from C-5 to C-4) in presence of *isomerase* produced 17-α-hydroxy progesterone.
4. In the next step, 17-α-hydroxy progesterone also reacts in two different ways. In one way it undergoes hydroxylation at C-21 position to produce 11-deoxycortisol in presence of *C_{21} hydroxylase* (Type of reaction is "hydroxylation" and position of hydroxylation is "C-21").
5. The formed 11-deoxycortisol undergoes hydroxylation at C-11β position to produce cortisol in presence of *C_{11}-β-hydroxylase* (Type of reaction is "hydroxylation" and position of hydroxylation is "C-11β").

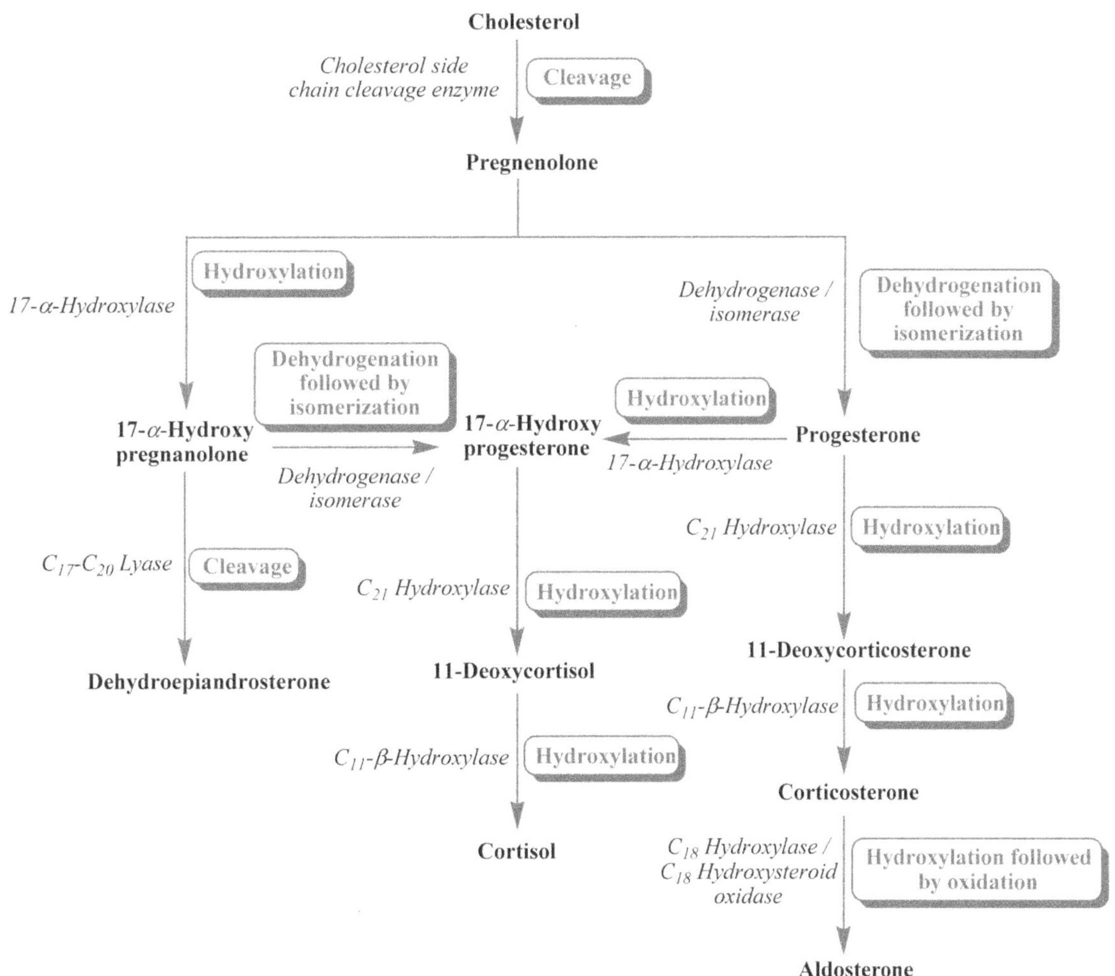

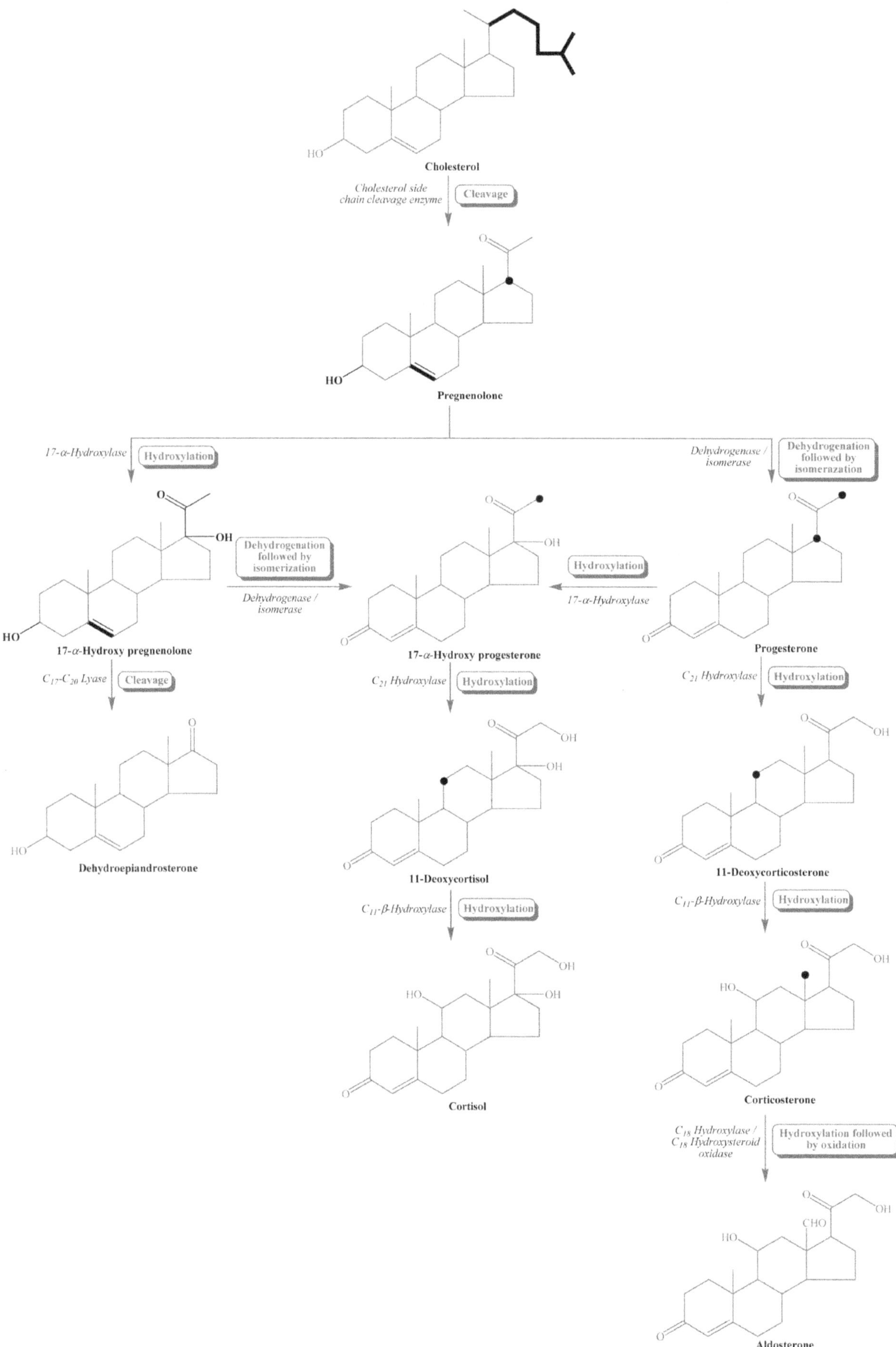
HO
Cholesterol
Cholesterol side chain cleavage enzyme
Cleavage
O
HO
Pregnenolone
17-α-Hydroxylase
Hydroxylation
Dehydrogenase / isomerase
Dehydrogenation followed by isomerazation
O
OH
HO
17-α-Hydroxy pregnenolone
Dehydrogenation followed by isomerization
Dehydrogenase / isomerase
O
OH
O
17-α-Hydroxy progesterone
Hydroxylation
17-α-Hydroxylase
O
O
Progesterone
C_{17}-C_{20} Lyase
Cleavage
C_{21} Hydroxylase
Hydroxylation
C_{21} Hydroxylase
Hydroxylation
O
HO
Dehydroepiandrosterone
O
OH
OH
O
11-Deoxycortisol
O
OH
O
11-Deoxycorticosterone
C_{11}-β-Hydroxylase
Hydroxylation
C_{11}-β-Hydroxylase
Hydroxylation
O
OH
HO
OH
O
Cortisol
O
OH
HO
O
Corticosterone
C_{18} Hydroxylase / C_{18} Hydroxysteroid oxidase
Hydroxylation followed by oxidation
O
OH
CHO
HO
O
Aldosterone

6. The pregnenolone formed in the first step may undergo another reaction also. In this reaction pregnenolone undergoes dehydrogenation at C-3 (secondary alcohol converted to ketone) in presence of *dehydrogenase* followed by isomerization (Position of double bond shifted from C-5 to C-4) in presence of *isomerase* produced progesterone.
7. In the succeeding reactions, progesterone reacts in two different ways. In one way, it is hydroxylated at C-17 position by *17-α-hydroxylase* (Type of reaction is "hydroxylation" and position of hydroxylation is "C-17α") results in the formation of 17-α-hydroxy progesterone. In the second type of reaction, progesterone is hydroxylated at C-21 position by *C_{21} hydroxylase* (Type of reaction is "hydroxylation", and position of hydroxylation is "C-21") results in the formation of 11-deoxycorticosterone.
8. The formed 11-deoxycorticosterone further undergoes hydroxylation at C-11β position to produce corticosterone in presence of *C_{11}-β-hydroxylase* (Type of reaction is "hydroxylation" and position of hydroxylation is "C-11β").
9. Finally, aldosterone is synthesized from corticosterone by hydroxylation at C-18 position in presence of *C_{18} hydroxylase* (Type of reaction is "hydroxylation" and position of hydroxylation is "C-18") followed by oxidation of that C-18 primary alcohol to aldehyde in presence of *C_{18} hydroxysteroid oxidase* (Substrate is "C_{18} hydroxy steroid" and the type of reaction is "oxidation").

2. Synthesis of steroid sex hormones:

The steroid sex hormones are responsible for growth, development, maintenance, and regulation of the reproductive system. Three different sex hormones are present. They are,

1. **Androgens:** These are male sex hormones that are C-19 steroids and are produced mainly by Leydig cells of the testes. In both sexes, adrenal glands produce a minor quantity of androgens. In addition, small amounts are produced by ovaries also.
2. **Estrogens:** These are female sex hormones which are C-18 steroids and are synthesized by follicles and corpus luteum of the ovary. The ring A of the steroid nucleus is phenolic in nature and is devoid of the C-19 methyl group. These hormones are responsible for maintenance of the menstrual cycle and reproductive process in women.
3. **Progesterone:** These are C-21 steroids produced during the luteal phase of menstrual cycle and also during pregnancy. It is synthesized and secreted by corpus luteum and placenta. Luteinizing hormone controls the production of progesterone.

   The various reactions involved in the synthesis of sex hormones are explained below.

   1. 17-α-Hydroxy progesterone and dehydroepiandrosterone are produced in the same way as mentioned in the synthesis of adrenocorticoids.
   2. Later, from both 17-α-hydroxy progesterone and dehydroepiandrosterone, androstenedione is produced. 17-α-Hydroxy progesterone losses the side chain attached at C-17 by C_{17} to C_{20} lyase enzyme followed by oxidation of alcohol group present in C-17 to ketone group results in formation of androstenedione. In addition, dehydroepiandrosterone undergoes dehydrogenation at C-3 (secondary alcohol converted to ketone) in presence of *dehydrogenase* followed by isomerization (Position of double bond shifted from C-5 to C-4) in presence of isomerase produced androstenedione.
   3. Androstenedione undergoes two different reactions. In one reaction, it undergoes aromatization, and the ring A of steroid nucleus is aromatized to produce estrone by *aromatase* enzyme (The type of reaction is "aromatization"). In another reaction, androstenedione undergoes reduction at C-17 position in presence of *reductase* enzyme (The type of reaction is "reduction") and produced testosterone. During this reaction, the keto group present at C-17 is reduced to a secondary alcohol.
   4. The estrone formed in the previous step undergoes hydroxylation at C-16α position to produce estriol in presence of 16-α-hydroxylase (The type of reaction is "hydroxylation" and position of hydroxylation is "C-16α").

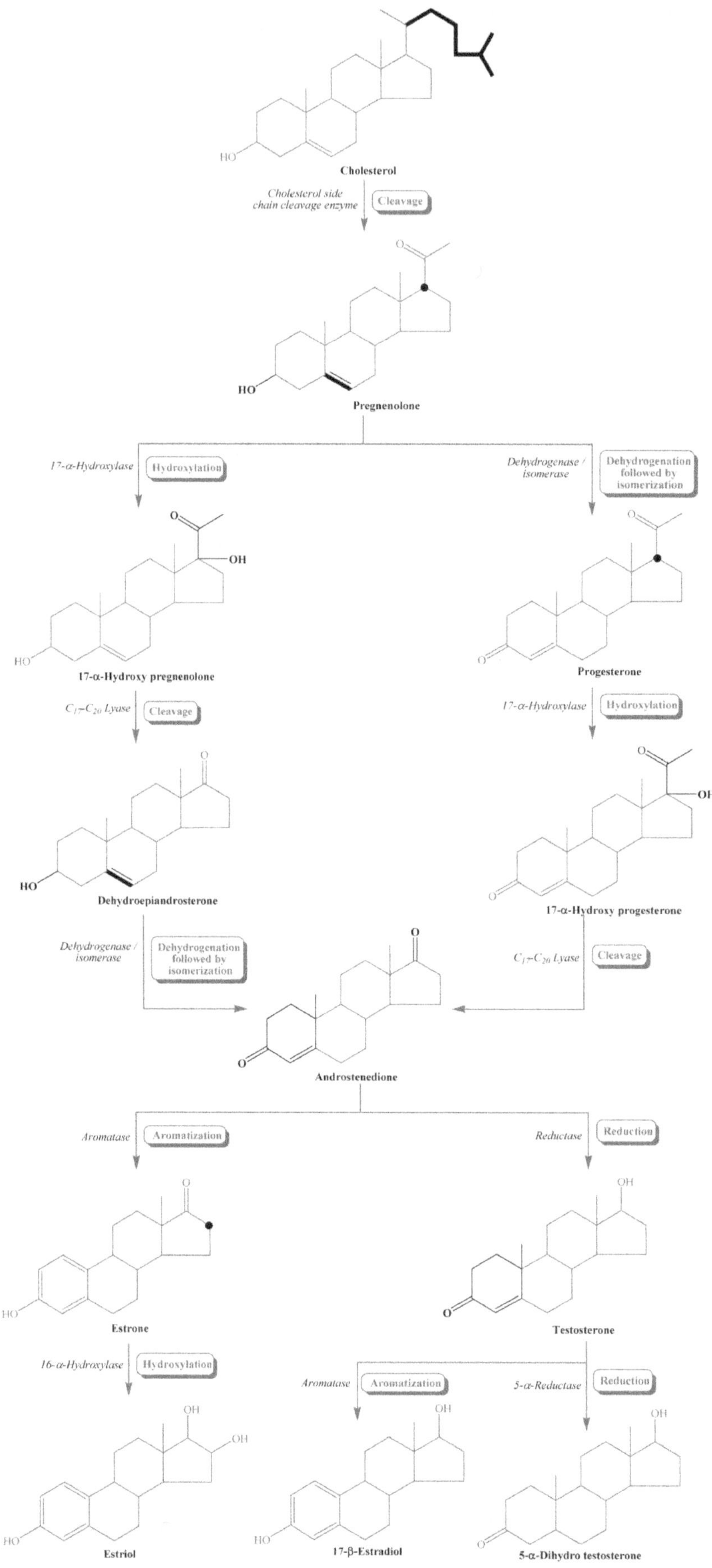
Cholesterol
Cholesterol side chain cleavage enzyme
Cleavage
Pregnenolone
17-α-Hydroxylase
Hydroxylation
Dehydrogenase / isomerase
Dehydrogenation followed by isomerization
17-α-Hydroxy pregnenolone
Progesterone
C_{17}-C_{20} Lyase
Cleavage
17-α-Hydroxylase
Hydroxylation
Dehydroepiandrosterone
17-α-Hydroxy progesterone
Dehydrogenase / isomerase
Dehydrogenation followed by isomerization
C_{17}-C_{20} Lyase
Cleavage
Androstenedione
Aromatase
Aromatization
Reductase
Reduction
Estrone
Testosterone
16-α-Hydroxylase
Hydroxylation
Aromatase
Aromatization
5-α-Reductase
Reduction
Estriol
17-β-Estradiol
5-α-Dihydro testosterone

5. Testosterone produced also undergoes two different reactions. At first, testosterone undergoes aromatization and the ring A of steroid nucleus is aromatized to produce 17-β-estradiol by *aromatase* enzyme (The type of reaction is "aromatization"). In another reaction, it undergoes reduction between C-4 and C-5 position in presence of *5-α-reductase* enzyme (The type of reaction is "reduction") and produced 5-α-dihydrotestosterone. During this reaction, double bond present between C-4 and C-5 is reduced.

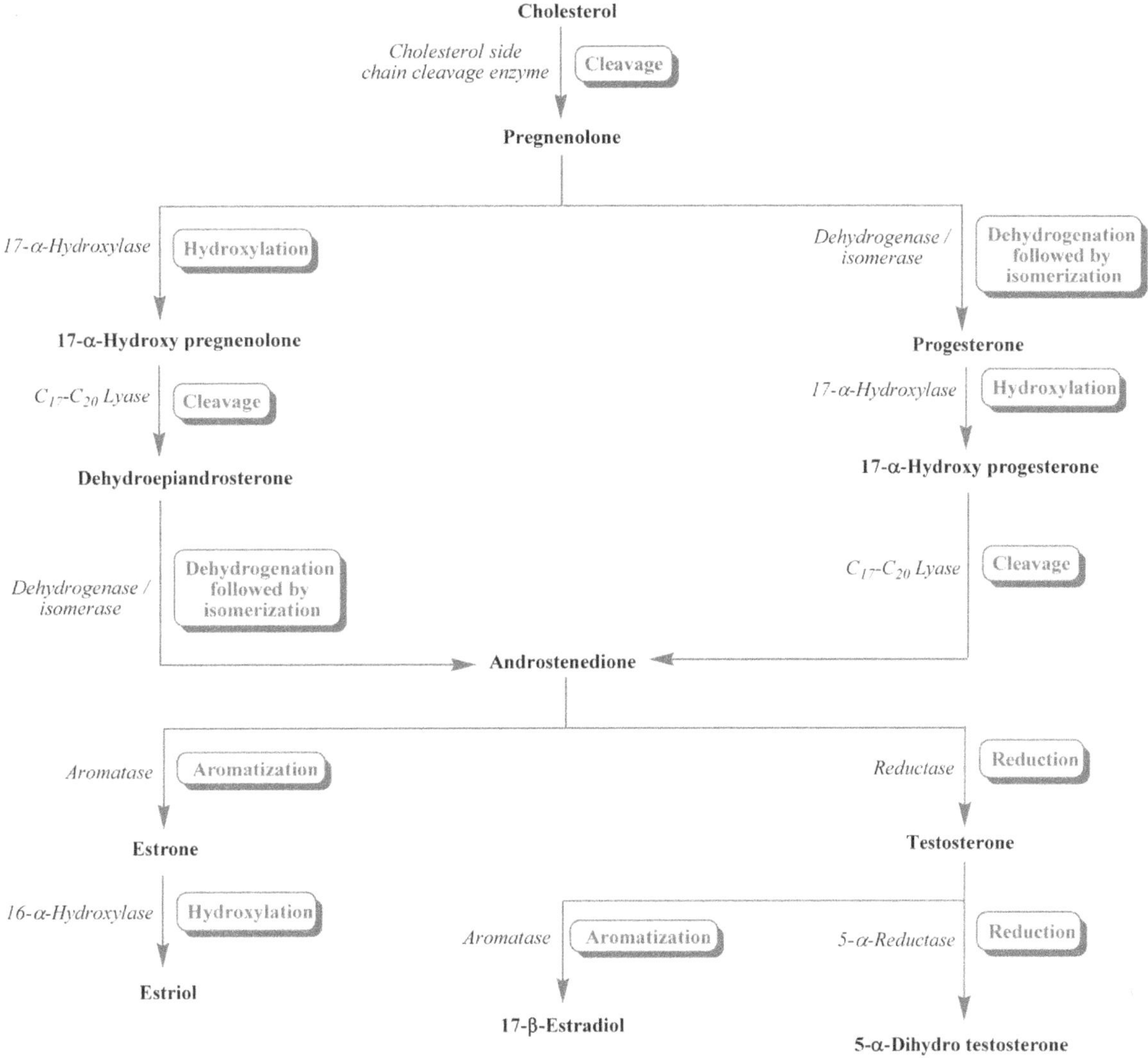

Conversion of Cholestrol into Vitamin-D

Vitamin D is synthesized in the body from cholesterol using ultraviolet (UV) rays present in sunlight. 7-Dehydrocholesterol is an intermediate compound present in cholesterol biosynthesis. The following are the sequence of reactions involved in the synthesis of active form of vitamin D.

1. When 7-dehydrocholesterol is exposed to UV rays present in sunlight converted to cholecalciferol or vitamin-D_3. The dietary source also contains vitamin-D as cholecalciferol only but it is inactive form. The active form of vitamin-D is biosynthesized from cholecalciferol.
2. In the next step, vitamin-D_3 undergoes hydroxylation at C-25 in the liver in presence of *calciol-25-hydroxylase* and produced 25-hydroxycholecalciferol or calcidiol.

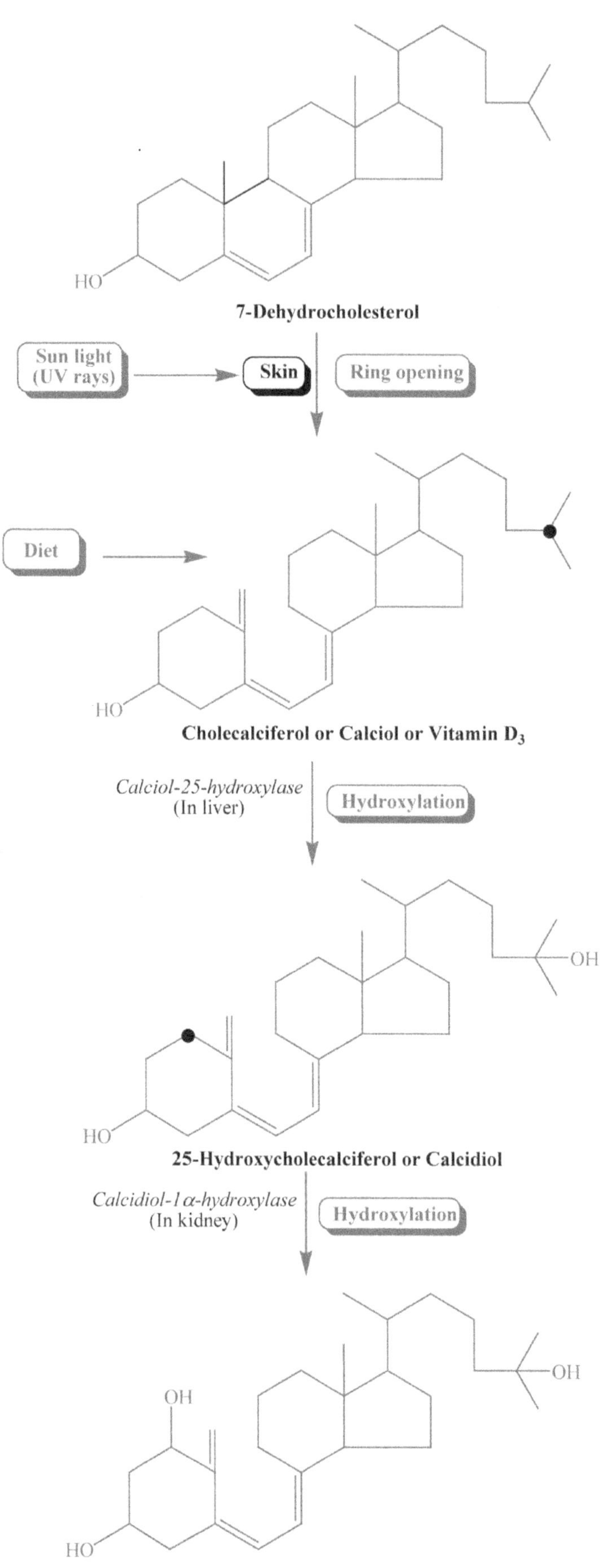

HO

7-Dehydrocholesterol

Sun light (UV rays) → Skin | Ring opening

Diet →

HO

Cholecalciferol or Calciol or Vitamin D_3

Calciol-25-hydroxylase (In liver) | Hydroxylation

OH

HO

25-Hydroxycholecalciferol or Calcidiol

Calcidiol-1α-hydroxylase (In kidney) | Hydroxylation

OH

OH

HO

1,25-Dihydroxycholecalciferol or Calcitriol or 1,25-DHCC (Active form of vitamin D)

3. This formed calcidiol in kidney further undergoes hydroxylation at C-1 in presence of *calcidiol-1α-hydroxylase* produced the active form of vitamin-D i.e., 1,25-dihydroxycholecalciferol or calcitriol or 1,25-DHCC.

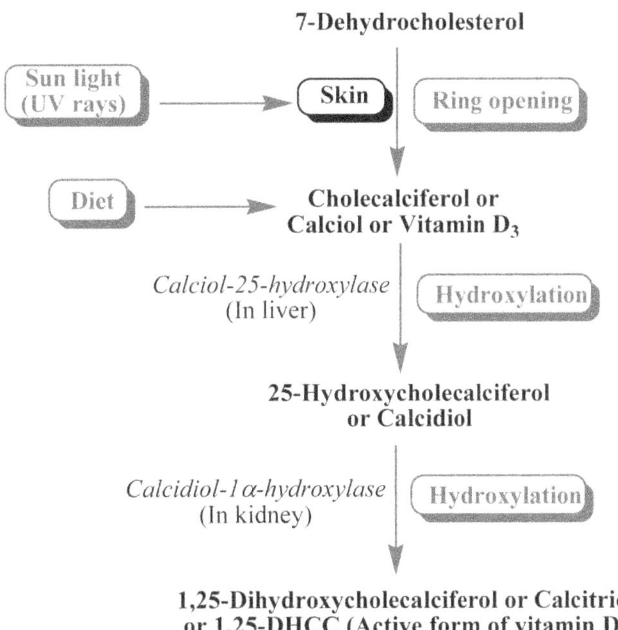

Metabolic Disorders of Lipid Metabolism

The following are the major metabolic disorders of lipid metabolism. They are,

1. Hypercholesterolemia
2. Atherosclerosis
3. Fatty liver
4. Obesity

1. Hypercholesterolemia:

Hypercholesterolemia is defined as an increased concentration of cholesterol in plasma (greater than 200 mg/dl). It is commonly observed in many disorders such as,

(a) **Diabetes mellitus:** In diabetes mellitus, increased glucose increases the concentration of acetyl CoA leads to increased cholesterol synthesis.

(b) **Hypothyroidism (Myxedema):** In hypothyroidism, cholesterol level is increased due to decreased HDL receptors on hepatocytes.

(c) **Obstructive jaundice:** In obstructive jaundice, cholesterol level is increased due to obstruction in cholesterol excretion through bile.

(d) **Nephrotic syndrome:** In nephrotic syndrome, cholesterol level is increased due to increased lipoprotein concentration in plasma. In nephrotic syndrome, plasma globulin concentration is increased.

In general, hypercholesterolemia is associated with atherosclerosis and coronary heart disease (CHD). With respect to CHD, LDL cholesterol is positively correlated and HDL cholesterol is negatively correlated. Cholesterol is a natural metabolite performing a wide variety of functions like membrane structure, a precursor for steroid hormones, bile acid, vitamin D, etc. If cholesterol is present in high concentrations as LDL is considered bad because LDL is involved in atherosclerosis. Hence, LDL or low-density lipoprotein may regard as lethally dangerous lipoprotein or simply bad cholesterol. The most dangerous fraction of LDL is small dense low-density lipoprotein (sdLDL) because it is associated with CHD. On the other hand, HDL cholesterol is considered as good because it counteracts atherogenesis. Hence, HDL or high-density lipoprotein may regard as highly desirable lipoprotein or simply good cholesterol.

In the development of CHD, individual lifestyle and habits influence due to its effect on serum cholesterol. Serum cholesterol level is increased by the parameters such as blood pressure, smoking, drinking of soft water against hard water, emotional stress, drinking of coffee, lack of exercise, obesity particularly abdomen, etc.

The plasma cholesterol levels can be lowered by following the below guidelines.

(a) **Consumption of polyunsaturated fatty acids (PUFA):** By *LCAT (Lecithin cholesterol acyltransferase)* mechanism PUFA is useful for the transport of cholesterol and its excretion from the body. PUFA is rich in cottonseed oil, soya bean oil, sunflower oil, corn oil, fish oil, etc. and it is poor in ghee and coconut oil.

(b) **Dietary cholesterol:** The influence of dietary cholesterol on plasma cholesterol is minimal. Even though it is advised to avoid cholesterol-rich foods and the advisable dietary cholesterol level is < 300 mg/day, drugs like ezetimide inhibit the absorption of cholesterol in the intestine.

(c) **Plant sterol:** Some plant sterol and their esters reduce plasma cholesterol by inhibiting cholesterol absorption in the intestine.

(d) **Dietary fiber:** Similar to plant sterol, dietary fibers also reduce plasma cholesterol by inhibiting cholesterol absorption from the intestine.

(e) **Avoiding a high carbohydrate diet:** It is better to avoid diets rich in carbohydrates to control hypercholesterolemia.

(f) **Impact of life styles:** Adequate changes in lifestyle may decrease plasma cholesterol because increased serum cholesterol level is seen in people with blood pressure, smoking, drinking of soft water against hard water, emotional stress, drinking of coffee, lack of exercise, obesity particularly abdomen, etc.

(g) **Moderate alcohol consumption:** Besides low alcohol content, red wine is beneficial due to its antioxidant properties. The ill-effects of chronic alcoholism mask the beneficial effect of consuming moderate alcohol.

(h) **Use of drugs:** Statins decrease plasma cholesterol by inhibiting the synthesis of cholesterol through *HMG CoA reductase* (*HMGCAR*) inhibition. Drugs like cholestyramine and colestipol bind with bile acids and decrease their intestinal absorption. Hence, more cholesterol is converted to bile acids and excreted through feces. The activity of lipoprotein *lipase* is increased and plasma cholesterol and triacylglycerol level are decreased by clofibrate.

2. **Atherosclerosis:**

In Greek, "athere" means "mush" and atherosclerosis is a complex cardiac disorder defined as hardening or thickening of inner arterial walls due to accumulation of lipids (particularly cholesterol in a free and esterified form), collagen, fibrous tissues, proteoglycans, calcium deposits, etc. Atherosclerosis is a progressive disorder, hence, it may lead to narrowing of blocks and at one stage it completely blocks the arteries. Death of affected tissue due to the stoppage of blood flow is termed as infarction. If the infarction is taking place in coronary arteries (supplying blood to the heart) it is known as myocardial infarction and it is the most common one.

The risk of CHD and the development of atherosclerosis are directly correlated with plasma LDL and cholesterol. Conversely, HDL is inversely correlated with CHD. Diseases like diabetes mellitus, hyperlipoproteinemia, hypothyroidism, nephrotic syndrome, etc., are generally associated with atherosclerosis. The various probable causes of atherosclerosis are obesity, high consumption of saturated fat, excessive smoking, lack of physical exercise, hypertension, stress, etc.

In general, increased plasma HDL i.e., good cholesterol is correlated with a low incidence of cardiovascular disorders. Compared to men, women are less prone to heart disease because they have higher HDL. Estrogen present in women is responsible for higher HDL. The risk of CHD is reduced by increasing the concentration of HDL in the following ways like doing strenuous physical exercise, consuming moderate alcohol, consumption of PUFA, reducing body weight, etc.

LDL and lipoprotein-a (Lp-a) are identical in structure. Additional apoprotein-a (Apo-a) is present in lipoprotein-a (Lp-a) compared to LDL. Fibrinolysis is inhibited by lipoprotein-a (Lp-a). CHD risk is increased when the plasma lipoprotein-a (Lp-a) is elevated to more than 30 mg/dl. It is assumed that interfering with the plasminogen activation reduces the breakdown of blood clots when lipoprotein-a (Lp-a) is elevated. This leads to intravascular thrombosis and an increased risk of heart attacks. Compared to western people, Indians have higher levels of lipoprotein-a (Lp-a).

In general, the oxidation of LDL is decreased by antioxidants. Some evidences suggest that taking antioxidants such as vitamin-C, vitamin-E or β-carotene decreases the risk of atherosclerosis and CHD.

3. **Fatty liver:**

About 5 % of lipid (mostly phospholipid) is present in the liver normally. Unlike adipose tissue, the liver is not a storage organ for fat. But in some conditions lipids particularly triglycerides are excessively accumulated in the liver leading to the fatty liver [deposition of lipids in liver]. Generally, lipids are present in the form of droplets in Kupffer cells. But in fatty liver droplets of triacylglycerols are present throughout the entire cytoplasm of the hepatic cell. Hence, fatty liver may lead to impairment in metabolic functions of the liver. Fatty liver is usually associated with fibrotic changes and cirrhosis. The two major causes of fatty liver are 1) Increased synthesis of triacylglycerols, 2) Impairment in lipoprotein synthesis.

Increased synthesis of triacylglycerols: Mobilization of free fatty acids from adipose tissue and their influx into the liver is much higher than their utilization. Hence, triacylglycerides are overproduced and accumulated in the liver. Free fatty acid mobilizations are increased in clinical conditions such as diabetes mellitus, starvation, alcoholism, and a high-fat diet which often causes fatty liver. Fat synthesis and its deposition are promoted by inhibiting fatty acid oxidation by alcohol.

Impairment in lipoprotein synthesis: Phospholipids and apoprotein-B are required for the production of VLDL in the liver. The reasons for fatty liver caused by impaired lipoprotein synthesis are,

(a) A defect in phospholipid synthesis.

(b) A block in apoprotein formation.

(c) A failure in the formation or secretion of lipoprotein.

Usually, a defect in phospholipid synthesis is associated with dietary deficiency of lipotropic factors such as choline, betaine, inositol, etc. Production of phospholipid is decreased due to essential fatty acids deficiency. In addition, phospholipid synthesis is impaired by competition of excessive cholesterol consumption with essential fatty acids.

Fatty liver can also be caused by some chemicals such as puromycin, chloroform, lead, phosphorous, etc. These chemicals inhibit the synthesis of protein due to the blockade in the synthesis of apoprotein-B required for VLDL production. ATP is required for the synthesis and secretion of lipoprotein. Sometimes, in pyridoxine and pantothenic acid deficiency lipoprotein formation is impaired due to decreased availability of ATP. Ethionine reduces the availability of ATP, thereby, it takes part in the development of the fatty liver. Available adenosine (as adenosylethionine) is trapped when ethionine competes with methionine leads to decreased ATP levels. The deficiency of vitamin-E is associated with fatty liver. In such a condition, selenium acts as a protective agent. Hormones like adrenocorticotropic hormone (ACTH), insulin, thyroid hormones, adrenocorticoids promote the deposition of fat in the liver.

4. **Obesity:**

Due to excessive fat deposition, an abnormal increase in body weight is known as obesity. When the weight of adipose tissue fat exceeds 20 % and 25 % of total body weight then the men and women are considered obese, respectively. Basically, obesity is a disorder of excess calorie intake or simply overeating. 1 g fat will deposit in the body and increases body weight for every 7 calories of excess intake. Obesity contributors are overeating coupled with a lack of physical exercise. Sometimes, a virus infection may be the reason for obesity. 15 % of people weighing more than 120 kg had antibodies to *adenovirus-36* in their blood. It implies that the virus infection by an unknown mechanism contributes to obesity. Surprisingly, serum cholesterol and other lipid parameters are normal in *adenovirus-36* infected peoples.

Body mass index (BMI): Body mass index (BMI) is generally used to represent clinical obesity. The following formula is used to estimate body mass index (BMI).

$$BMI\left(\frac{kg}{m^2}\right) = \frac{\text{Weight (in kg)}}{\text{Height (in m}^2\text{)}}$$

The healthy reference range for BMI is usually between 18.5 and 24.8 kg/m^2. Based on the body mass index (BMI), obesity is broadly classified into three different classes as follows.

(a) **Overweight or Grade – I obesity:** In this class, BMI is between 25 to 30 kg/m^2.

(b) **Clinical obesity or Grade – II obesity:** In this class, BMI is > 30 kg/m^2.

(c) **Morbid obesity or Grade – III obesity:** In this class, BMI is > 40 kg/m^2.

Generally, obesity is associated with many health issues like CHD, type – II diabetes mellitus, stroke, hypertension, arthritis, and gall bladder disease. The ratio between waist and hip sizes is more efficient than BMI for representing obesity. Hence, recently waist to hip ratio is used to represent the risk of heart disease. For men, the normal waist to hip ratio is < 0.9 and for women, it is < 0.85. If the waist to hip ratio is less then, the risk for health complications is less and leads to better health.

Obesity has genetic basis and there is a 75 % chance of being obese if a child born to two obese people. ob gene expressed in adipocytes (of white adipose tissue) producing a protein called leptin (16000 daltons molecular weight) is associated with obesity. Leptin is considered as a body weight regulatory hormone. It functions as a lipostat by binding with specific receptors in the brain. Leptin levels are high when the fat stores in adipose tissues are adequate. This leads to a restriction of feeding behavior and limits fat deposition. Also, lipolysis is stimulated and lipogenesis is inhibited by leptin. Any genetic defect in leptin or its receptor will lead to extreme overeating and obesity. In this case, the people can be treated by leptin to reverse obesity. Leptin levels fall during starvation which promotes feeding and fat production and its deposition.

Both the size and number of adipocytes (adipose tissues) are increased in obesity. Adipose tissues are two types namely white adipose tissue and brown adipose tissue. White adipose tissue is metabolically less active but stored fats is more; whereas, brown adipose tissue is metabolically very active but stored fats is less. The reason for high activity of brown adipose tissue is attributed to their high mitochondria and cytochrome proportion and low activity of *ATP synthase*. It is responsible for the diet induced thermogenesis and it is an active center for the oxidation of fat and glucose. The unique feature of brown adipose tissue mitochondria is that the oxidation and phosphorylation are not coupled. More heat and less ATP are produced in mitochondrial oxidation. In the inner membrane of these mitochondria, a specific protein known as thermogenin has been isolated. This thermogenin acts like an uncoupler and dissipiates the energy in the form of heat and blocks the formation of ATP. Mostly, brown adipose tissue is found in hibernating animals, and the animals exposed to cold, besides the newborn. In human adults it is located in the thoracic region though not a permanent tissue. In obese peoples this brown adipose tissue is almost absent. Fortunately, some people have active brown adipose tissue. They do not become obese due to eat and liberate it as heat.

Olestra and orlistat are the synthetic lipids used recently for the treatment of obesity. They are not digested, excreted unchangingly and taste like natural lipids.

Amino Acid Metabolism

Amino acid metabolism differs from other biomolecule metabolisms due to the presence of nitrogen. The nitrogen present in amino group of amino acid can be transferred from one amino acid to another keto acid [**transamination**] or removal of amino group from amino acid [**deamination**]. The carbon skeletons of amino acids are usually metabolized like carbohydrate and fat. The amino acid undergoes some common reactions like transamination followed by deamination to liberate ammonia. The liberated ammonia is utilized for the formation of **urea which is the excretory end product of protein metabolism**. The overview of amino acid metabolism is presented in Figure 3.3. Through transamination the carbon skeleton of amino acid is converted to keto acid. The produced keto acids may meet any one or more of the following fates.

1. Keto acid is used for generation of energy.
2. Keto acid is utilized for the production of glucose.
3. Keto acid is used for the synthesis of fat or ketone bodies.
4. Keto acid is involved in the synthesis of non-essential amino acid also.

General Reactions of Amino Acid Metabolism

The following are the three major metabolic reactions taking place in amino acid metabolism.

1. Transamination
2. Deamination
3. Decarboxylation

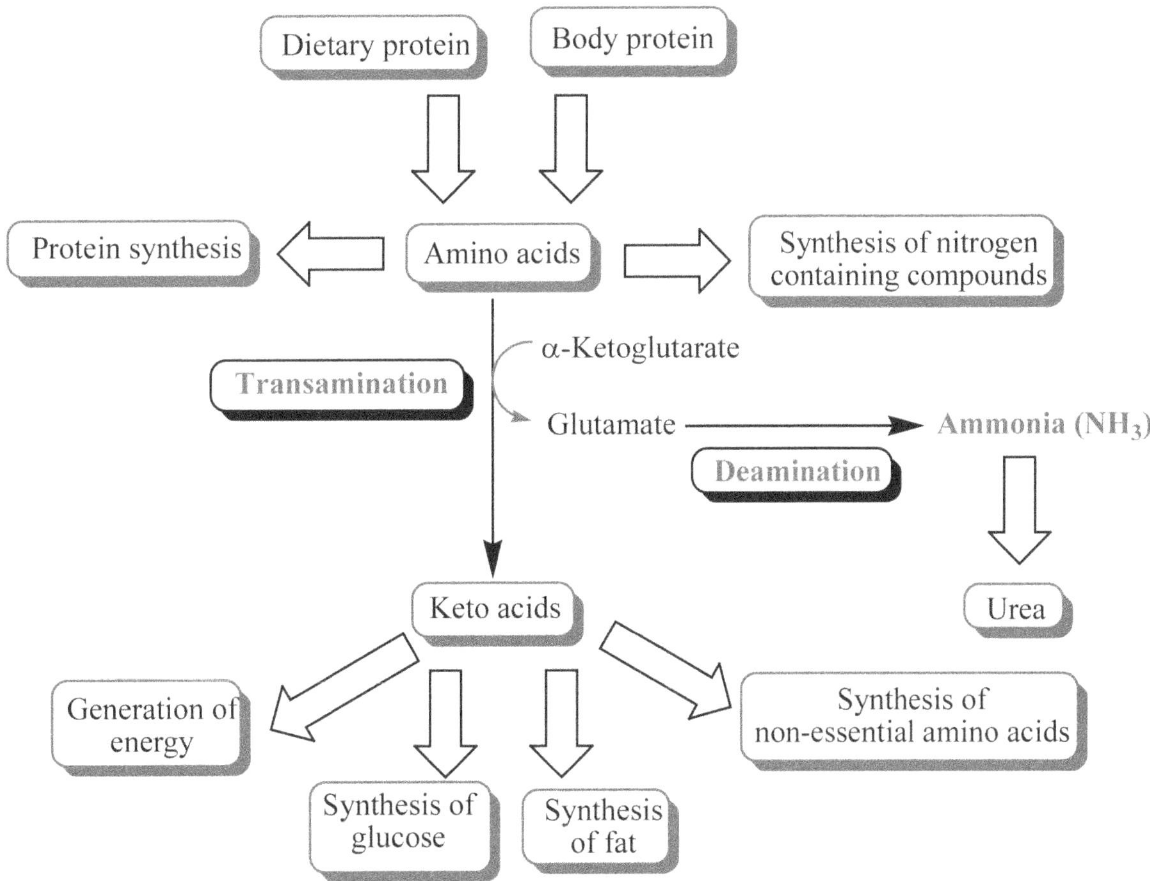

Figure 3.3 Overview of amino acid metabolism.

Transamination

Definition:

Transamination is defined as the transfer of amino (NH_2) group from amino acids to keto acids. Transamination takes place in the presence of the enzyme known as *transaminase* or *aminotransferase* (In transfer involved reactions the enzymes acted are "*transferase*" and the substrate is "amine"). *Transaminase* enzyme needs pyridoxal phosphate (PLP) as co-enzyme. Transamination involves the inter conversion of pair of amino acids and a pair of keto acids.

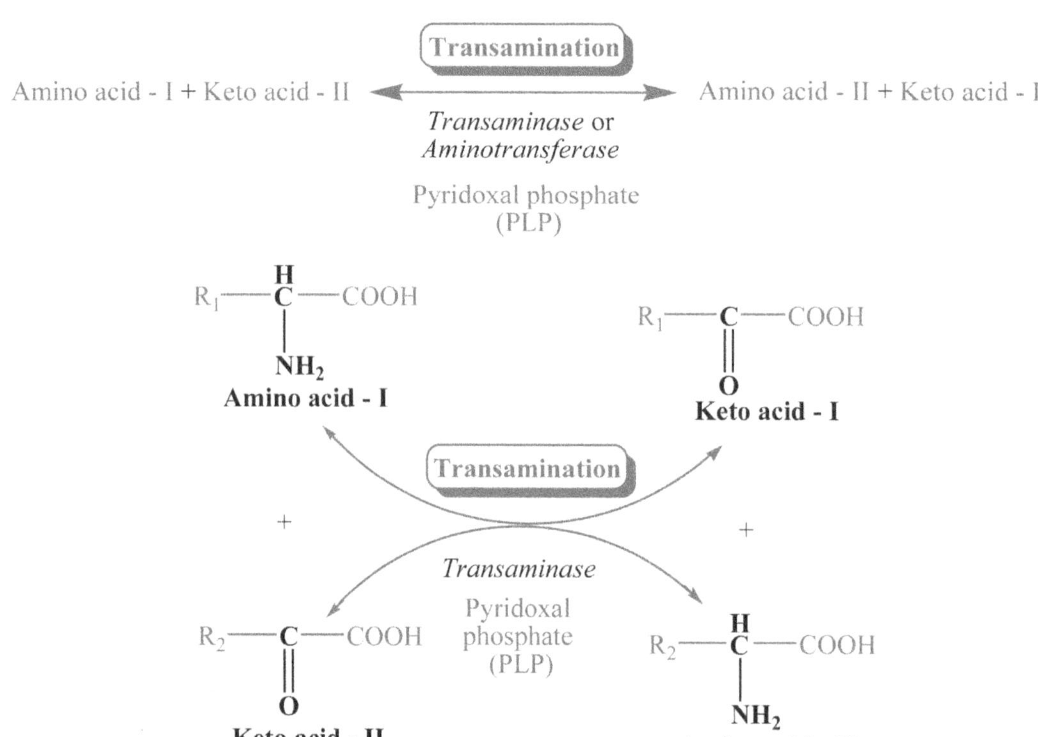

Most important features:

1. Generally, transamination reactions are reversible in nature.
2. No free ammonia (NH_3) is liberated in transamination reaction and only amino groups are transferred from one amino acid to other keto acid.
3. For each pair of amino acids and keto acids specific *transaminase* enzyme exists. Out of several *transaminase* known only two namely *aspartate transaminase (AST)* and *alanine transaminase (ALT)* made significant contribution for transamination reactions.
4. Except lysine, threonine, proline and hydroxyproline, rest all amino acids undergo transamination reaction.
5. Based on the need of cell, transamination reaction is useful for the synthesis of non-essential amino acids and for redistribution of amino groups.
6. Both synthesis (anabolism) and degradation (catabolism) of amino acids are involved in transamination reactions.
7. Some of the *transaminase* enzymes are useful clinically for the diagnosis of various diseases. **Example:** *SGPT (Serum glutamate pyruvate transaminase)* is useful for diagnosis of liver diseases and *SGOT (Serum glutamate oxaloacetate transaminase)* is useful for diagnosis of heart diseases.
8. A vitamin B_6 or pyridoxine derived co-enzyme pyridoxal phosphate (PLP) is required for the activity of all *transaminases*.
9. Excess amino acids are diverted for the production of energy by transamination reactions.

10. The nitrogen of amino acids is finally concentrated as glutamate through transamination reactions. Glutamate is the only amino acid which liberates free ammonia for the synthesis of urea by oxidative deamination reaction.
11. Transamination reactions is not only restricted for α-amino groups. δ-amino group of ornithine may also undergo transamination.

Deamination

Deamination is defined as removal of amino group from amino acid as ammonia and results in formation of corresponding keto acids. The enzyme responsible for deamination is *deaminase* (In removal reactions the enzymes acted are "*de*" and the substrate is "amine"). The liberated ammonia is utilized for the production of urea. Meanwhile carbon skeleton of amino acid is converted to keto acid.

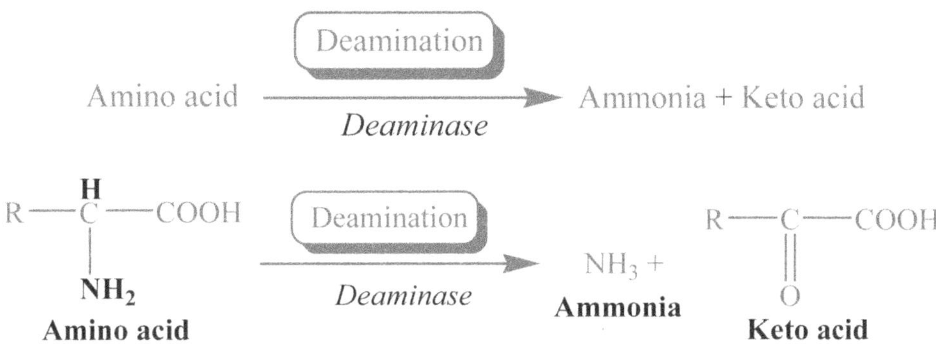

Generally, transamination and deamination occur simultaneously with glutamate as the central molecule. Hence transamination and deamination involving glutamate is commonly known as **trans deamination**. Deamination is broadly classified into two major reactions as 1) Oxidative deamination, 2) Non-oxidative deamination.

1. **Oxidative deamination:**

   In this type, the amino group of amino acid is lost as ammonia coupled with oxidation. This is a major type of deamination reaction. Glutamate is the only substrate which undergoes oxidative deamination reaction. It takes place mainly in liver and kidney and the purpose is to provide ammonia for urea synthesis and keto acids for many reactions particularly energy production.

   Glutamate dehydrogenase (GDH): Most of amino acids transfer its amino group to α-ketoglutarate and produce glutamate through transamination. Hence in biological systems glutamate is called as collection centre for amino groups. This glutamate rapidly releases free ammonia by oxidative deamination in presence of enzyme called *glutamate dehydrogenase (GDH)* (In NAD^+ or $NADP^+$ involved reactions the enzymes acted are "*dehydrogenase*" and the substrate is "glutamate") and also produces α-ketoglutarate. The unique feature of *glutamate dehydrogenase (GDH)* is it can use either NAD^+ or $NADP^+$ as co-enzyme. The α-iminoglutarate is formed as intermediate during the conversion of glutamate to α-ketoglutarate by oxidative deamination.

   The *glutamate dehydrogenase (GDH)* catalyzed reaction is reversible and it linked with TCA cycle through α-ketoglutarate. In both anabolic and catabolic reactions *glutamate dehydrogenase (GDH)* is involved. *Glutamate dehydrogenase (GDH)* is complex mitochondrial enzyme containing zinc and six identical units with 56,000 as molecular weight each. It is allosterically regulated (GTP and ATP inhibits and GDP and ADP activate). It is also inhibited by hormones like steroid and thyroid hormone. Liver glutamate level is increased after protein rich meal and it is converted to α-ketoglutarate and free ammonia. The degradation of glutamate is increased when the cellular energy is low to provide α-ketoglutarate to citric acid cycle for production of energy.

Glutamate ⇌ (NAD⁺ or NADP⁺ / NADH + H⁺ or NADPH + H⁺; Reduction; Glutamate dehydrogenase (GDH)) α-Imino glutarate ⇌ (H_2O / NH_3; Deamination; Glutamate dehydrogenase (GDH)) α-Keto glutarate

2. **Non-oxidative Deamination:** In this amino group is removed from amino acid without oxidation; hence it is known as non-oxidative deamination.

***Amino acid dehydratase*:** The hydroxyl (OH) group containing amino acids such as serine, homoserine and threonine undergo non-oxidative deamination in the presence of *dehydratase* enzyme (Type of reaction involved is "dehydration"). This enzyme is dependent on pyridoxal phosphate (PLP).

Serine or Homoserine or Threonine → (Dehydration; NH_3; *Dehydratase*; PLP) **Corresponding α-keto acids**

***Amino acid desulfhydrase*:** The sulphur (S) group containing amino acids such as cysteine and homocysteine undergo non-oxidative deamination coupled with desulfhydration in presence of *desulfhydrase* enzyme (Type of reaction involved is "desulfhydration").

Desulfhydration

$SH-CH_2-CH(NH_2)-COOH$ (**Cysteine**) → (H_2O; $NH_3 + H_2S$; *Desulfhydrase*) $CH_3-C(=O)-COOH$ (**Pyruvate**)

***Histidase*:** Histidine undergoes non-oxidative deamination in presence of *histidase* enzyme (Substrate is "histidine") and produce uroconate.

Histidine (imidazole ring $-CH_2-CH(NH_2)-COOH$) → (Non-oxidative deamination; NH_3; *Histidase*) **Uroconate** (imidazole ring $-CH=CH-COOH$)

Decarboxylation

Decarboxylation is defined as removal of carboxyl group from amino acid as carbondioxide results in formation of corresponding amines. The enzyme responsible for decarboxylation is *decarboxylase* (Type of reaction involved is "decarboxylation"). Like *transaminase, decarboxylase* also needs pyridoxal phosphate (PLP) as co-enzyme.

Enzyme – PLP Schiff base → Transamination → Amino acid – PLP Schiff base

$$R-CH(COOH)-NH_2 \xrightarrow[\text{Decarboxylase, Pyridoxal phosphate (PLP)}]{\text{Decarboxylation}} R-CH_2-NH_2 + CO_2$$

Amino acid → **Primary amine**

Histamine: The biologically important biogenic amine "histamine" is biosynthesized in biological system by decarboxylation in presence of *histidine decarboxylase* (Substrate is "histidine" and the type of reaction involved is "decarboxylation").

Histidine $\xrightarrow[\text{Histidine decarboxylase, Pyridoxal phosphate (PLP)}]{\text{Decarboxylation}}$ **Histamine** + CO_2

Tyramine: Aromatic amino acid tyrosine undergoes decarboxylation in presence of *tyrosine decarboxylase* (Substrate is "tyrosine" and the type of reaction involved is "decarboxylation") and produces tyramine.

Tyrosine $\xrightarrow[\text{Tyrosine decarboxylase, Pyridoxal phosphate (PLP)}]{\text{Decarboxylation}}$ **Tyramine** + CO_2

Urea Cycle or Kreb's-Henseleit Cycle

The end excretory product of amino acid or protein metabolism is urea. The ammonia produced through transamination and oxidative deamination by nitrogen of amino acids are toxic to the biological system. Hence, it is detoxified by converting into urea. Among various nitrogen containing substances excreted in urine, 80 to 90 % are accounted by urea only. It is the first metabolic cycle discovered in the year 1932 by Hans Krebs and Kurt Henseleit.

Urea cycle is defined as a series of chemical reactions occurring in biological system to convert toxic ammonia to urea. Urea cycle is very important metabolic cycle because it directly removes the toxic ammonia into urea. Urea synthesis takes place in liver and transported to kidney for excretion in urine.

$$\underset{\textbf{Ammonia (Toxic)}}{NH_3} + \underset{\textbf{Carbondioxide}}{CO_2} \xrightarrow{\text{Liver}} \underset{\text{Urea}}{NH_2-\overset{\overset{\displaystyle O}{\|}}{C}-NH_2}$$

Pathway:

Urea contains two amino groups and one carbonyl group. The sources of two amino and carbonyl group are as follows:

1. One amino group is derived from ammonia.
2. Carbonyl group is derived from carbondioxide.
3. Another amino group is derived from amino acid aspartate.

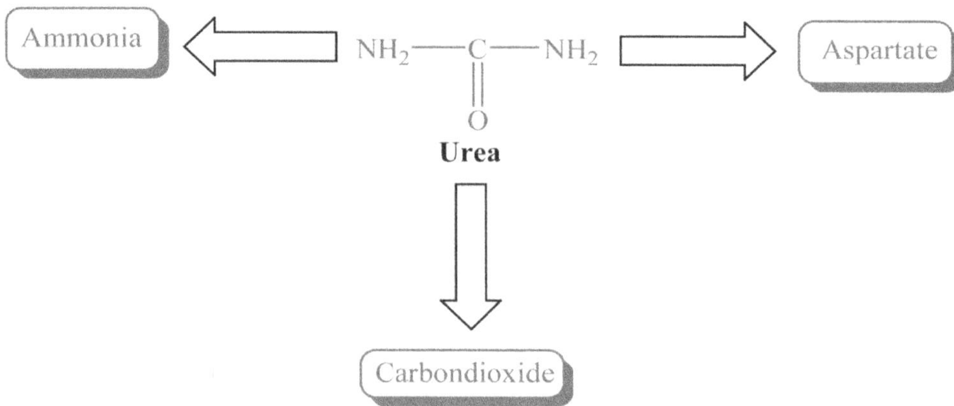

There are five important metabolic reactions in urea cycle with five distinguished enzymes. Out of that first two enzymes are present in mitochondria whereas rests of three enzymes are present in cytosol.

1. *Cabomoyl phosphate synthase – I (CPS-I)* (Product formed is "carbamoyl phosphate" and the type of reaction involved is "synthesis") present in mitochondria condense the toxic ammonia and carbon dioxide into carbamoyl phosphate. Ammonia and carbon dioxide needed for this step is obtained from trans deamination and TCA cycle, respectively. **It is a rate limiting enzyme of urea cycle** and this reaction is irreversible. Hence, ***CPS-I* regulates urea cycle**. *CPS-II* is an enzyme involved in the synthesis of pyrimidine nucleus. *CPS-I* needs N-acetylglutamate (NAG) for its activity whereas *CPS-II* doesn't need NAG for its activity. The first amino group and carboxyl group are incorporated in this step. 2 ATPs are converted into 2 ADP and one inorganic phosphate & other phosphate are taken by carbamoyl group **(2 ATP is utilized).**
2. Carbamoyl phosphate then reacts with ornithine and produce citrulline in presence of *ornithine trans carbamoylase* (Substrate is "ornithine" and the type of reaction involved is "transfer of carbamoyl group"). This reaction is similar to **aldol condensation** and takes place in mitochondria only. **Ornithine plays a catalytic role in urea cycle** as it is later regenerated (Like oxaloacetate in TCA cycle). Then, formed citrulline is transported from mitochondria to cytosol by transporter system. Both ornithine and citrulline are basic amino acids.
3. In third step, aspartate is reacting with citrulline by dehydration condensation and produce argininosuccinate. The reaction is catalyzed by the enzyme *argininosuccinate synthase* (Product formed is "argininosuccinate" and the type of reaction involved is hydrolysis [in reverse manner]). Aspartate needed for this step is obtained from TCA cycle. In this step, the second amino group of urea is incorporated. One ATP is breakdown into AMP and pyrophosphate and the latter one is immediately breakdown into two inorganic phosphate by *pyrophosphatase* (Substrate is "pyrophosphate" and the type of reaction involved is "hydrolysis") **[2 ATP is utilized].**

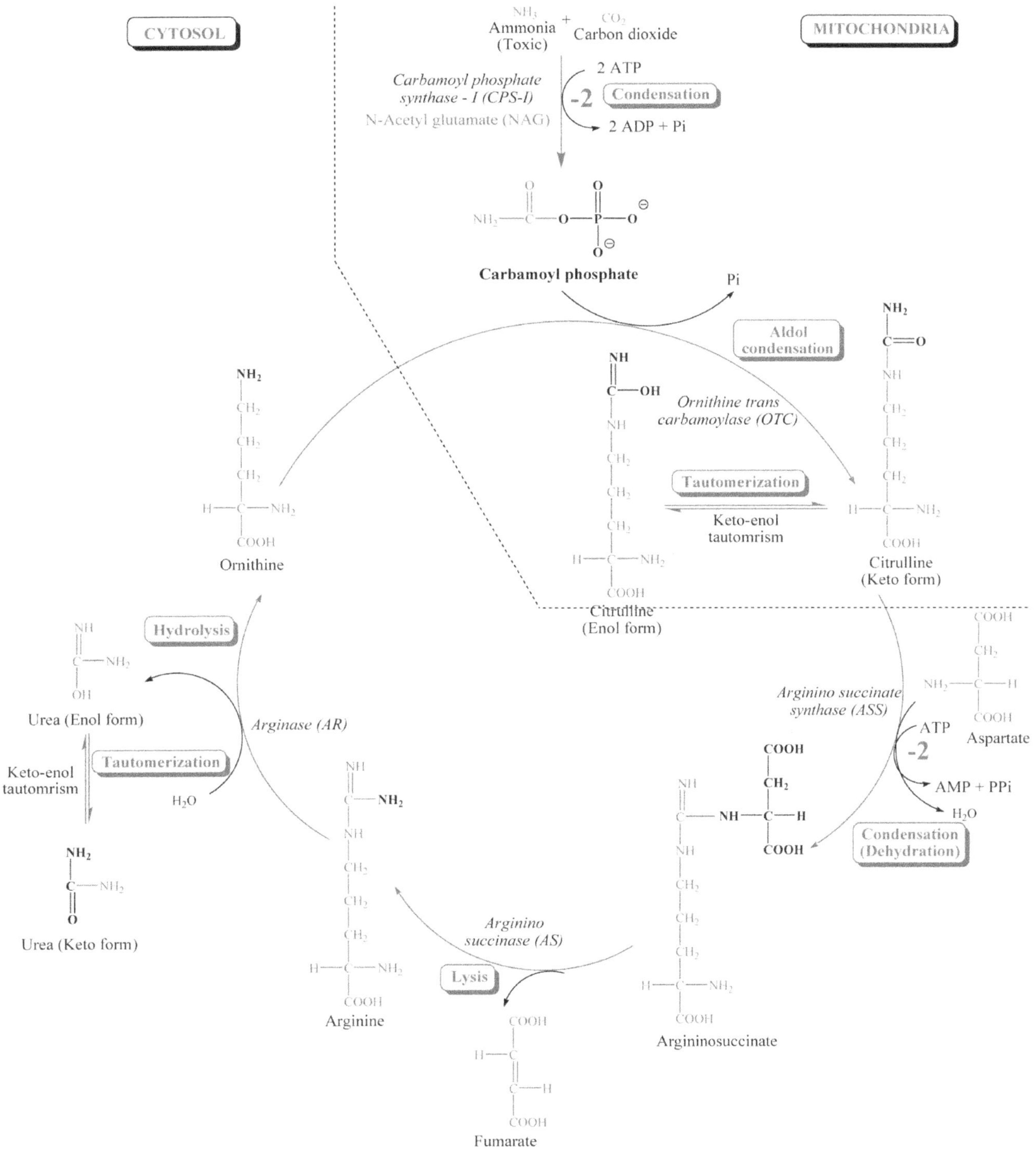
CYTOSOL
MITOCHONDRIA
NH3 + CO2
Ammonia (Toxic)
Carbon dioxide
2 ATP
Carbamoyl phosphate synthase - I (CPS-I)
N-Acetyl glutamate (NAG)
-2
Condensation
2 ADP + Pi
Carbamoyl phosphate
Pi
Aldol condensation
Ornithine trans carbamoylase (OTC)
Ornithine
Tautomerization
Keto-enol tautomrism
Citrulline (Enol form)
Citrulline (Keto form)
Aspartate
Arginino succinate synthase (ASS)
ATP
-2
AMP + PPi
H2O
Condensation (Dehydration)
Argininosuccinate
Arginino succinase (AS)
Lysis
Fumarate
Arginine
Arginase (AR)
Hydrolysis
Urea (Enol form)
Tautomerization
Keto-enol tautomrism
H2O
Urea (Keto form)

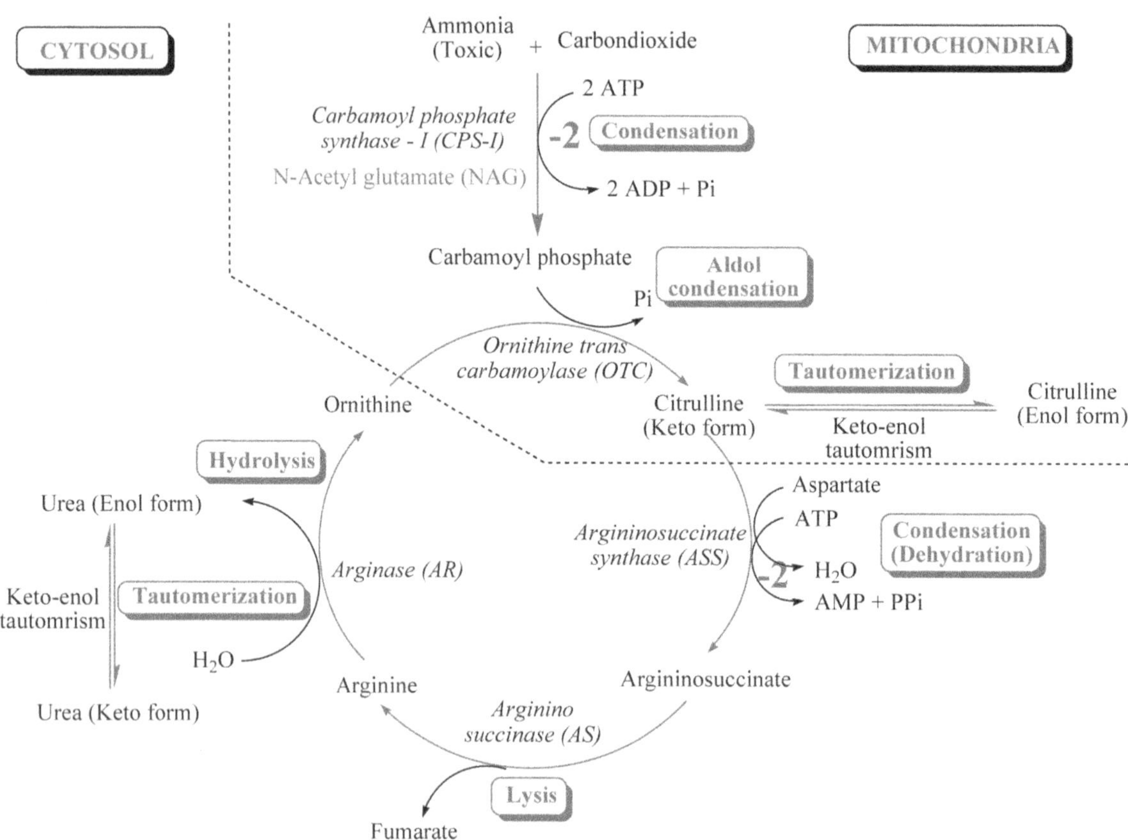

4. In the next step argininosuccinate is cleaved into arginine and fumarate in presence of *argininosuccinase*. (Substrate is "argininosuccinate" and the type of reaction involved is "lysis or cleavage"). Fumarate liberated in this step is entering into TCA cycle, gluconeogenesis, etc.
5. In last step, ornithine is regenerated with production of urea when arginine is hydrolyzed in presence of *arginase* (Substrate is "arginine" and the type of reaction involved is "hydrolysis"). Regenerated ornithine enters into mitochondria for its reuse in urea cycle. Co^{2+} and Mn^{2+} activates *arginase* enzyme.

Except *arginase* all other four enzymes of urea cycle is present in all tissues. *Arginase* is mainly present in liver only. Hence, in many tissues arginine synthesis may occur in varying degree but in liver only it can ultimately converted into urea. The first two enzymes of urea cycle are present in mitochondria whereas the rest of three enzymes are present in cytosol part of the cell. Urea cycle is irreversible in nature and totally for the synthesis of one urea molecule 4 ATPs are utilized (2 ATP in first step and another 2 ATP in third step). The overall reactions of urea cycle can be written as follows.

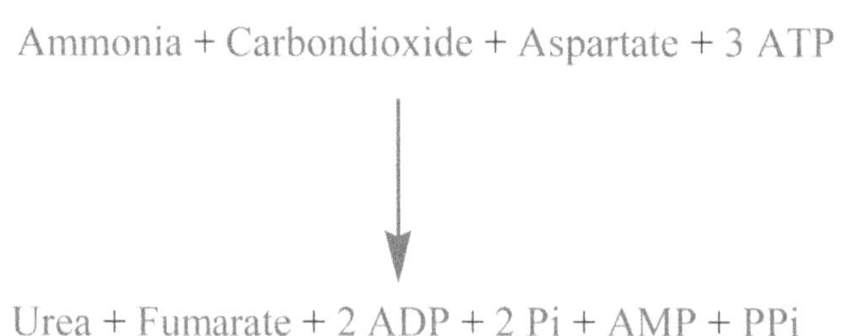

Metabolic disorders of urea cycle:

In the Table 3.2. metabolic disorders associated with the five enzymes of urea cycle are summarized. The clinical symptoms associated with urea cycle metabolic disorders are vomiting, lethargy, irritability, ataxia and mental retardation. Blood ammonia level is increased invariably in all the disorders which leads to toxicity. The other metabolites also accumulate depending on the specific enzyme defects.

Table 3.2 Metabolic disorders of urea cycle.

S. No.	Metabolic disorder name	Characteristics	Enzyme responsible
1	Hyperammonemia type -I	Increased ammonia level in blood	*Carbamoyl phosphate synthase – I (CPS-I)*
2	Hyperammonemia type - II	Increased ammonia level in blood	*Ornithine trans carbamoylase (OTC)*
3	Citrullinemia	Increased citrulline level in blood	*Argininosuccinate synthase (ASS)*
4	Argininosuccinic aciduria	Increased argininosuccinate level in blood	*Argininosuccinase (AS)*
5	Hyperargininemia	Increased arginine level in blood	*Arginase (AR)*

Phenylalanine and Tyrosine

Phenylalanine and tyrosine are aromatic amino acids which are structurally related because tyrosine is chemically *p*-hydroxyphenylalanine. Out of these two amino acids phenylalanine is essential amino acid and tyrosine is non-essential amino acid because tyrosine is biosynthesized from phenylalanine. Overview of phenylalanine and tyrosine metabolism is presented in Figure 3.4.

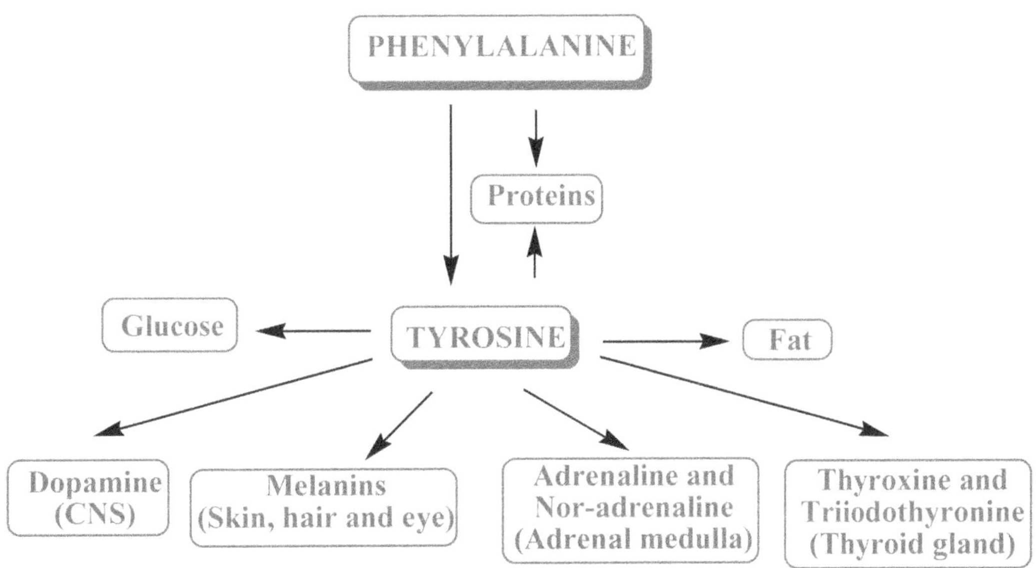

Figure 3.4 Overview of phenylalanine & tyrosine metabolism.

The major functions of phenylalanine is biosynthesis of tyrosine and incorporation into proteins. Tyrosine is invo lved in incorporation of proteins and synthesis of some different biologically important compounds such as a) Melanin (in skin, hair and eye), b) Dopamine (in CNS), c) Adrenaline and nor-adrenaline (in adrenal medulla), d) Thyroxine and triiodothyronine (in thyroid gland) e) Glucose & fat. Ingestion of tyrosine reduces dietary requirement of phenylalanine is referred as **sparing action of tyrosine and phenylalanine**. Tyrosine is both glucogenic and ketogenic amino acid because metabolites of tyrosine serves as a precursor for the synthesis of glucose and fat.

Catabolism of Phenylalanine & Tyrosine

Phenylalanine and tyrosine metabolism are considered together. These amino acids are degraded into fumarate and acetoacetate which is a precursor for the synthesis of carbohydrates and fats, respectively. The various reactions involved in this degradation are described here.

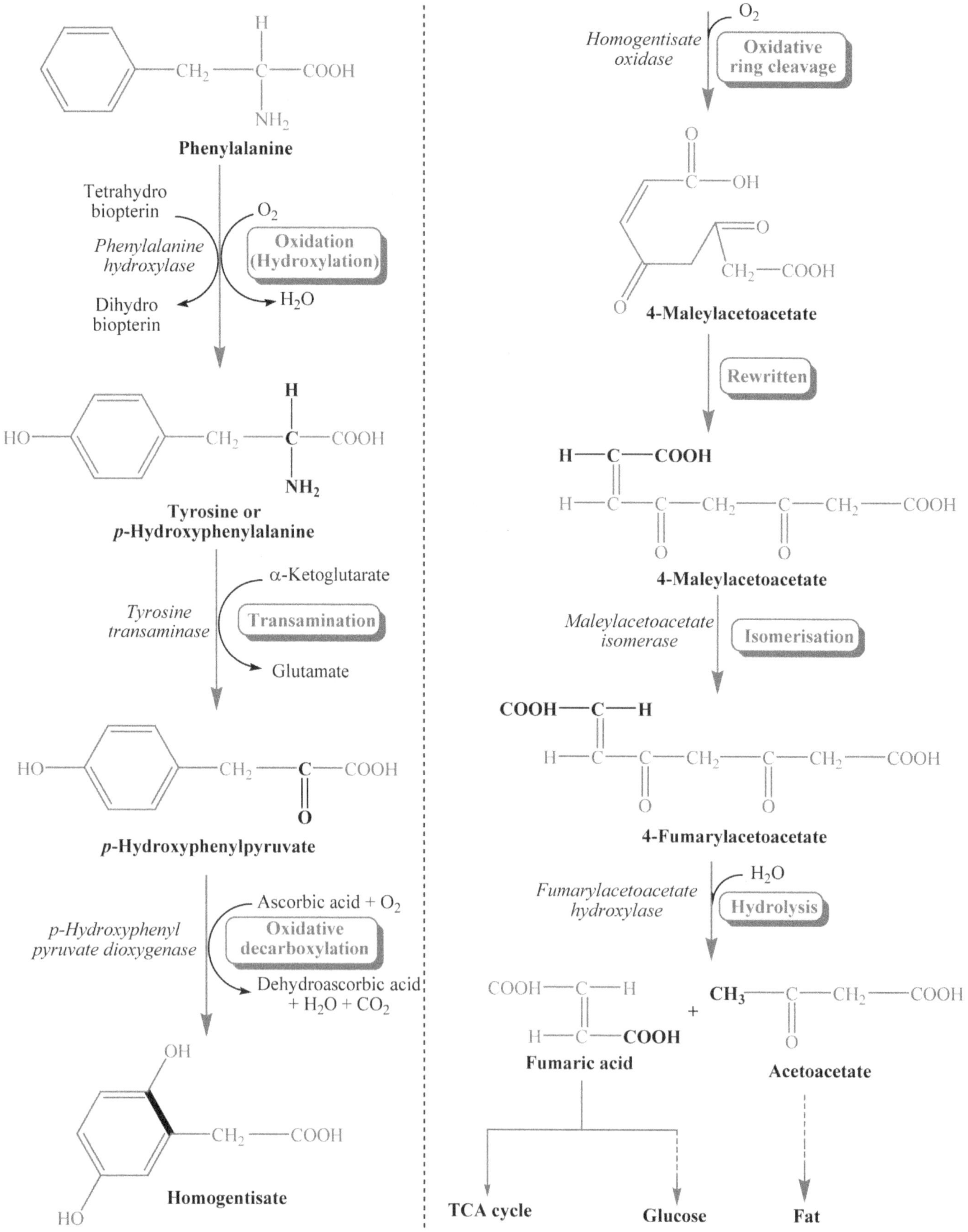

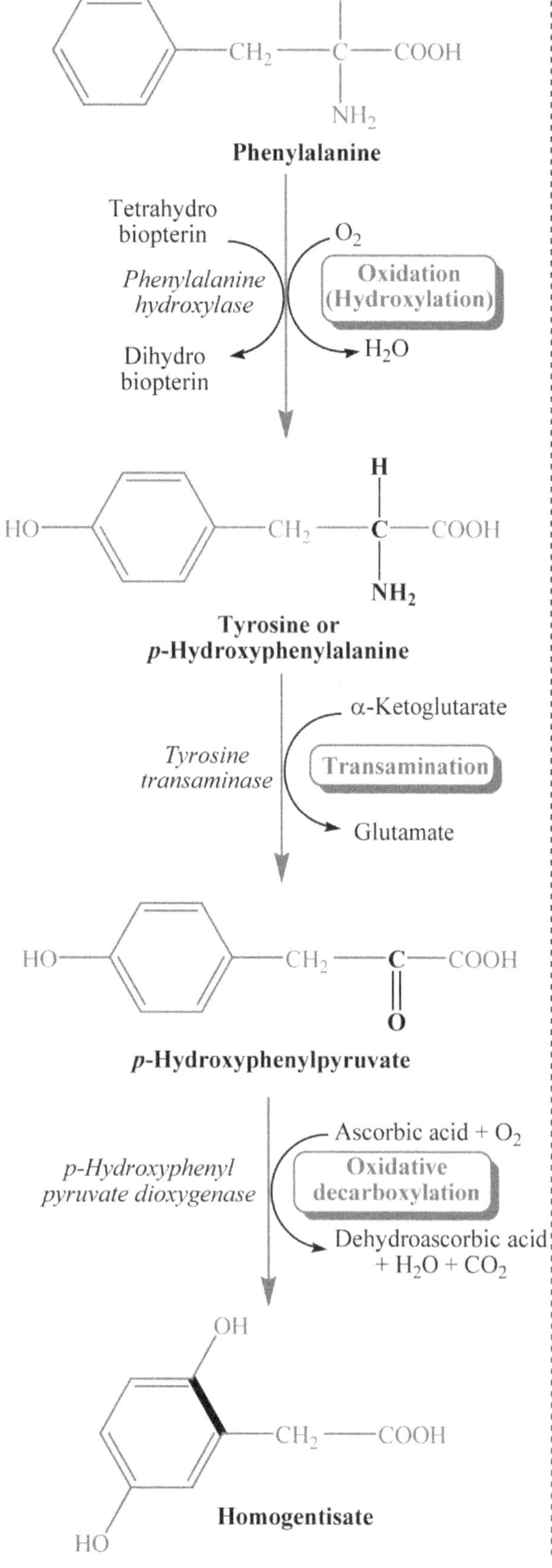

H
CH_2 — C — COOH
NH_2
Phenylalanine
Tetrahydro biopterin
O_2
Phenylalanine hydroxylase
Oxidation (Hydroxylation)
Dihydro biopterin
H_2O
H
HO — CH_2 — C — COOH
NH_2
Tyrosine or p-Hydroxyphenylalanine
α-Ketoglutarate
Tyrosine transaminase
Transamination
Glutamate
HO — CH_2 — C — COOH
O
p-Hydroxyphenylpyruvate
Ascorbic acid + O_2
p-Hydroxyphenyl pyruvate dioxygenase
Oxidative decarboxylation
Dehydroascorbic acid + H_2O + CO_2
OH
CH_2 — COOH
HO
Homogentisate
O_2
Homogentisate oxidase
Oxidative ring cleavage
O
C — OH
O
CH_2 — COOH
O
4-Maleylacetoacetate
Rewritten
H — C — COOH
H — C — C — CH_2 — C — CH_2 — COOH
O
O
4-Maleylacetoacetate
Maleylacetoacetate isomerase
Isomerisation
COOH — C — H
H — C — C — CH_2 — C — CH_2 — COOH
O
O
4-Fumarylacetoacetate
H_2O
Fumarylacetoacetate hydroxylase
Hydrolysis
COOH — C — H
H — C — COOH
+
CH_3 — C — CH_2 — COOH
O
Fumaric acid
Acetoacetate
TCA cycle
Glucose
Fat

Phenylalanine

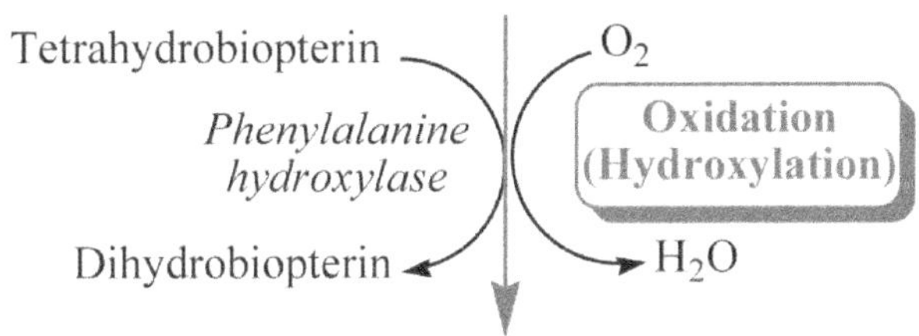

Tyrosine or *p*-Hydroxyphenylalanine

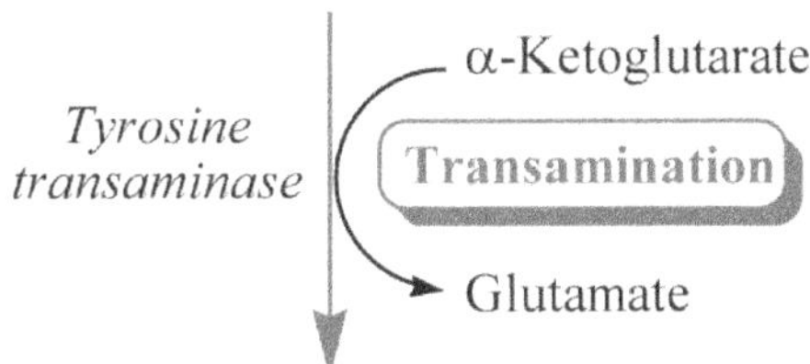

***p*-Hydroxyphenylpyruvate**

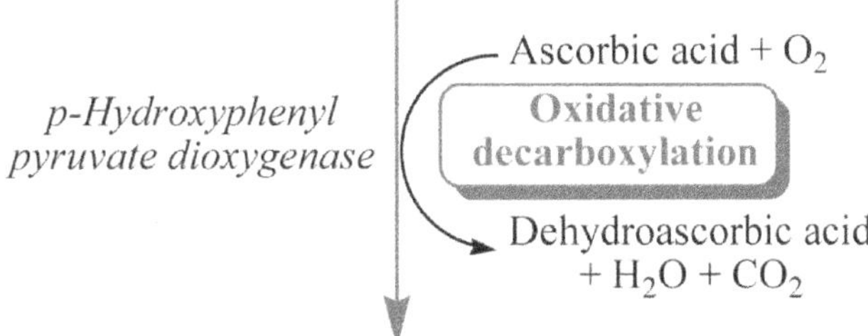

Homogentisate

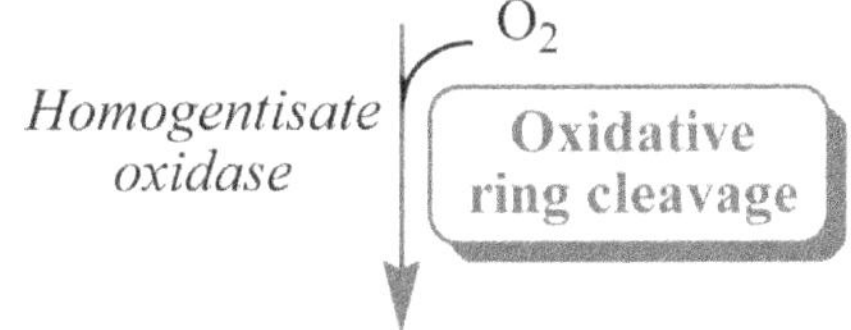

4-Maleylacetoacetate

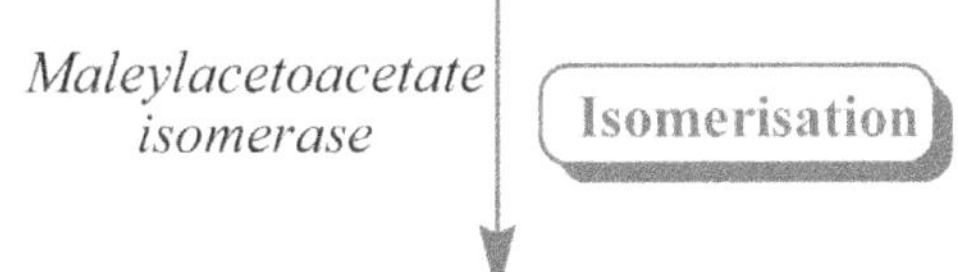

4-Fumarylacetoacetate

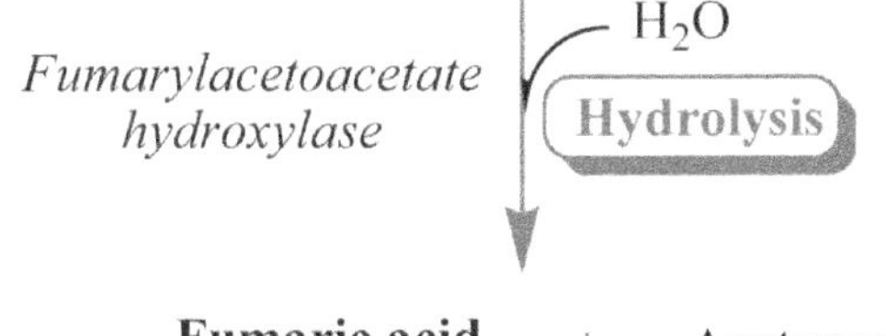

Fumaric acid + **Acetoacetate**

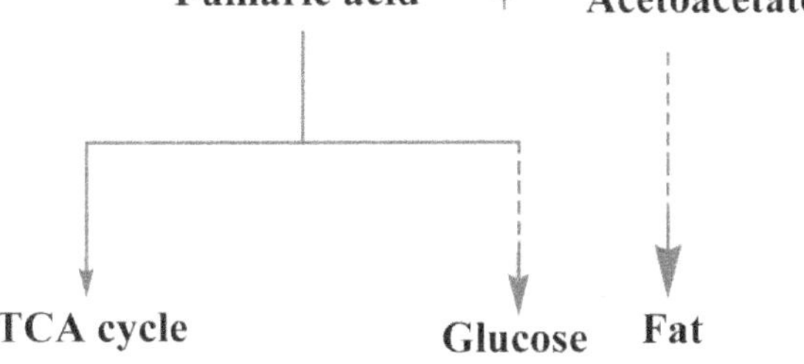

1. Initially, phenylalanine is converted into tyrosine by hydroxylation or oxidation at aromatic carbon atom in the presence of *phenylalanine hydroxylase* (The substrate is "phenylalanine" and the type of reaction involved is "hydroxylation"). In this reaction, one mole of oxygen is involved. In that one of the oxygen atoms is incorporated in phenylalanine at *para* position and the another oxygen atom coupled with two hydrogen atoms of tetrahydrobiopterin are removed as water molecule. The tetrahydrobiopterin is converted into dihydrobiopterin as it loses two hydrogen atoms.
2. In the next step, tyrosine undergoes transamination reaction by reacting with α-ketoglutarate and produces *p*-hydroxyphenylpyruvate in presence of *tyrosine transaminase* (The substrate is "tyrosine" and the type of reaction involved is "transamination") & liberates glutamate. *Tyrosine transaminase* needs PLP (pyridoxal phosphate) as co-enzyme.
3. *p*-Hydroxyphenylpyruvate undergoes oxidative decarboxylation (oxidation at ortho position of phenyl ring and side chain) to produce homogentisate in presence of copper containing enzyme *p-hydroxyphenylpyruvate dioxygenase or p-hydroxyphenylpyruvate hydroxylase* (The substrate is "*p*-hydroxyphenylpyruvate" and the type of reaction involved is "hydroxylation"). During this reaction carboxyl group is removed as carbondioxide results in corresponding aldehyde which is further oxidized to carboxylic acid. In addition, one mole of oxygen is involved in this reaction. In that one of the oxygen atoms is incorporated in phenylalanine at *ortho* position and the other oxygen atom coupled with two hydrogen atoms of ascorbic acid and removed as water molecule. The ascorbic acid is converted into dehydroascorbic acid as it loses two hydrogen atoms. In the mean time *para* hydroxyl group of *p*-hydroxyphenylpyruvate is transferred to *meta* position (C-5) in order to get stable configuration.
4. 4-Maleylacetoacetate is produced from homogentisate by oxidative ring cleavage reaction and the reaction is catalyzed by iron containing enzyme "*homogentisate oxidase*" (The substrate is "homogentisate" and the type of reaction involved is "oxidation" with incorporation of both oxygen of molecular oxygen). The benzene ring is opened between C-1 and C-2 and produce dicarboxylic acid derivatives.
5. In the next step 4-fumarylacetoacetate is produced from 4-maleylacetoacetate by isomerization and the reaction takes place in the presence of *4-maleylacetoacetate isomerase* (The substrate is "4-maleylacetoacetate" and the type of reaction involved is "isomerization").
6. 4-Fumarylacetoacetate is hydrolyzed in the next step and produces fumarate and acetoacetate. The reaction is catalyzed by *4-fumarylacetoacetate hydroxylase* (The substrate is "4-fumarylacetoacetate" and the type of reaction involved is "hydrolysis").
7. In TCA cycle, fumarate is one of the intermediate and also it serves as a precursor for gluconeogenesis for the synthesis of glucose. The ketone body acetoacetate is used as a precursor for the synthesis of fat.

Biosynthesis of Catecholamines

Biologically important amines i.e., catecholamines such as dopamine, adrenaline or epinephrine and nor-adrenaline or nor-epinephrine are biosynthesized from tyrosine. Catecholamines are the amine derivatives of catechol or *o*-hydroxy phenol and its synthesis is takes place in adrenal medulla and CNS. The various reactions involved in the synthesis of catecholamines are described here.

1. Tyrosine is converted into DOPA (3,4-dihydroxyphenylalanine) by hydroxylation or oxidation at *meta* position in presence of *tyrosine hydroxylase* (The substrate is "tyrosine" and the type of reaction involved is "hydroxylation"). In this reaction, one mole of oxygen is involved. In that one of the oxygen atom is incorporated in phenylalanine at *meta* position and another oxygen atom coupled with two hydrogen atoms of tetrahydrobiopterin are removed as water molecule. The tetrahydrobiopterin is converted into dihydrobiopterin as it loses two hydrogen atoms. **It is the rate limiting step in the biosynthesis of catecholamines**. Two different enzyme systems i.e., *tyrosine hydroxylase* and *tyrosinase* exist for conversion of tyrosine to DOPA.

2. In second step, DOPA undergoes decarboxylation and produce its corresponding amine i.e., dopamine by losing carboxylic group as carbondioxide. This reaction is catalyzed by *aromatic amino acid decarboxylase* (The substrate is "DOPA" which is aromatic amino acid analog and the type of reaction involved is "decarboxylation") which requires PLP for its activity.
3. Dopamine further hydroxylated at β-position of side chain in the presence of *dopamine-β-hydroxylase* (The substrate is "dopamine" and the type of reaction involved is "β-hydroxylation") and produces nor-adrenaline or nor-epinephrine. In this reaction one mole of oxygen is involved. In that one of the oxygen atoms is incorporated in β-position of side chain in dopamine and another oxygen atom coupled with two hydrogen atoms of ascorbic acid are removed as water molecule. The ascorbic acid is converted into dehydroascorbic acid as it loses two hydrogen atoms.
4. Adrenaline or epinephrine is synthesized from nor-adrenaline or nor-epinephrine by N-methylation reaction in presence of *phenylethanolamine-N-methyl transferase* (The substrate is "nor-adrenaline or nor-epinephrine" which is phenylethanolamine derivative) and the type of reaction is "methyl group transfer"). In this reaction methyl group is donated by S-adenosyl methionine (SAM) and it is converted to S-adenosyl homocysteine after donating methyl group.

Tissue specificity exists in biosynthesis of catecholamines. Epinephrine and nor-epinephrine are prominently synthesized in adrenal medulla. In some part of the brain nor-epinephrine is synthesized but dopamine is specifically synthesized in substantia nigra and coeruleus of brain.

Biological significance of catecholamines:

1. Two catecholamines, nor-epinephrine and dopamine, act as neuromodulators in the central nervous system and as hormones in the blood circulation. The catecholamine nor-epinephrine is a neuromodulator of the peripheral sympathetic nervous system but is also present in the blood.
2. Catecholamines, including dopamine and nor-epinephrine, are the principal neurotransmitters that mediate a variety of the central nervous system functions, such as motor control, cognition, emotion, memory processing, and endocrine modulation.
3. Both epinephrine and nor-epinephrine modulate metabolism to increase blood glucose levels by stimulating glycogenolysis in the liver (via β_2 receptors), increased glucagon secretion (via β_2 receptors) and decreased insulin secretion (via α_2 receptors) from the pancreas.
4. Both epinephrine and nor-epinephrine produce lipolysis in adipose tissue (via β_3 receptors).
5. Epinephrine and nor-epinephrine increases blood pressure.
6. Decreased dopamine is linked with Parkinson's disease.
7. Epinephrine and nor-epinephrine are frequently used as vasopressor agents to treat acute hypotensive states, as well as in treatment algorithms for cardiac arrest.
8. Affinity of epinephrine and nor-epinephrine to the α-1 receptor also is used to induce localized vasoconstriction to reduce bleeding during procedures such as wound closure.
9. Catecholamine releasing agents in the form of sprays or ointments are used as nasal decongestants.
10. The pharmacodynamic inhibition of catecholamine reuptake is commonly used in the psychiatric treatment of some depressive disorders, post-traumatic stress disorder, anxiety disorders, attention deficit disorder, and panic disorders.
11. Catecholamine reuptake inhibitors may be used to treat neuropathic and chronic musculoskeletal pain.
12. Epinephrine is the universal treatment for anaphylaxis and is also used to treat other causes of laryngeal edema or bronchospasm.
13. The blockage of adrenergic receptors otherwise activated by catecholamines is an integral part of the treatment of hypertension, congestive heart failure, and other cardiovascular diseases.
14. The "fight or flight" response of the sympathetic nervous system is a direct result of the multisystem action of catecholamines.
15. Epinephrine also inhibits release of mediators from mast cells and basophils in type-I hypersensitivity reactions.
16. Urine testing for catecholamine is used to detect pheochromocytoma.

17. High catecholamine levels in blood are associated with stress, which can be induced from psychological reactions or environmental stressors such as elevated sound levels, intense light, or low blood sugar levels.

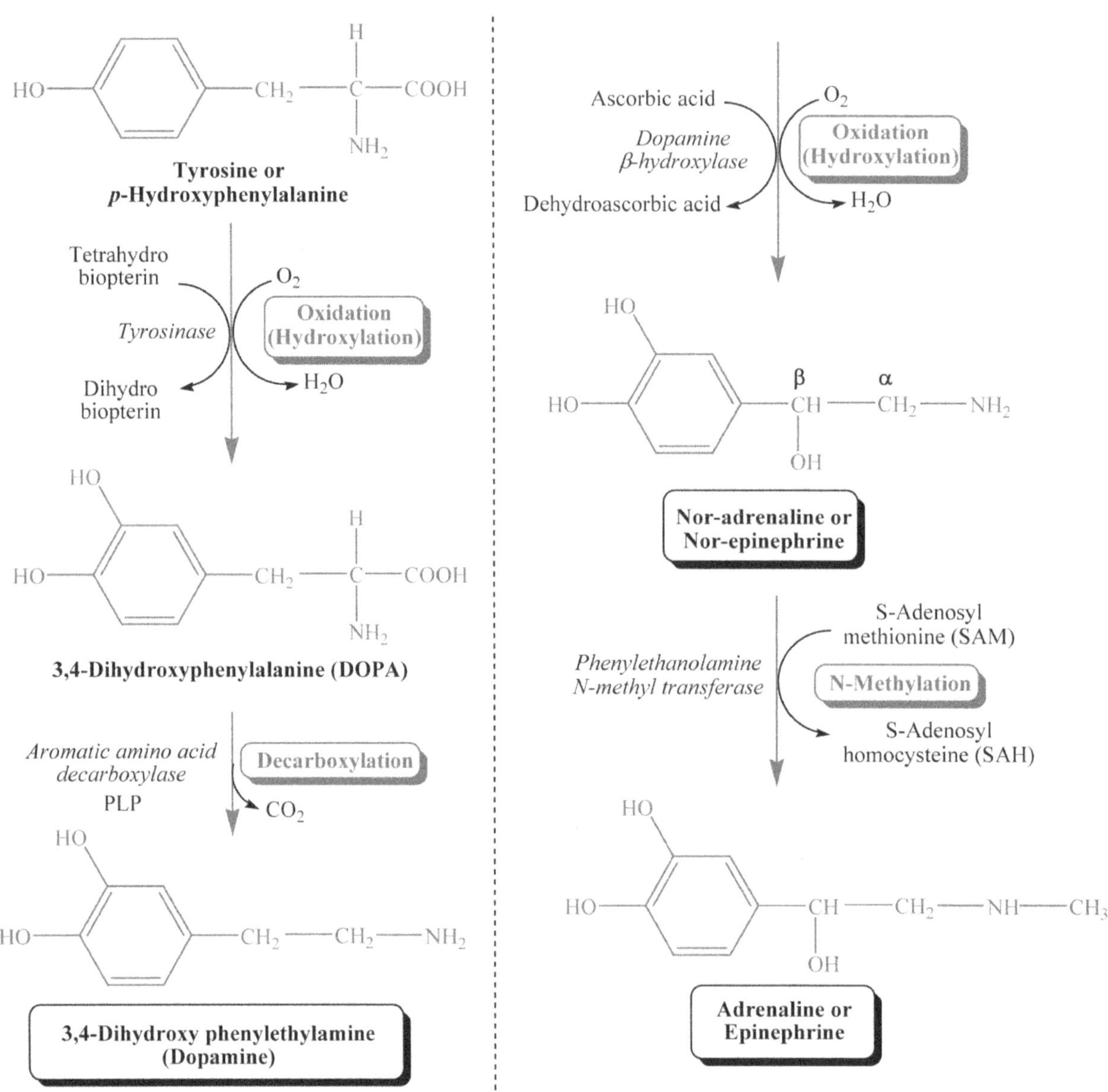

Biosynthesis of 5-hydroxytryptamine (5-HT) or Serotonin and Melatonin

5-Hydroxytryptamine (5-HT) & melatonin is biosynthesized from tryptophan. 5-HT is commonly known as serotonin which is a neurotransmitter. In general, 1 % of tryptophan is utilized for the production of serotonin. In the target tissues serotonin is biosynthesized. largest amount of serotonin is biosynthesized in mammals in intestinal cells. As such platelets cannot synthesize serotonin but it contains high concentration of serotonin and the significance is not known. The serotonin synthesis is usually compared with the synthesis of catecholamines. Melatonin is a hormone biosynthesized mostly in pineal gland. Light controls the synthesis and secretion of melatonin in pineal gland. The various reactions involved in the synthesis of serotonin and melatonin are described here.

1. Tryptophan is converted into 5-hydroxytryptophan by hydroxylation or oxidation at *meta* position in presence of *tryptophan hydroxylase* (The substrate is "tryptophan" and the type of reaction is

"hydroxylation"). In this reaction one mole of oxygen is involved. In that one of the oxygen atoms is incorporated in tryptophan at C-5 position and another oxygen atom is coupled with two hydrogen atoms of tetrahydrobiopterin are removed as water molecule. The tetrahydrobiopterin is converted into dihydrobiopterin as it loses two hydrogen atoms. ***Tryptophan hydroxylase* is the rate limiting enzyme of serotonin synthesis.**

2. In second step, 5-hydroxytryptophan undergoes decarboxylation and produce its corresponding amine i.e., 5-hydroxytryptamine (5-HT) or serotonin by losing carboxylic group as carbondioxide. This reaction is catalyzed by *aromatic amino acid decarboxylase* (The substrate is "5-hydroxytryptophan" which is aromatic amino acid analog and the type of reaction involved is "decarboxylation") which requires PLP for its activity.
3. Serotonin is further acetylated at amino group of side chain in presence of *serotonin-N-acetyl transferase* (The substrate is "serotonin" and the type of reaction involved is "acetyl group transfer to nitrogen") and produces N-acetylserotonin. In this reaction one mole of acetyl CoA is converted to co-enzyme A after transferring acetyl group to serotonin. ***Serotonin-N-acetyl transferase* is the rate limiting enzyme of melatonin synthesis**. In another way, serotonin is deaminated in presence of *monoamine oxidase (MAO)* (The substrate is "serotonin" which is monoamine analog and the type of reaction involved is "oxidative deamination") and produces 5-hydroxyindoleacetate which is excreted in urine. In this reaction amino group is lost as ammonia.
4. Finally, melatonin is synthesized from N-acetylserotonin by *O*-methylation reaction in presence of *N-acetylserotonin-O-methyl transferase* (The substrate is "N-acetylserotonin" and the type of reaction involved is "methyl group transfer to oxygen"). In this reaction methyl group is donated by S-adenosyl methionine (SAM) and it is converted to S-adenosyl homocysteine (SAH) after donating methyl group.
5. In other way, tryptophan is converted to indoleacetate and excreted in urine. This takes place in two different ways.
   (a) In first process initially tryptophan undergoes deamination in presence of *monoamine oxidase (MAO)* (The substrate is "tryptophan" which is monoamine analog and the type of reaction involved is "oxidative deamination") and produces indole-3-pyruvate. In this reaction amino group is lost as ammonia. In the succeeding step, indole-3-pyruvate undergoes oxidative decarboxylation and produce indoleacetate by losing carboxylic group as carbondioxide. This reaction is catalyzed by *aromatic keto acid decarboxylase* (The substrate is "indole-3-pyruvate" which is aromatic keto acid analog and the type of reaction involved is "decarboxylation") which requires PLP for its activity.
   (b) In second process initially tryptophan undergoes decarboxylation and produce its corresponding amine i.e., tryptamine by losing carboxylic group as carbondioxide. This reaction is catalyzed by *aromatic amino acid decarboxylase* (The substrate is "tryptophan" which is aromatic amino acid and the type of reaction involved is "decarboxylation") which requires PLP for its activity. In the next step, tryptamine undergoes deamination in presence of *monoamine oxidase (MAO)* (The substrate is "tryptamine" which is monoamine analog and the type of reaction involved is "oxidative deamination") and produces indoleacetate. In this reaction amino group is lost as ammonia.

Biological significance of serotonin:

1. Serotonin is a neurotransmitter and produces smooth muscle contraction in arterioles and bronchioles due to powerful vasoconstrictor activity.
2. Cerebral activity (excitation) is closely regulated with the involvement of serotonin.
3. In psychosis patient's serotonin level is decreased in brain because serotonin is primarily stimulator of brain activity.
4. It is involved in the control of behavioral patterns, blood pressure, body temperature and sleep.
5. From gastrointestinal tract peptide hormone release is evoked by serotonin.
6. Motility of GIT or peristalsis needs serotonin.

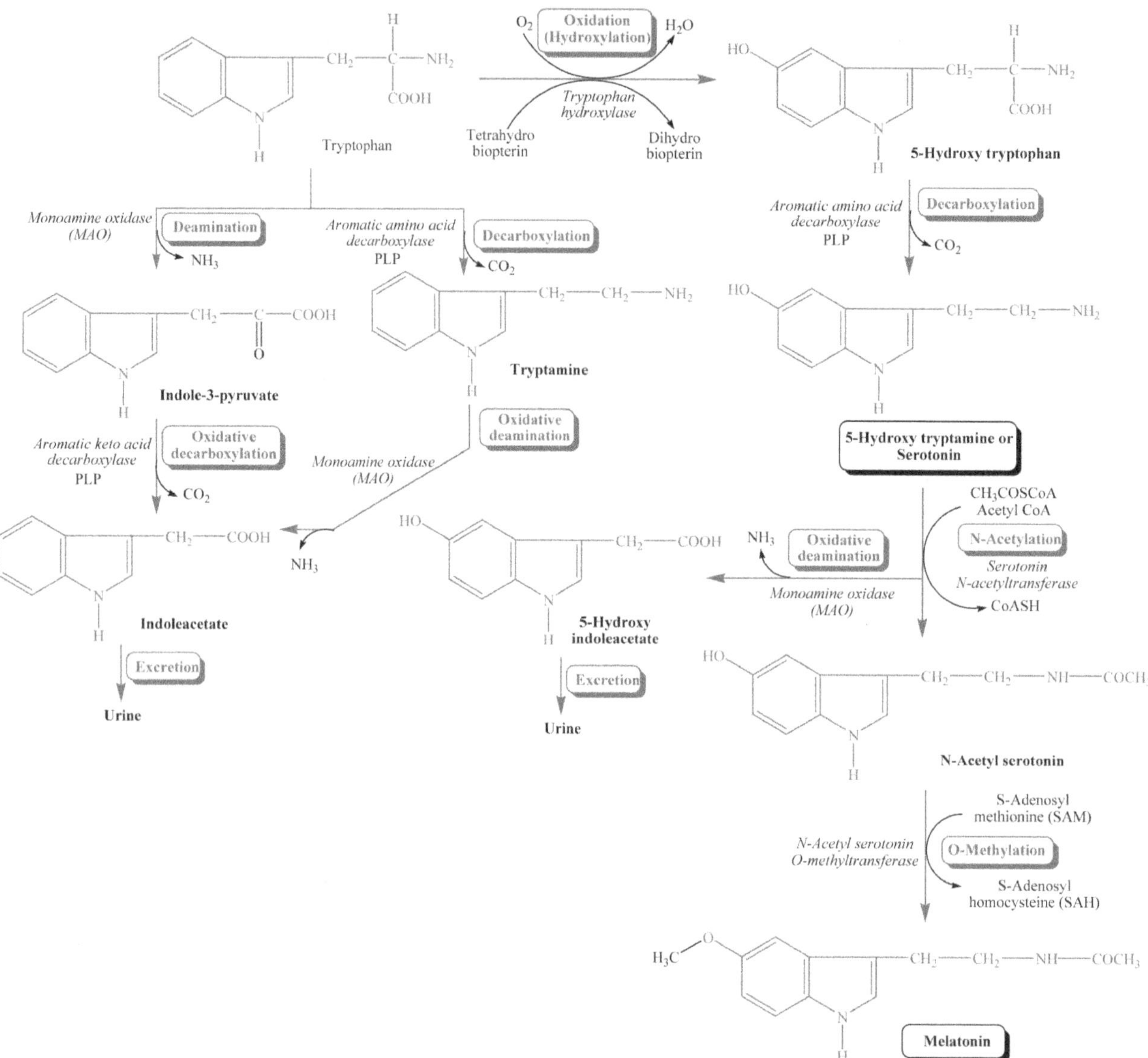

7. Serotonin inhibitors are clinically used as depressant drugs. **Example:** Reserpine increases the degradation of serotonin, Lysergic acid diethylamide (LSD) competes with serotonin.
8. Serotonin stimulators are psychic stimulant. **Example:** Iproniazid inhibits *MAO* and elevates serotonin level.
9. Estimation of 5-hydroxyindoleacetate (5-HIA) in urine is used for the diagnosis of malignant carcinoid syndrome. 5-HIA level is increased in malignant carcinoid syndrome due to increased synthesis of serotonin.

Biological significance of melatonin:

1. Melatonin plays an important role in sleep and wake process. Because it is involved in diurnal variations or circadian rhythms.
2. It is safe and non-addictive sleep-inducing drug, which can eliminate disruptions in our circadian rhythm, in such situations as shift working, changing of time zones (during intercontinental air travelling) or insomnia.
3. Neurotransmitter function is also performed by melatonin.
4. On ovarian function melatonin exhibits some inhibitory effects.
5. Production of adrenocorticotropic hormone (ACTH) and melanocyte stimulating hormone is inhibited by melatonin.

6. Melatonin is a potent antioxidant and free radical scavenger.
7. Melatonin may be used in prophylaxis of cardiovascular system diseases, neoplastic diseases and other functional disorders of organisms.
8. Melatonin makes the immune system stronger, decreases susceptibility of the organism to stress and improves mood and general feeling.

Metabolic Disorders of Amino Acid Metabolism

Several enzyme defects in amino acid metabolism may lead to various metabolic disorders of amino acid metabolism. The following are some important metabolic disorders of amino acid metabolism.

1. Phenylketonuria
2. Albinism
3. Alkaptonuria
4. Tyrosinemia
5. Hyperbilirubinemia
6. Jaundice

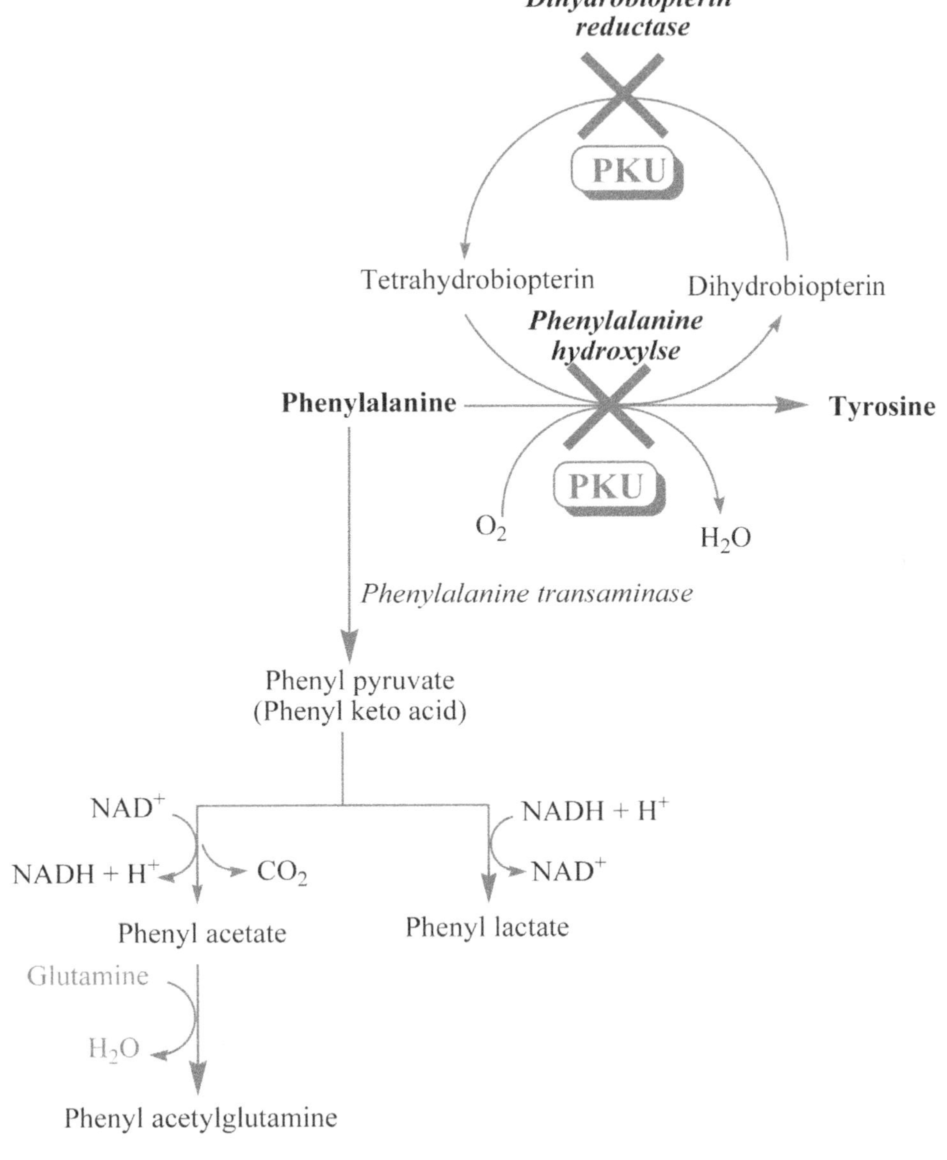

1. **Phenylketonuria (PKU):**

   Phenylketonuria is defined as increased excretion of phenyl keto-acid like phenyl pyruvate in urine due to deficiency of hepatic enzyme *phenylalanine hydroxylase*. In PKU, high concentration of other phenylalanine metabolites such as phenyl acetate, phenyl lactate and phenyl acetyl glutamine also excreted in urine.

   In amino acid metabolism this is the most common metabolic disorder. The prevalence of phenylketonuria is 1 in 10,000. This disorder is due to deficiency of hepatic enzyme *phenylalanine hydroxylase* (The substrate is "phenylalanine" and the type of reaction involved is "hydroxylation") caused by an autosomal recessive gene. Recently less common another type of PKU due to defect of *dihydrobiopterin reductase* is reported. This deficiency leads to impaired synthesis of tetrahydrobiopterin which is necessary for the activity of *phenylalanine hydroxylase*. Ultimately tyrosine is not produced form phenylalanine.

   Primarily PKU causes increased phenylalanine concentration in blood and tissues which leads to increased excretion in urine. In PKU, conversion of phenylalanine to tyrosine is blocked, hence phenylalanine is diverted for other alternate pathways. This leads to increased production of phenyl pyruvate, phenyl acetate, phenyl lactate and phenyl acetylglutamine. Hence, high concentrations of these metabolites are excreted in urine. Mousey odor of urine is due to phenyl acetate only. The followings are the various clinical manifestation of PKU.

   1. Mental retardation, failure to talk or walk, failure of growth, seizure and tremor.
   2. Defect in myelin formation.
   3. Impaired synthesis of serotonin due to competition of phenylalanine and its metabolite with tryptophan.
   4. Hypopigmentation due to competitive inhibition of *tyrosinase* by phenylalanine causes light skin color, fair hair, blue eyes, etc.

   Guthrie test (Bacterial particularly *Bacillus substilis* bioassay for phenylalanine) is used for the diagnosis of PKU. In addition, ferric chloride test is used for the detection of phenyl pyruvate in urine. PKU is treated generally by taking foods with low phenylalanine and / or feeding synthetic amino acid preparations low in phenylalanine. In serious PKU cases, 5-hydroxy tryptophan and DOPA is administered to restore the synthesis of serotonin and catecholamines. PKU with tetrahydrobiopterin deficiency needs tetrahydrobiopterin supplementation.

2. **Albinism:**

   In Greek albino means "white". Albinism is also related to albinos. Albinism is due to lack of synthesis of pigment melanin and it is an inborn disorder. 1 in 20,000 is the frequency of this autosomal recessive disorder. The most common cause of albinism is defect in *tyrosinase* which is mostly responsible for the synthesis of melanin.

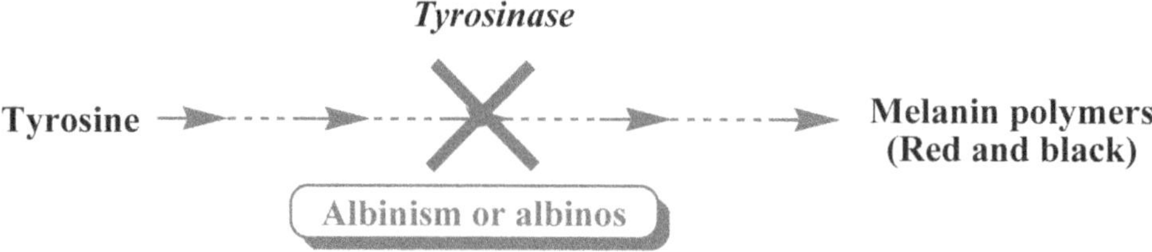

   Many genes control the color of the skin and hair. Many factors influence the synthesis of melanin from tyrosine. The following are the most possible causes for albinism.

   1. Lack of deficiency of enzyme "*tyrosinase*".
   2. Decreased melanosomes in melanocytes.
   3. Defect in melanin polymerization.
   4. Protein matrix lack in melanosomes.
   5. Limitation of tyrosine availability.
   6. Presence of *tyrosinase* inhibitors.

Melanin protects the body from sun radiation which is the most important functions of melanin. The followings are the clinical manifestation of albinism.

1. Sensitive to sun light.
2. Increased susceptibility to carcinoma (skin cancer).
3. Photophobia (intolerance to light) is associated with lack of pigment in eyes. But there is no impairment in the eyesight.

3. **Alkaptonuria:**

It is otherwise known as **black urine disease**. The prevalence of this autosomal recessive disorder is 1 in 25,000. Alkaptonuria is defined as increased excretion of homogentisate in urine (due to lack of *homogentisate oxidase*) which on standing produces pigment alkapton in urine.

This disorder is tyrosine metabolic disorder due to lack of *homogentisate oxidase*. This is an enzyme responsible for the conversion of homogentisate into 4-maleylacetoacetate. Hence, lack of *homogentisate oxidase* increases the concentration of homogentisate in blood which accumulates and excreted in urine. On standing homogentisate undergoes oxidation and produces respective quinone derivative which further polymerized and give black or brown color. Hence alkaptonuria patient's urine looks coke in color, hence it is also known as black urine disease.

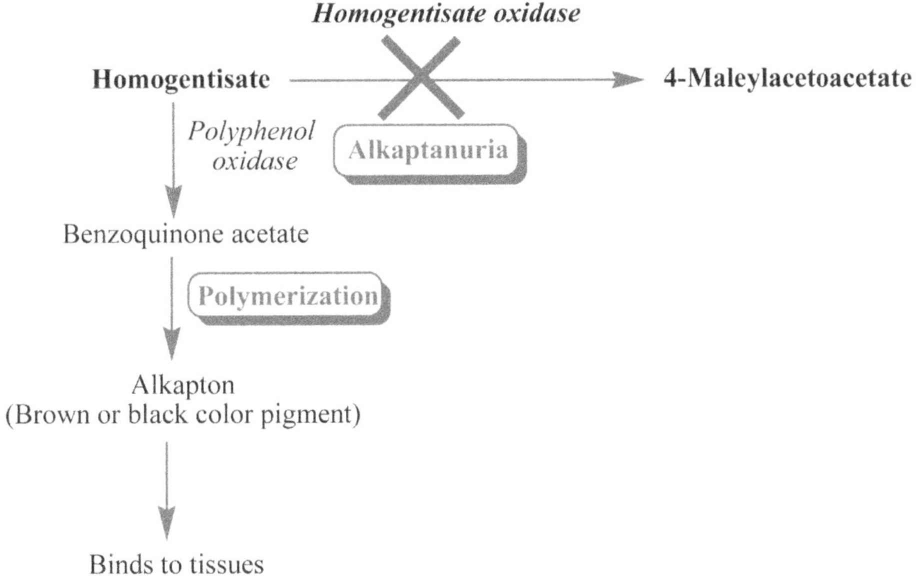

The followings are the clinical manifestation of alkaptonuria.

1. Production of pigment alkapton through benzoquinone acetate from homogentisate by oxidation in presence of *polyphenol oxidase* followed by polymerization.
2. Ochronosis is a clinical condition due to deposition of alkapton in connective tissues, bones and various organs like ear, nose, etc.
3. Arthritis in many patients due to deposition of alkapton pigment in the joints.

Alkaptonuria is easily diagnosed from urine color change on standing to brown or block. The urine gives positive test with ferric chloride, silver nitrate, Benedict's test and other reducing test due to strong reducing activity of homogentisate. No treatment is needed as it is not a dangerous disease. Even though, it is treated by consuming protein diet with relatively low phenylalanine content.

4. **Tyrosinemia:**

Tyrosinemia is defined as increased concentration of tyrosine in blood and excretion of tyrosine and its metabolic products in urine due to deficiency of enzymes involved in tyrosine degradation pathway. There are two different types of tyrosinemia. They are,

1. Tyrosinemia type - I or Tyrosinosis
2. Tyrosinemia type - II or Hanhart syndrome

Tyrosinemia type – I or Tyrosinosis: It is a rare but serious disorder due to deficiency of the enzymes *fumarylacetoacetate hydroxylase* and/or *maleylacetoacetate isomerase*. Tyrosine, its metabolites and many other amino acids are excreted in urine. Infant exhibits diarrhea, vomiting and cabbage like odor in acute tyrosinosis. Generally, tyrosinemia type – I may cause liver failure, rickets, renal tubular dysfunction and polyneuropathy. Within one-year death may occur due to liver failure. It is treated by consuming diets containing less phenylalanine, tyrosine and methionine.

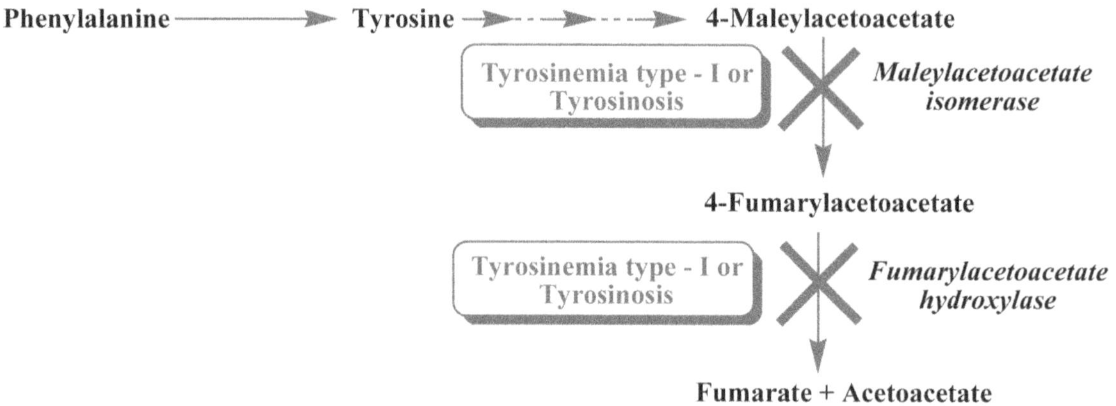

Tyrosinemia type – II or Hanhart syndrome: It is due to the deficiency of *tyrosine transaminase* which is involved in the conversion of tyrosine into *p*-hydroxyphenyl pyruvate. Hence tyrosine degradative pathway is blocked leads to accumulation and excretion of tyrosine and its metabolites such as *p*-hydroxyphenyl pyruvate, *p*-hydroxyphenyl acetate, *p*-hydroxyphenyl lactate, N-acetyl tyrosine and tyramine. In general, it is characterized by dermatitis, eye lesions and rarely mental disorder. In these patients disturbed self coordination is seen.

5. **Hyperbilirubinemia:**

Hyperbilirubinemia is defined as the increased concentration of bilirubin in blood. **Bilirubin is the excretory end product of heme metabolism** and it is a yellow color bile pigment. In liver bilirubin undergoes conjugation and produces bilirubin diglucuronide. Later, it enters in intestine where it is converted to urobilinogen further to urobilin and stercobilin (urobilin is the substances which is responsible for yellow color of urine and stercobilin is the substance which is responsible for brown color of feces).

The normal serum bilirubin levels are 0.2 to 1 mg/dl. Bilirubin can be available in both conjugated and unconjugated form in liver. The normal conjugated bilirubin serum level is 0.2 to 0.4 mg/dl. In that conjugated form 75 % are diglucuronide and 25 % are monoglucuronide. The normal unconjugated bilirubin level in serum is 0.2 to 0.6 mg/dl. Hyperbilirubinemia is characterized by increased bilirubin in the blood, increased color of urine due to more concentration of urobilin excretion and dark brown color feces due to more concentration of stercobilin excretion.

6. **Jaundice:**

When the level of bilirubin is more in blood it may leads to deposition of bile pigments in skin and white part of the eye (sclerae). Exactly speaking jaundice is not a disease; it is a symptom which denotes the increased level of bilirubin in biological system. In French, "Jaune" means "yellow". Jaundice is also known as icterus. It is a clinical condition characterized by yellow color of the white of the eyes (sclerae) and skin due to deposition of bilirubin. Jaundice is due to increased level of serum bilirubin beyond 2 mg/dl (Normal bilirubin level is < 1 mg/dl). Jaundice is caused due to multiple factors; hence it is difficult to classify jaundice. Even though for convenience jaundice are broadly classified into three major types as a) Hemolytic jaundice, b) Hepatic jaundice or hepatocellular jaundice, c) Obstructive jaundice or regurgitation jaundice.

(a) **Hemolytic jaundice:** Generally, hemolytic jaundice is associated with increased hemolysis of erythrocytes (**Example:** Malaria, sickle cell anemia and incompatible blood transfusion). If erythrocytes breakdown more it leads to more production of bilirubin. Hence, more bilirubin is excreted in bile leads to increased production of urobilinogen and stercobilinogen. Hemolytic jaundice is characterized by a) increased serum unconjugated bilirubin, b) increased excretion of urobilinogen in urine, c) dark color of feces due to high amount of stercobilinogen.

(b) **Hepatic jaundice or hepatocellular jaundice:** It is caused by liver dysfunction due to parenchymal cell damage. This may be due to presence of toxic substances such as poisons and toxins like chloroform, carbon tetrachloride, phosphorous, etc., viral infection (viral hepatitis), liver cirrhosis, heart failure, etc. The most common one is viral hepatitis. Liver damage affects bilirubin uptake and its conjugation by liver cells. Hence, hepatic jaundice is characterized by a) increased serum conjugated and unconjugated bilirubin, b) dark color urine due to increased excretion of bilirubin and urobilinogen, c) increased activity of *serum glutamate pyruvate transaminase* (*SGPT*) and *serum glutamate oxaloacetate transaminase* (*SGOT*) due to hepatocyte damage, d) pale, clay colored stools due to absence of stercobilinogen, e) nausea and anorexia (loss of appetite).

(c) **Obstructive jaundice or regurgitation jaundice:** It is due to obstruction in the bile ducts which prevents the passage of bile into the intestine. Gall stones, tumors, etc. may be the reasons for obstructions. From the liver, the conjugated bilirubin enters into the circulation due to the blockage. Obstructive jaundice is characterized by a) increased level of conjugated bilirubin in serum, b) elevated *serum alkaline phosphatase* due to release from damaged bile ducts, c) increased activity of *serum glutamate pyruvate transaminase (SGPT) and serum glutamate oxaloacetate transaminase* (*SGOT*) d) dark color urine due to increased excretion of bilirubin and urobilinogen, e) pale, clay colored stools due to absence of stercobilinogen, f) excess fat in feces indicates fat digestion impairments and absorption in the absence of bile particularly bile salts, g) nausea and GIT pain.

Jaundice may also cause due to some hereditary abnormalities also. The following are some type of jaundice due to genetic defects. They are,

1. Neonatal physiologic jaundice
2. Crigler-Najjar syndrome type - I
3. Crigler-Najjar syndrome type - II

Catabolism of Heme

The life span of erythrocytes is only 120 days. After 120 days the erythrocytes are removed from the circulation and taken up by the macrophages of the reticuloendothelial (RE) system in the spleen and liver. In macrophages erythrocytes are degraded into non-protein heme and the protein part globin by cleaving. This protein part globin may be degraded into individual amino acids or as such it is reutilized for the formation of hemoglobin. The formed amino acids may undergo its own metabolism including participation in fresh globin synthesis. About 80 % of the heme subjected for degradations is obtained from erythrocytes only. The remaining 20 % are obtained from immature RBC, cytochromes and myoglobin.

Later, heme is converted into biliverdin (**Green pigment**) in the presence of enzyme *heme oxygenase* which utilizes NADPH + H^+ and oxygen and breaks the methenyl bridges present in between two pyrrole rings (A and B ring). In the mean time ferrous (Fe^{2+}) is oxidized into ferric (Fe^{3+}) ion. Carbon monoxide is also released during this reaction. In amphibian and birds, the biliverdin is excreted as such, whereas in mammals it further undergoes degradations.

In the next step, the methenyl bridge present between pyrrole ring C and D of biliverdin is reduced to methylene group and forms bilirubin (**Yellow pigment**). *Biliverdin reductase* catalyzes this reaction which is a NADPH + H^+ dependent soluble enzyme. The term bile pigments are used to collectively represent bilirubin and its derivatives like biliverdin.

Bilirubin is insoluble in aqueous solution because it is lipophilic in nature. Hence it is transported into plasma in a non-covalently bound form to albumin as bilirubin-albumin complex. Albumin has two binding sites namely high affinity site (about 25 mg of bilirubin per 100 ml of plasma tightly binds at this site) and low affinity sites (Rest of bilirubin binds loosely at this site). The later one easily detaches from the albumin and enters into the tissues. Some times bilirubin may enter into the CNS and cause damage to the neurons because certain drugs like sulfonamides and salicylates can displace the bilirubin from albumin.

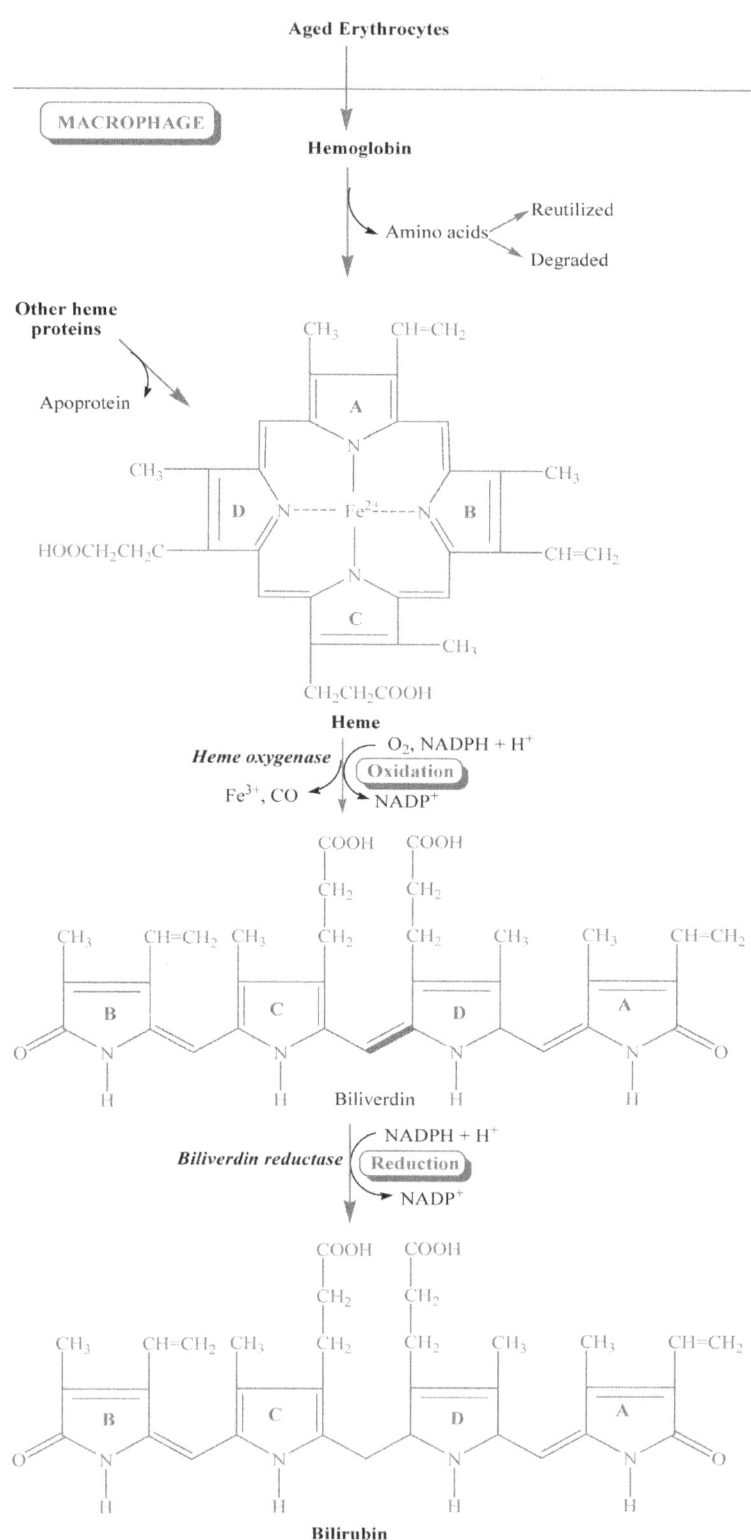

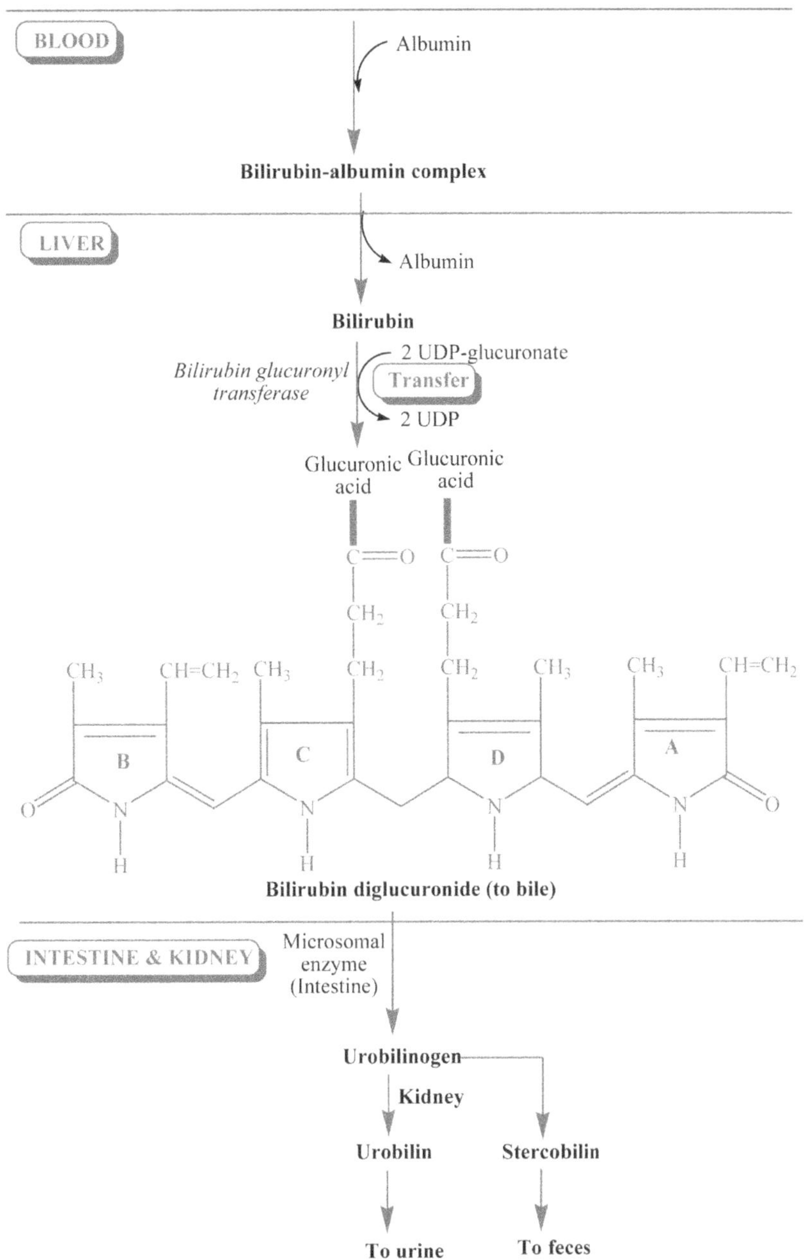

Once albumin-bilirubin complex enters into the liver, the dissociated bilirubin was taken up the sinusoidal surface of the hepatocytes through a carrier mediated active transport system. In liver, bilirubin binds with a specific intracellular protein namely ligandin. More over bilirubin in liver undergoes glucuronic acid conjugation by reacting with two moles of UDP glucuronate and produces bilirubin diglucuronide which is water soluble and liberates free UDP. This reaction is catalyzed by the enzyme called *bilirubin glucuronyl transferase* of smooth endoplasmic reticulum. This enzyme can be induced by number of drugs such as phenobarbital. When excess bilirubin is there bilirubin monoglucuronide may also accumulate in the body.

Later, conjugated bilirubin is excreted into the bile canaliculi against a concentration gradient which then enters into the bile. This transport of bilirubin diglucuronide is an energy dependent, active and rate limiting process. Almost all the bilirubin (> 98 %) enters into the bile are conjugated form only.

The specific bacterial enzymes present in the intestine namely β-*glucuronidase* hydrolyzes the bilirubin glucuronide into bilirubin. Latter, bilirubin is converted into urobilinogen which is a colorless compound and a small part of it may reabsorb into the circulation. In the kidney, urobilinogen can be converted into yellow color compound urobilin and excreted in urine. The characteristic yellow color of the urine is due to urobilin only. A major part of the urobilinogen is converted into stercobilin by the intestinal bacteria. This formed stercobilin is excreted along with feces. The characteristic brown color of the feces is due to stercobilin only.

PROBABLE QUESTIONS

PART – A: Multiple Choice Questions

1. Which of the following is two-carbon fragment removed during β-oxidation of fatty acids?
   (a) Malonyl CoA (b) Formyl CoA
   (c) Acyl CoA (d) Acetyl CoA
2. Which compound is the active form of fatty acid that participated in β-oxidation?
   (a) Malonyl CoA (b) Formyl CoA
   (c) Acyl CoA (d) Acetyl CoA
3. Hypercholesterolemia is observed in which of the following(s) disorder(s).
   (a) Hypothyroidism (b) Diabetes mellitus
   (c) Nephrotic syndrome (d) All of them
4. Which hormone inhibits the hormone sensitive lipase activity.
   (a) Epinephrine (b) Insulin
   (c) Thyroxine (d) Glucocorticoids
5. What are two final products obtained in the β-oxidation of odd chain fatty acids.
   (a) Acetyl CoA & Malonyl CoA (b) Acetyl CoA & Acetyl CoA
   (c) Acetyl CoA & Propionyl CoA (d) Acetyl CoA & Succinyl CoA
6. Complete oxidation of one mole palmitate liberates how many ATPs?
   (a) 5 (b) 133
   (c) 131 (d) 129
7. Carnitine transport systems is very good example for which of the following?
   (a) Active transport (b) Passive transport
   (c) Facilitated diffusion (d) Simple diffusion
8. How any ATPs are needed for the activation of fatty acid in cytosol?
   (a) 1 (b) 2
   (c) 3 (d) 4
9. 10 % SIDS may be due to the deficiency of which of the following enzyme?
   (a) Thiokinase (b) Enoyl CoA hydratase
   (c) Thiolase (d) Acyl CoA dehydrogenase
10. Which enzyme regulates the fatty acid synthesis?
    (a) Enoyl reductase (b) Palmityl
    (c) Acetyl transacylase (d) Acetyl CoA carboxylase
11. Which of the following is an example for multi enzyme complex?
    (a) Plamitylthioesterase (b) Ketoacyl reductase
    (c) Enoyl reductase (d) FAS
12. In which part of the cell, the enzyme machinery or fatty acid production is present.
    (a) Mitochondria (b) Cytosomal fraction
    (c) Golgi apparatus (d) Lysosome

13. Which of the following is not a ketone bodies metabolic disorder?
    (a) Ketonemia (b) Ketonurea
    (c) Ketoacidosis (d) Refsum's disease
14. Which of the following are primary bile acids?
    (a) Deoxycholic acid (b) Lithocholic acid
    (c) Chenodexycholic acid (d) Taurocholic acid
15. Which of the following is not synthesized from cholesterol?
    (a) Ketone bodies (b) Bile acids
    (c) Steroid hormones (d) Vitamin D
16. Which of the following is not true in transamination reaction?
    (P) Reversible reaction
    (Q) Requires PLP
    (R) Important for production of non-essential amino acid
    (S) Free ammonia liberated

    Choose the correct option.
    (a) P, Q & R is correct; S is wrong (b) Q, R & S is correct; P is wrong
    (c) P, Q & S is correct; R is wrong (d) P, R & S is correct; Q is wrong
17. Which of the following is obtaining when ketogenic amino acids are degraded?
    (a) Succinyl CoA (b) Fumarate
    (c) Acetyl CoA (d) Pyruvate
18. Which of the following amino acid undergoes transamination reaction?
    (a) Lysine (b) Alanine
    (c) Threonine (d) Proline
19. All *transaminase* reaction requires which coenzyme?
    (a) PLP (b) NAD^+
    (c) FAD (d) TPP
20. Which of the following reaction converts amino acids to corresponding amine?
    (P) Transamination (Q) Deamination
    (R) Decarboxylation (S) Transmethylation

    Choose the correct option.
    (a) P & Q only (b) R & S only
    (c) R only (d) S only
21. What is the other name of urea cycle?
    (a) Krebs cycle (b) Henseleit cycle
    (c) Krebs-Henseleit cycle (d) Embde-Meyerhof cycle
22. N-acetyl glutamate is required for the activation of which enzyme?
    (a) *CPS-I* (b) *CPS-II*
    (c) *Arginase* (d) *Arginino-succinase*
23. Which of the following enzyme is mitochondrial enzyme?
    (a) *Arginase* (b) *Arginino-succinate synthase*
    (c) *Arginino-succinase* (d) *CPS-I*

24. Which of the following compound doesn't donate any atom in the formation of urea?
   (a) CO_2 (b) Ornithine
   (c) NH_3 (d) Aspartate
25. Citrullinemia is metabolic disorder of urea cycle which is due to the defects of which enzyme?
   (a) *Arginase* (b) *Arginino-succinate synthase*
   (c) *Arginino-succinase* (d) *CPS-I*
26. Which of the following compound serves as a collection center for amino groups in the biological system?
   (a) Glycine (b) Alanine
   (c) Aspartate (d) Glutamate
27. Which enzyme regulates urea cycle?
   (a) *Arginase* (b) *Arginino-succinate synthase*
   (c) *Arginino-succinase* (d) *CPS-I*
28. How many ATPs are utilized in urea cycle?
   (a) Two (b) Three
   (c) Four (d) Five
29. Which of the following products are not biosynthesized from tyrosine?
   (a) Dopamine (b) Choline
   (c) Thyroxine (d) Melanin
30. Kynurenine and serotonin pathway are metabolic pathways of which amino acid?
   (a) Phenylalanine (b) Methionine
   (c) Tryptophan (d) Valine
31. Glutamate is metabolically converted to α-ketoglutarate and NH_4^+ by a process __________
   (a) Oxidative deamination (b) Transamination
   (c) Reductive deamination (d) Deamination
32. Free ammonia combined with glutamate to yield glutamine by the action of __________
   (a) *Glutaminase* (b) *Glutamine synthase*
   (c) *Glutamate dehydrogenase* (d) *Amino transferase*
33. Pyridoxal phosphate and its aminate form, pyridoxamine phosphate are tightly bound co-enzymes of __________
   (a) *Amino transferase* (b) *Glutaminase*
   (c) *Glutamine synthase* (d) *Glutamate dehydrogenase*
34. The combined action of *aminotransferase* and *glutamate dehydrogenase* is referred as __________
   (a) Oxidative deamination (b) Transamination
   (c) Reductive deamination (d) Transdeamination
35. Urea cycle converts __________
   (a) Keto acids into amino acids (b) Amino acids into keto acids
   (c) Ammonia into a less toxic form (d) Ammonia into a more toxic form
36. Which is the end product of heme metabolism?
   (a) Urea (b) Uric acid
   (c) Bilirubin (d) Amino acid

37. Which of the following is a metabolic disorder of heme synthesis characterized by increased excretion of porphyrins and precursors of porphyrins?
    (a) Porphyria
    (b) Jaundice
    (c) Alkaptonuria
    (d) Hyperbilirubinemia

Key for Multiple Choice Questions

1. (d)	2. (c)	3. (d)	4. (c)	5. (b)
6. (d)	7. (c)	8. (b)	9. (d)	10. (d)
11. (d)	12. (b)	13. (d)	14. (c)	15. (a)
16. (a)	17. (c)	18. (b)	19. (a)	20. (c)
21. (c)	22. (a)	23. (d)	24. (b)	25. (b)
26. (d)	27. (d)	28. (c)	29. (b)	30. (c)
31. (a)	32. (b)	33. (a)	34. (d)	35. (c)
36. (c)	37. (a)			

PART – B: Short Answers

1. Explain the terms: a) Hypoglycemia; b)Fatty liver.
2. What is fatty liver? Write the different causes of fatty liver.
3. What is atherosclerosis? Explain briefly its pathogenesis.
4. Note on a) Obesity; b) Hypercholesterimia.
5. Explain the terms: a) Ketosis; b)Ketonemia.
6. Define Denovo synthesis of fatty acids.
7. Sketch the biosynthesis of ketone bodies.
8. What is carnitine transport system?
9. Explain the conversion of cholesterol to bile acids.
10. Short notes on bile salts.
11. Write the synthesis of steroid hormones from cholesterol.
12. Write the conversion of cholesterol to vitamin-D.
13. What is hemolytic jaundice? How is it diagnosed?
14. What are transamination reactions? Give one example.
15. How urea cycle is regulated?
16. Explain the term "oxidative deamination".
17. What is non-oxidative deamination ?
18. What are decarboxylation reactions? Give one example.
19. Define and list out various types of jaundice.
20. What is the relationship between hyperbilirubinemia and jaundice?
21. Write a note on urea cycle metabolic disorders.
22. Write a note on phenylketonuria.
23. What is albinism?
24. Explain alkaptonuria.
25. Define and explain tyrosinemia.

26. List out the biological significance of catecholamines.
27. What is the importance of melatonin?

PART - C: Long Answers

1. Explain β-oxidation of saturated fatty acids and write the total energy yield from one molecule of palmitic acid.
2. Explain the synthesis of bile salts from cholesterol.
3. Write the steps involved in ketogenesis and explain its regulation. Add a note on ketoacidosis.
4. Note on metabolism of cholesterol.
5. Describe the biosynthesis of fatty acids.
6. Describe cholesterol levels and atherosclerosis in human body.
7. Write a note on lipid metabolism. Explain various lipid metabolic disorders.
8. Write in detail about β-oxidation of saturated fatty acids.
9. What are ketone bodies? Explain biosynthesis of ketone bodies.
10. Write a note on ketone bodies metabolism.
11. Write in detail about the general aspects of amino acid metabolism.
12. Explain in detail about three major metabolic reactions taking place in amino acid metabolism.
13. Write a note on transamination & deamination of amino acid metabolism.
14. Write about catabolism of amino acids.
15. Explain urea cycle and its metabolic disorders.
16. Write about the urea cycle. Discuss about transamination and decarboxylation.
17. Describe the general metabolic pathways of amino acids.
18. Note on Kreb's-Henseleit cycle.
19. Detailed note on metabolism of phenylalanine.
20. How catecholamines are biosynthesized in biological system. Add a note on biological significance of catecholamines.
21. Explain the metabolism of tryptophan.
22. How serotonin and melatonin is biosynthesized? Explain their biological significance also.
23. Write a detailed note on metabolic disorders of amino acid metabolism.
24. Explain a) Jaundice b) Tyrosinemia ?
25. Write about hyperbilirubinemia & phenylketonuria.
26. Write a note on metabolism of heme.
27. Explain β-oxidation of palmitic acids.
28. Add a detailed note on degradation of cholesterol.
29. Write the biosynthesis of steroid sex hormones.
30. Discuss the mechanism of β-oxidation of a molecule of palmitic acid, its regulation & energy yield in it.
31. Sketch the Denovo synthesis of a molecule of palmitic acid and how is it regulated.
32. Sketch the complete oxidation of one molecule of palmitic acid in a mitochondrion & indicate the energy yield in this process.
33. Discuss the biosynthesis of long chain saturated fatty acids and write a note on the regulation of this phenomenon.

UNIT 4

Nucleic Acid Metabolism

Nucleic Acid Metabolism

Nucleic acid metabolism is the process by which nucleic acids (DNA & RNA) are synthesized and degraded. Nucleic acids are the polymers of nucleotides. Nucleotide synthesis is an anabolic process.

Biosynthesis of Purine Nucleotides

Purine rings of the nucleotides are contributed by many compounds. Sources of individual atoms in purine ring are presented in Figure 4.1. They are,

1. N_1 of purine is derived from the amino group of aspartate.
2. C_2 and C_8 of purine are derived from N^{10}-formyl THF.
3. N_3 and N_9 of purine are derived from the amide group of glutamine.
4. C_4, C_5 and N_7 of purine are derived from glycine.
5. C_6 of purine is derived from carbondioxide.

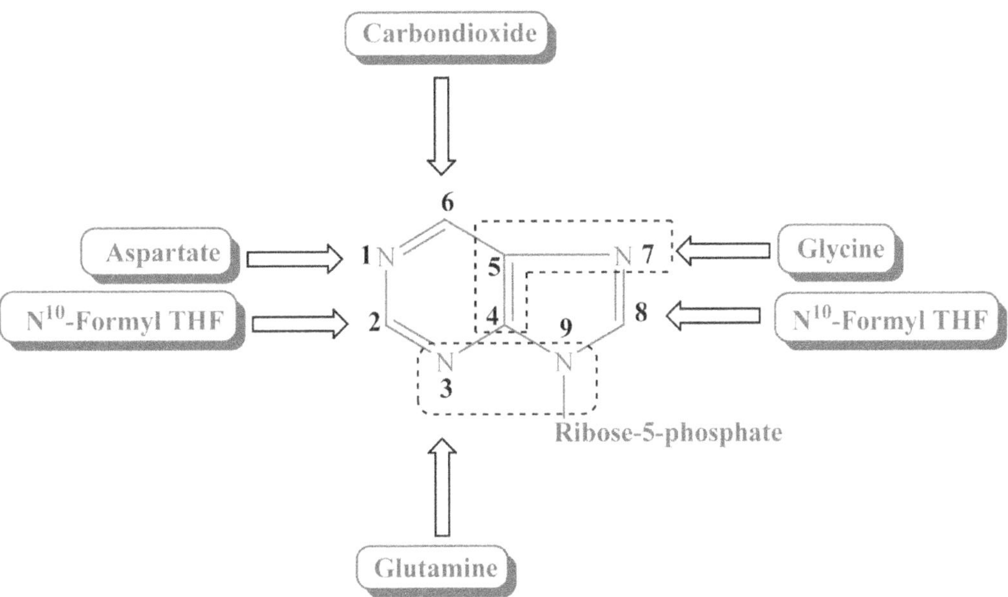

Figure 4.1 Sources of individual atoms in purine ring.

Pathway:

Purine bases are synthesized as ribonucleotides and not as a free base. Hence, biosynthesis of purine nucleotides in the body is a complex process. In the pre-existing ribose-5-phosphate, purines are built and synthesized. Purine nucleotides are mainly synthesized in the liver. Purine nucleotides are not synthesized in erythrocytes, polymorphonuclear leukocytes and the brain. The parent purine nucleotide is inosine monophosphate (IMP) and is synthesized by the following ways from α-D-ribose-5-phosphate.

1. The HMP shunt pathway of carbohydrate metabolism produces pentose sugar ribose-5-phosphate which acts as a precursor for the synthesis of purine nucleotides. In the first step, ribose-5-phosphate is reacted with ATP in presence of *phosphoribosyl pyrophosphate (PRPP) synthetase* (Product formed is "phosphoribosyl pyrophosphate (PRPP)"and the type of reaction involved is "synthesis") and produces 5-phosphoribosyl-α-pyrophosphate (PRPP) with liberation of AMP by simple pyro phosphorylation reaction. In this reaction, one ATP is converted to AMP **(2 ATP is utilized)**.
2. In the next step, PRPP initially undergoes hydrolysis followed by reaction with glutamine and gains amide nitrogen by replacing with pyrophosphate at C-1 of ribose sugar results in formation of β-5-phosphoribosylamine. The reaction is catalyzed by *PRPP glutamyl amido transferase* (Substrate is "PRPP" and the type of reaction involved is "amide transfer") and **it is a committed step (rate limiting step) of purine nucleotide biosynthesis**. By feedback inhibition of nucleotides such as IMP, AMP and GMP, the enzyme *PRPP glutamyl amido transferase* is controlled.
3. Later, the formed β-5-phosphoribosylamine undergoes amidation by reacting with glycine and produces glycinamide ribosyl-5-phosphate with one water molecule in the presence of *synthetase* (The type of reaction involved is "synthesis"). During this reaction, the energy needed is provided by breakdown of ATP into ADP and inorganic phosphate **(1 ATP is utilized)**.
4. In the succeeding step, formyl group from N^{10}-formyl THF is transferred to glycinamide ribosyl-5-phosphate by formylation reaction in presence of *formyl transferase* (Group transferred is "formyl" and the type of reaction involved is "transfer") produces formylglycinamide ribosyl-5- phosphate.
5. Then, obtained formylglycinamide ribosyl-5- phosphate reacts with glutamine and gains amide nitrogen to produce formylglycinamidine ribosyl-5-phosphate with a loss of water molecule in presence of *synthetase* (The type of reaction involved is "synthesis"). The energy needed by this reaction is provided by breakdown of ATP into ADP and inorganic phosphate **(1 ATP is utilized)**.
6. In the next step, formylglycinamidine ribosyl-5-phosphate in enol form undergoes cyclization with a loss of water molecule to produce 5-aminoimidazole ribosyl-5- phosphate in presence of *synthetase* (The type of reaction involved is "synthesis"). The energy needed for this reaction is obtained from the breakdown of ATP into ADP and inorganic phosphate **(1 ATP is utilized)**.
7. Through carboxylation, 5-aminoimidazole ribosyl-5-phosphate is converted to 5-aminoimidazole carboxylate ribosyl-5-phosphate by reacting with carbondioxide in the presence of *carboxylase* enzyme (The type of reaction involved is "carboxylation"). Unlike other carboxylation reactions, this carboxylation doesn't need biotin and / or ATP.
8. In this step, aspartate is condensed with the formed 5-aminoimidazole carboxylate ribosyl-5-phosphate to produce 5-aminoimidazole-4-succinyl carboxamide ribosyl-5-phosphate with loss of water molecule. *Synthetase* enzyme (The type of reaction involved is "synthesis") catalyzes this reaction and it needs energy which is derived from breakdown of ATP into ADP and inorganic phosphate **(1 ATP is utilized)**.
9. Later, the obtained 5-aminoimidazole-4-succinyl carboxamide ribosyl-5-phosphate undergoes lysis reaction with the removal of fumarate and produces 5-aminoimidazole-4-carboxamide ribosyl-5-phosphate. *Adenosuccinate lyase* (Substrate is "5-aminoimidazole-4-succinyl carboxamide ribosyl-5-phosphate" which is adenosuccinate derivative and the type of reaction involved is "lysis") is an enzyme responsible for this reaction.

α-D-Ribose 5-phosphate

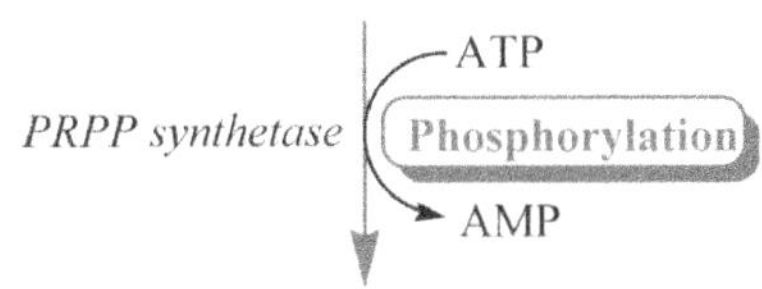

5- Phosphoribosyl-α-pyrophosphate (PRPP)

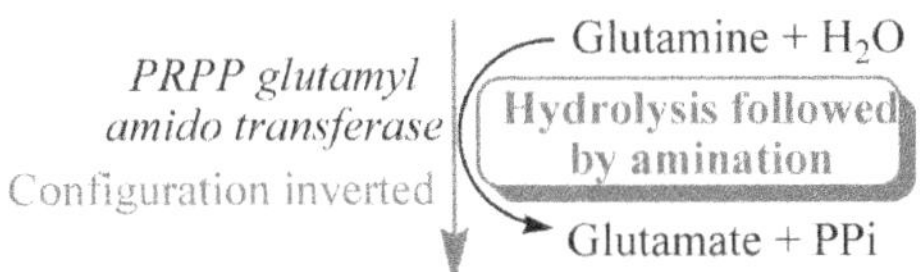

β-5-Phosphoribosylamine

Synthetase — NH_2CH_2COOH + ATP (Glycine) — Amidation or Condensation — H_2O + ADP + Pi

Glycinamide ribosyl-5-phosphate

Formyl transferase — N^{10}- Formyl THF — Formylation — THF

Ribose-5-phosphate

Formylglycinamide ribosyl-5-phosphate

Synthetase — Glutamine + ATP — Amidation — Glutamate + H_2O + ADP + Pi

Ribose-5-phosphate

Formylglycinamidine ribosyl-5-phosphate (Keto form)

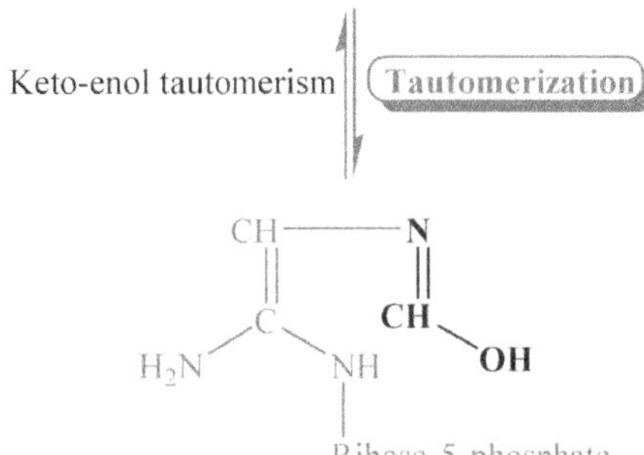

Formylglycinamidine ribosyl-5-phosphate (Enol form)

Synthetase — ATP — Cyclization — ADP + Pi + H_2O

Ribose-5-phosphate

5- Aminoimidazole ribosyl-5-phosphate

Carboxylase — CO_2 — Carboxylation

Ribose-5-phosphate

5- Aminoimidazole carboxylate ribosyl-5-phosphate

Synthetase — $COOHCH(NH_2)CH_2COOH$ + ATP (Aspartate) — Condensation — ADP + Pi + H_2O

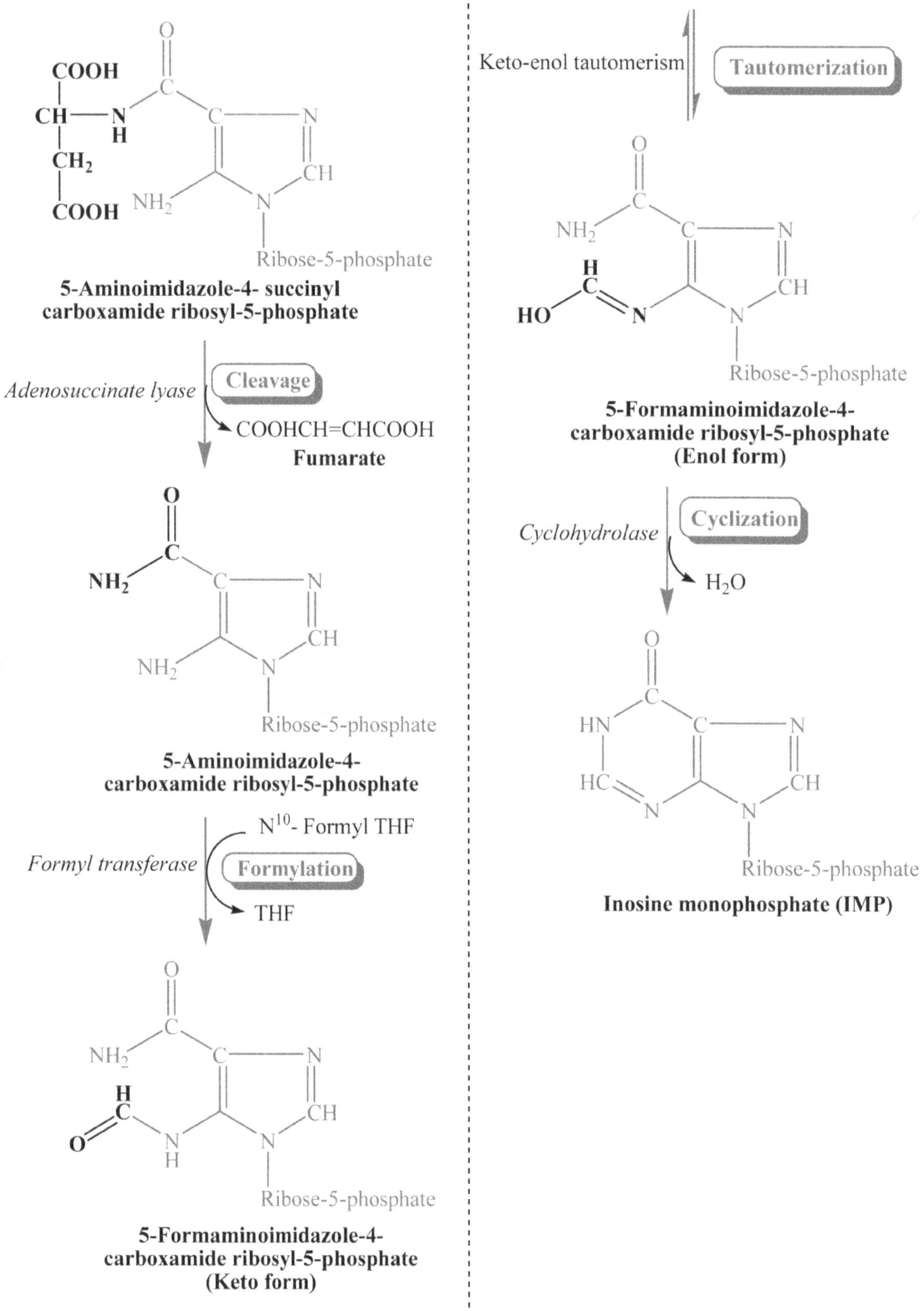

5-Aminoimidazole-4- succinyl carboxamide ribosyl-5-phosphate

Adenosuccinate lyase — Cleavage → COOHCH=CHCOOH **Fumarate**

5-Aminoimidazole-4-carboxamide ribosyl-5-phosphate

Formyl transferase — N^{10}- Formyl THF → Formylation → THF

5-Formaminoimidazole-4-carboxamide ribosyl-5-phosphate (Keto form)

Keto-enol tautomerism — Tautomerization

5-Formaminoimidazole-4-carboxamide ribosyl-5-phosphate (Enol form)

Cyclohydrolase — Cyclization → H_2O

Inosine monophosphate (IMP)

10. In the pre final step, 5-aminoimidazole-4-carboxamide ribosyl-5-phosphate undergoes formylation reaction by reacting with N^{10}-formyl THF in presence of *formyl transferase* (Group transferred is "formyl" and the type of reaction involved is "transfer") to produce 5-formaminoimidazole-4-carboxamide ribosyl-5-phosphate. All the carbon and nitrogen atoms of purine rings are contributed by the respective sources with this step.
11. Finally, 5-formaminoimidazole-4-carboxamide ribosyl-5-phosphate in enol form undergoes cyclization in presence of *cyclohydrolase* (The type of reaction involved is "cyclization with removal of water molecule") produces parent purine ribonucleotide i.e., inosine monophosphate (IMP) with loss of water molecule. The other purine ribonucleotides are synthesized from this inosine monophosphate (IMP).

Inhibitors of purine nucleotide synthesis

For the synthesis of purine nucleotides, folic acid is necessary. Sulfonamides are the drugs which inhibit the synthesis of folic acid in microorganisms due to structural similarities with *p*-aminobenzoic acid (PABA). Hence, indirectly, sulfonamides inhibit the synthesis of purine nucleotides there by synthesis of nucleic acid such as DNA and RNA. The sulfonamide is not producing any effect in the human because folic acid is not synthesized in humans and is supplied through diet.

Methotrexate is the analog of folic acid and it is used to control the cancer. Methotrexate inhibit *formyl transferase* (the steps in which N^{10}-formyl THF is involved) leads to inhibition of purine nucleotide synthesis there by synthesis of nucleic acid. In this reaction one carbon moiety (formyl group) is transferred. Proliferations of normal growing cells are also affected by these inhibitors which lead to several side effects such as anemia, baldness, scaly skin, etc.

Synthesis of AMP and GMP from IMP

The immediate precursor for the production of adenosine monophosphate (AMP) and guanosine monophosphate (GMP) is inosine monophosphate (IMP).

1. In the enol form IMP reacts with aspartate to produce adenyl succinate or adenylosuccinate with loss of water molecule by condensation in presence of *adenyl succinate synthase* or *adenylosuccinate synthase* (The product formed is "adenyl succinate" and the type of reaction involved is "synthesis"). The energy needed for this reaction is derived from breakdown of GTP into GDP and inorganic phosphate **(1 ATP is utilized)**.
2. Later, the obtained adenyl succinate breakdown with the removal of fumarate and produces adenosine monophosphate (AMP). *Adenyl succinase* (The substrate is "adenyl succinate" and the type of reaction involved is "lysis") is an enzyme responsible for this reaction.
3. In other ways, inosine monophosphate (IMP) undergoes oxidation by reacting with reducing equivalent NAD^+ and water molecules produce xanthosine monophosphate (XMP) and the reaction is catalyzed by *IMP dehydrogenase* (In NAD^+ / $NADP^+$ / FAD involved reactions, the enzymes acted are "*dehydrogenase*" and the substrate is "IMP").
4. Finally, xanthosine monophosphate (XMP) in enol form reacts with glutamine and gains amide nitrogen to produce guanosine monophosphate (GMP) with a loss of water molecule in presence of *GMP synthetase* (The product formed is "GMP" and the type of reaction involved is "synthesis"). The energy needed by this reaction is provided by breakdown of ATP into AMP and pyrophosphate **(2 ATP is utilized).**

Drugs such as 6-mercaptopurine acts on *adenyl succinase* of AMP pathway and *IMP dehydrogenase* of IMP pathway leads to inhibition of AMP and GMP synthesis. Hence, 6-mercaptopurine is considered as AMP and GMP synthesis inhibitors.

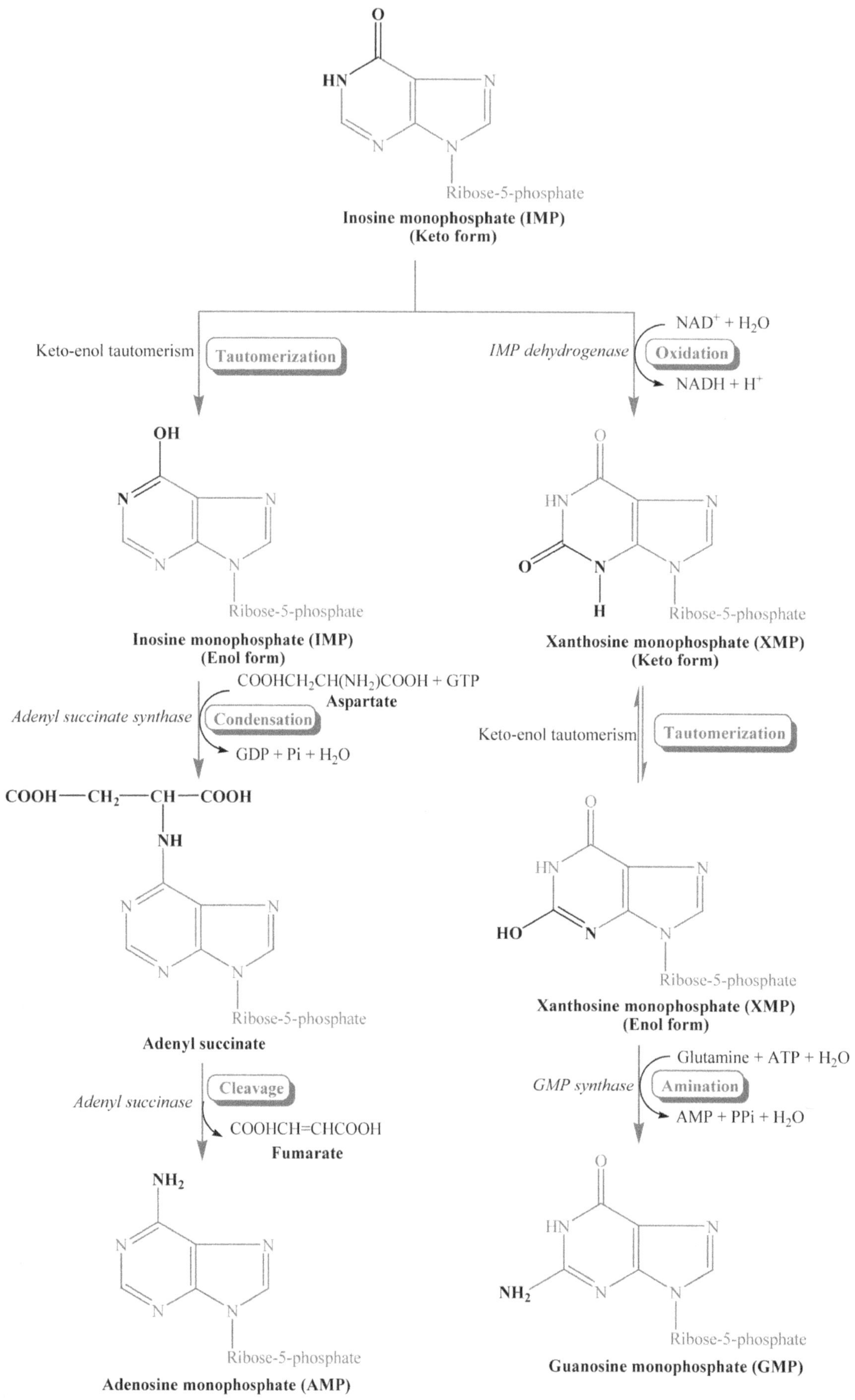

Ribose-5-phosphate
Inosine monophosphate (IMP)
(Keto form)

Keto-enol tautomerism — **Tautomerization**

IMP dehydrogenase — **Oxidation** ($NAD^+ + H_2O$ → $NADH + H^+$)

Ribose-5-phosphate
Inosine monophosphate (IMP)
(Enol form)

Ribose-5-phosphate
Xanthosine monophosphate (XMP)
(Keto form)

Adenyl succinate synthase — **Condensation** ($COOHCH_2CH(NH_2)COOH$ + GTP, **Aspartate** → GDP + Pi + H_2O)

Keto-enol tautomerism — **Tautomerization**

$COOH—CH_2—CH—COOH$
NH

Ribose-5-phosphate
Adenyl succinate

Ribose-5-phosphate
Xanthosine monophosphate (XMP)
(Enol form)

Adenyl succinase — **Cleavage** (→ COOHCH=CHCOOH **Fumarate**)

GMP synthase — **Amination** (Glutamine + ATP + H_2O → AMP + PPi + H_2O)

NH_2

Ribose-5-phosphate
Adenosine monophosphate (AMP)

Ribose-5-phosphate
Guanosine monophosphate (GMP)

α-D-Ribose 5-phosphate

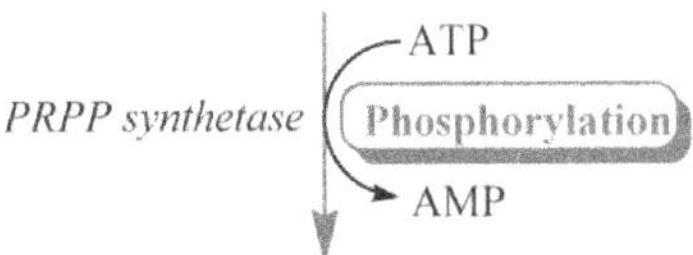

5- Phosphoribosyl-α-pyrophosphate (PRPP)

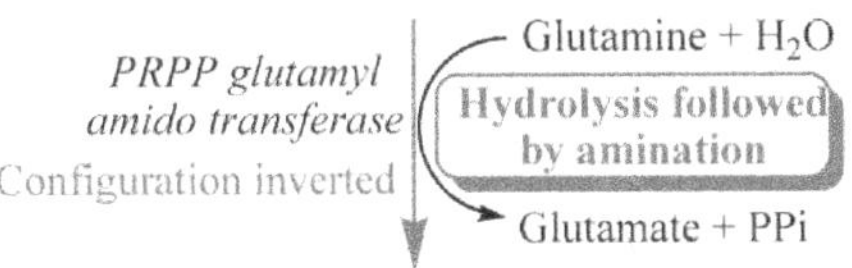

β-5-Phosphoribosylamine

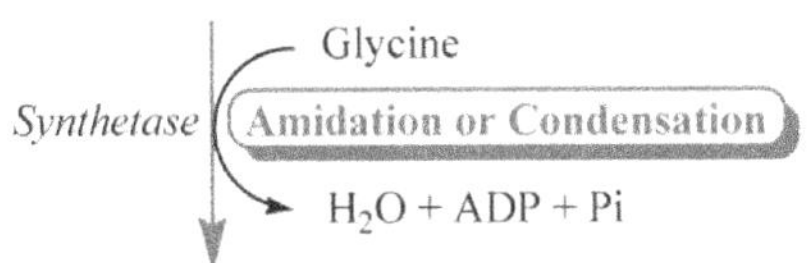

Glycinamide ribosyl-5-phosphate

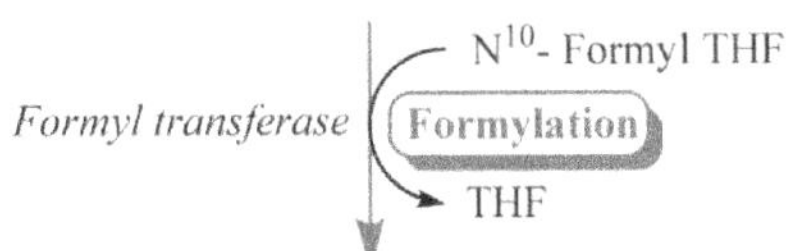

Formylglycinamide ribosyl-5-phosphate

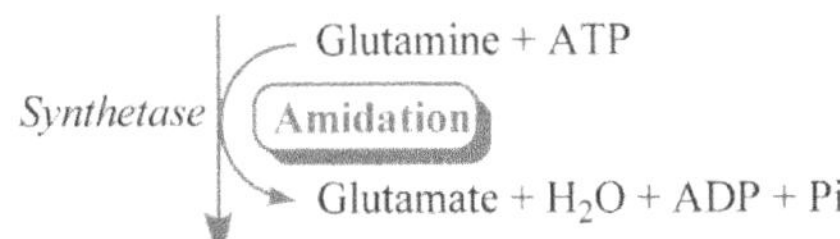

Formylglycinamidine ribosyl-5-phosphate (Keto form)

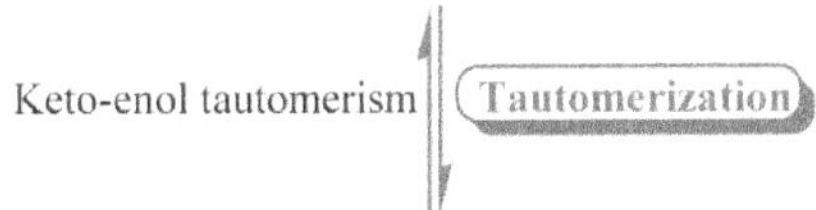

Formylglycinamidine ribosyl-5-phosphate (Enol form)

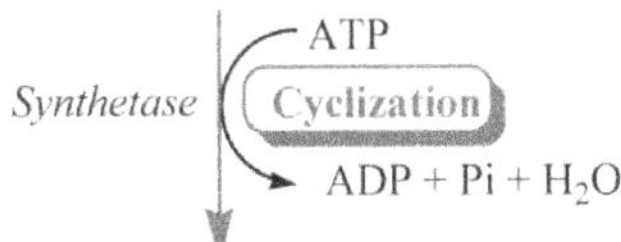

5- Aminoimidazole ribosyl-5-phosphate

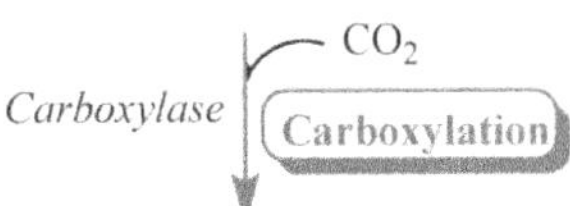

5- Aminoimidazole carboxylate ribosyl-5-phosphate

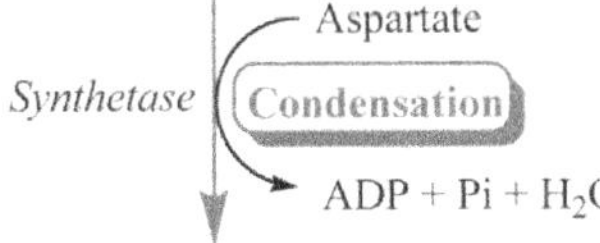

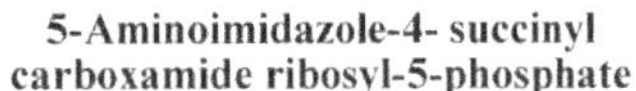

5-Aminoimidazole-4- succinyl carboxamide ribosyl-5-phosphate

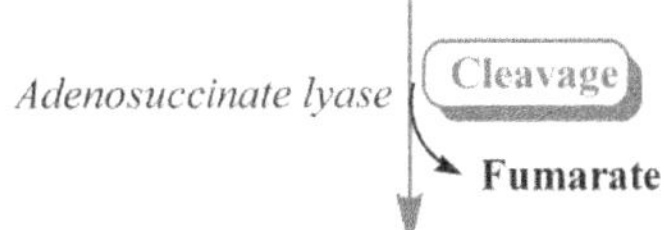

5-Aminoimidazole-4-carboxamide ribosyl-5-phosphate

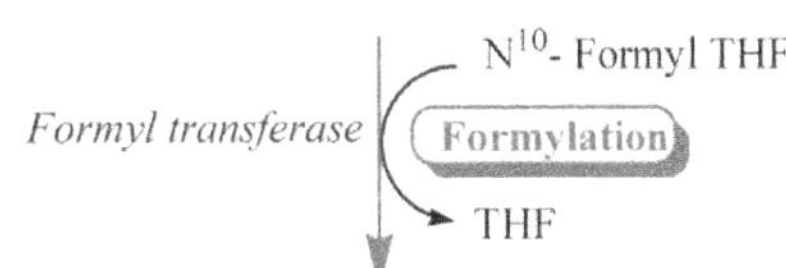

5-Formaminoimidazole-4-carboxamide ribosyl-5-phosphate (Keto form)

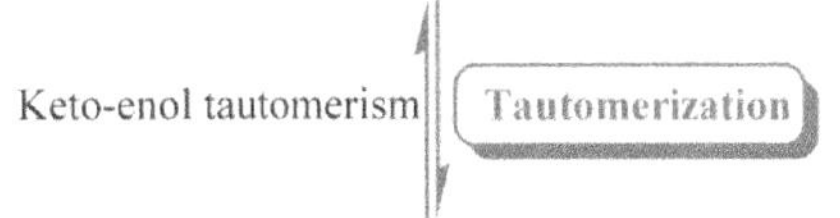

5-Formaminoimidazole-4-carboxamide ribosyl-5-phosphate (Enol form)

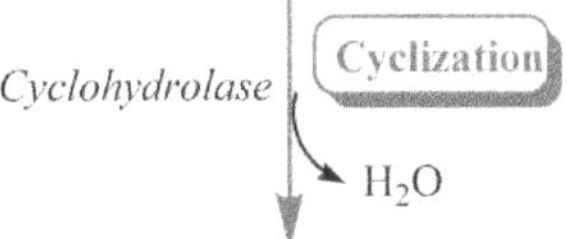

Inosine monophosphate (IMP) (Keto form)

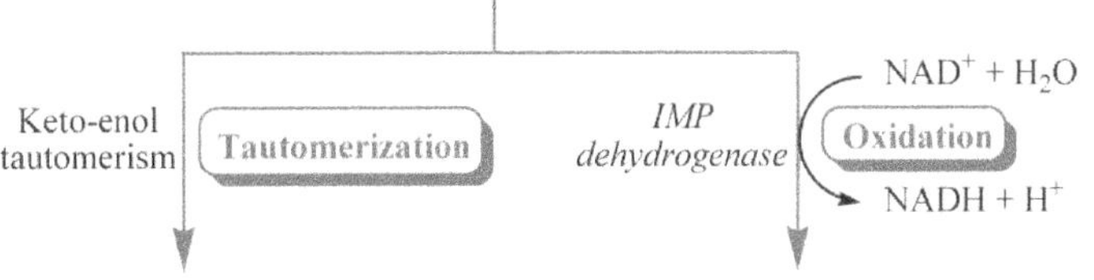

Inosine monophosphate (IMP) (Enol form)

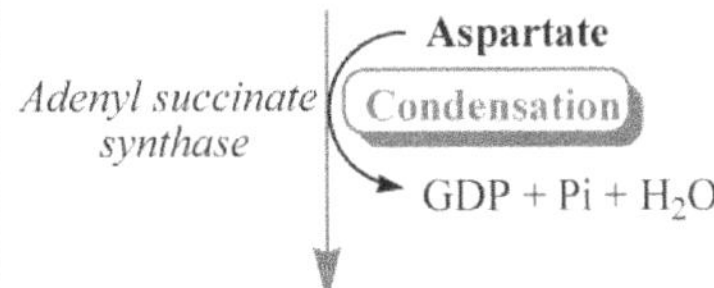

Adenyl succinate

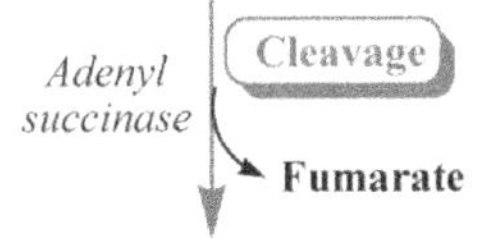

Adenosine monophosphate (AMP)

Xanthosine monophosphate (XMP) (Keto form)

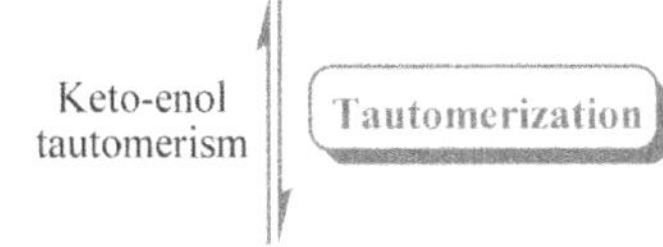

Xanthosine monophosphate (XMP) (Enol form)

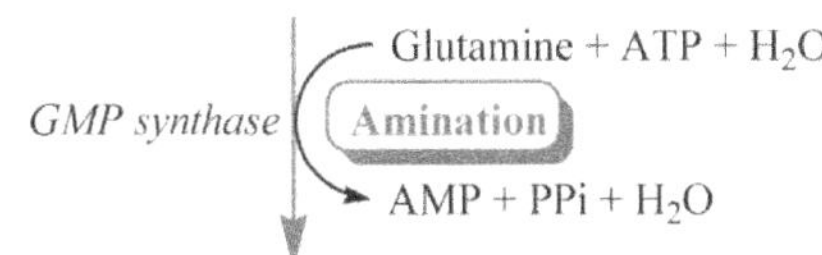

Guanosine monophosphate (GMP)

Degradation of Purine Nucleotides

Uric acid is the end product of purine metabolism. The various reactions involved in the degradation of purine nucleotides are as follows.

1. Firstly, all the purine nucleotides (AMP, IMP and GMP) are converted to their corresponding purine nucleoside (adenosine, inosine and guanosine) by simple hydrolysis with the loss of inorganic phosphate in presence of *nucleotidase* (The substrate is "nucleotide" and the type of reaction involved is "hydrolysis").
2. AMP and adenosine undergo deamination by reacting with water in presence of *AMP deaminase* (The substrate is "AMP" and the type of reaction involved is "deamination") and *adenosine deaminase* (The substrate is "adenosine and the type of reaction involved is "deamination") and produced IMP and inosine, respectively with a loss of ammonia.
3. In the presence of *purine nucleoside phosphorylase* (The substrate is "purine nucleoside" and the type of reaction involved is "phosphorylation"), inosine and guanosine undergoes phosphorylation reaction by reacting with inorganic phosphate to produce their corresponding nitrogen base such as hypoxanthine and guanine, respectively. During this reaction, sugar molecule ribose is removed as ribose-1-phosphate. Adenosine is not degraded by this *purine nucleoside phosphorylase,* hence, it is converted to inosine by the above-mentioned deamination reaction.
4. Guanine undergoes deamination by reacting with water in the presence of *guanine deaminase* (The substrate is "guanine" and the type of reaction involved is "deamination") and produces xanthine with a loss of ammonia.
5. Finally, hypoxanthine is reacted with water and oxygen to produce xanthine with the liberation of hydrogen peroxide in the presence of *xanthine oxidase* (The product formed is "xanthine" and the type of reaction involved is "oxidation"). The reaction involved in this process is simple oxidation. In a similar manner, xanthine is reacted with water and oxygen to produce uric acid with the liberation of hydrogen peroxide in the presence of *xanthine oxidase* (The substrate is "xanthine" and the type of reaction involved is "oxidation"). *Xanthine oxidase* is exclusively found in the liver and small intestine and it contains FAD, molybdenum and iron. The hydrogen peroxide liberated in this reaction is very harmful to the tissues because it is capable to produce free radicals. *Catalase* is an enzyme which cleaves hydrogen peroxide into water and oxygen.

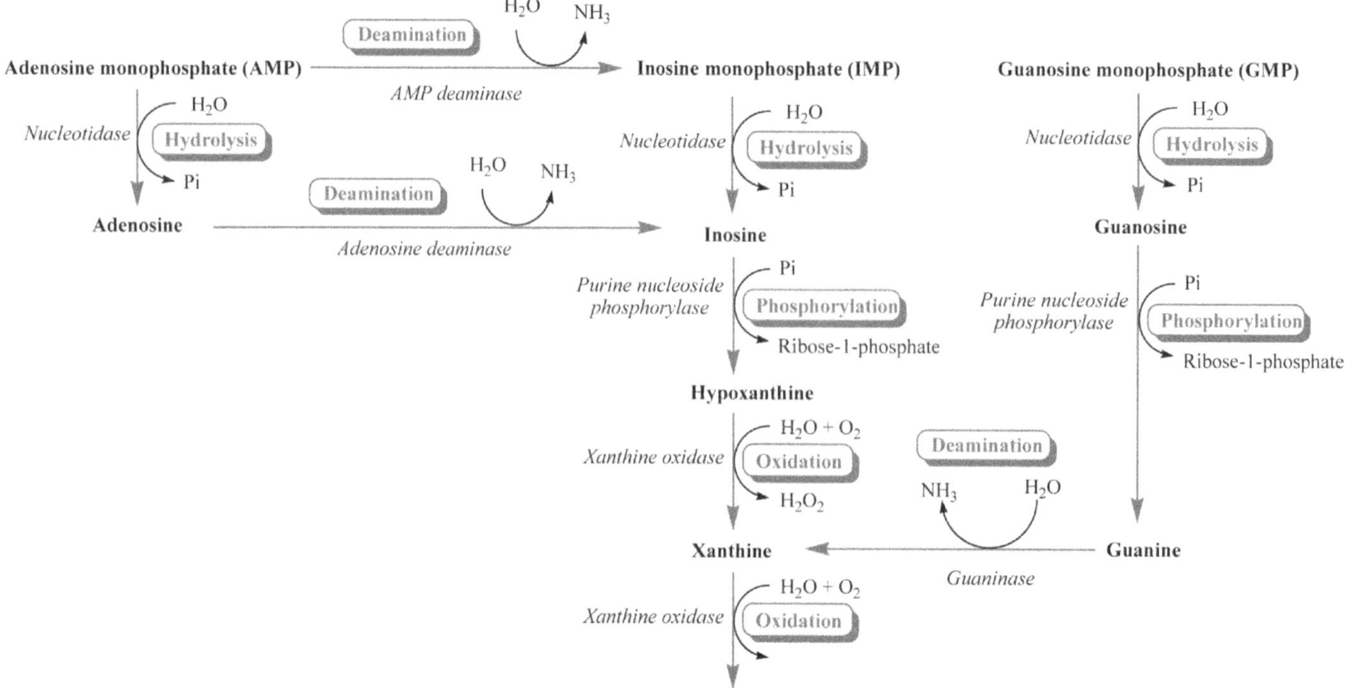

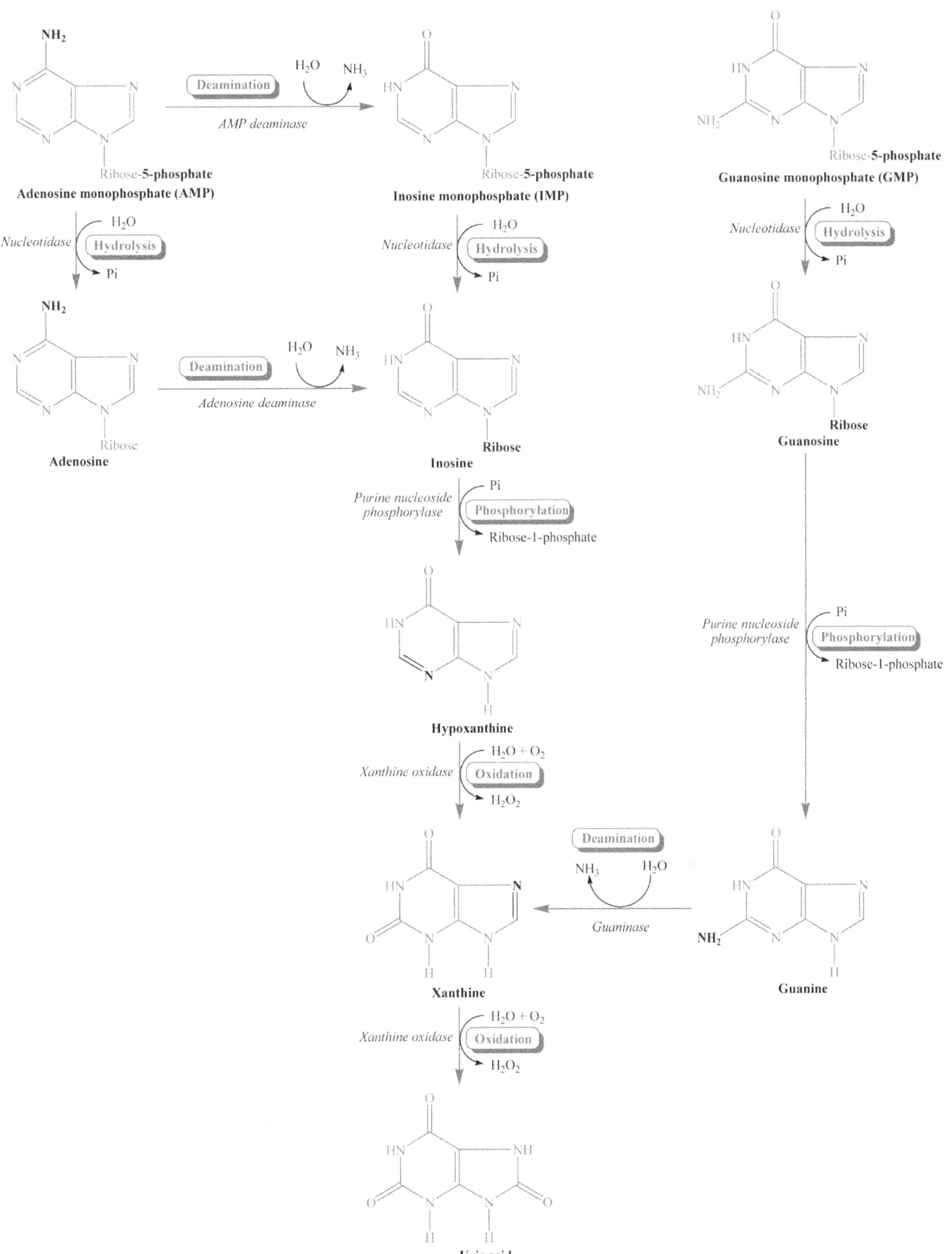
NH2
Deamination
H2O
NH3
AMP deaminase
Ribose-5-phosphate
Adenosine monophosphate (AMP)
Ribose-5-phosphate
Inosine monophosphate (IMP)
Ribose-5-phosphate
Guanosine monophosphate (GMP)
Nucleotidase
Hydrolysis
Pi
Adenosine deaminase
Ribose
Adenosine
Ribose
Inosine
Ribose
Guanosine
Purine nucleoside phosphorylase
Phosphorylation
Ribose-1-phosphate
Hypoxanthine
Xanthine oxidase
H2O + O2
Oxidation
H2O2
Guaninase
Xanthine
Guanine
Uric acid

Uric acid is chemically 2,6,8-trioxypurine and is the end product of purine metabolism excreted through urine in humans. Non-enzymatically, uric acid gets itself converted to allantoin and serves as an important antioxidant. In primates, the antioxidant role of ascorbic acid is replaced by uric acid because ascorbic acid is not synthesized in primates due to lack of enzyme responsible for the synthesis of ascorbic acid i.e., *gulonolactone oxidase*.

Other than primates, in most animals, uric acid is further degraded. Initially, in the presence of *uricase* (The substrate is "uric acid" and the type of reaction involved is "oxidation"), uric acid is converted to allantoin by oxidative ring cleavage. In the next step, allantoin is further converted to allantoic acid in presence of *allantoinase* (The substrate is "allantoin" and the type of reaction involved is "oxidation") by oxidative ring cleavage. In some fishes, this allantoic acid is excreted. In most fishes, amphibians and some molluscs, allantoic acid further degraded to urea with the liberation of glyoxylic acid in the presence of *allantoicase* (The substrate is "allantoic acid" and the type of reaction involved is "oxidation") by oxidative cleavage; whereas in marine invertebrates, urea is further hydrolyzed to produce ammonia and carbondioxide in the presence of *urease* (The substrate is "urea" and the type of reaction involved is "hydrolysis").

Metabolic Disorders of Purine Metabolism

The following are some important metabolic disorders of purine metabolism. They are,

1. Hyperuricemia
2. Uricosuria
3. Gout
   (a) Primary gout
   (b) Secondary gout
4. Pseudogout
5. Lesch-Nyhan syndrome
6. Severe combined immune deficiency (SCID)
   (a) B-cell dysfunction
   (b) T-cell dysfunction
7. Hypouricemia

Hyperuricemia:

In humans, the end excretory product of purine metabolism is uric acid. In adults, the normal serum concentration of uric acid is 3 to 7 mg/dl. Compared to men, in women, it is slightly lower by about 1 mg/dl. Per day about 500 to 700 mg of uric acid is excreted in the body through urine.

Hyperuricemia is defined as the increased concentration of uric acid in serum. Sometimes hyperuricemia is associated with uricosuria.

Uricosuria:

Uricosuria is defined as the increased excretion of uric acid in urine and it is sometimes associated with hyperuricemia.

Gout:

It is a metabolic disorder of purine metabolism and is associated with the overproduction of uric acid. Sodium urate is the more soluble form of uric acid at physiological pH. In severe hyperuricemia, the sodium urate crystals are deposited in the soft tissues, particularly in joints. Tophi are the common name for such deposition in the body. A painful gouty arthritis is produced due to the inflammation in the joints because of sodium urate crystals deposition. In the kidney, and ureter also, uric acid and / or sodium urate may precipitate which leads to stone formation and renal damage. Gout is most common in alcohol consumption, over eating and high living. In the previous centuries, during the manufacture and storage, lead contaminates alcohol. This lead poisoning leads to kidney damage and the decreased uric acid excretion causes gout. In general, the risk of gout is increased with consumption of a diet rich in meat and sea foods. Mostly, it affects males and the prevalence is 3 in 1000 people. Like men, post-menopausal women are susceptible for this disorder. Gout is broadly classified into two major types as,

(a) Primary gout
(b) Secondary gout

Primary gout: This type of gout is an inborn error of metabolism due to overproduction of uric acid. The reason behind over production of uric acid is increased synthesis of purine nucleotides. The following are the major metabolic defects associated with primary gout.

1. Elevation of *phosphoribosyl pyrophosphate (PRPP) synthetase*
2. Elevation of *PRPP glutamyl amidotransferase*
3. Deficiency of *hypoxanthine-guanine phospho ribosyl transferase (HGPRT)*
4. Deficiency of *glucose-6-phosphatase*
5. Elevation of *glutathione reductase*

Secondary gout or secondary hyperuricemia: This type of gout is due to various diseases causing increased production or decreased excretion of uric acid. In various cancers such as leukemia, polycythemia, lymphomas, etc., psoriasis and increased tissue breakdown conditions such as trauma, starvation, etc. nucleic acid degradation is increased leads to increased production of uric acid. In case of renal function impairment, excretion of uric acid is decreased leading to accumulation of uric acid, resulting in gout.

Diagnosis of gout: The miscible uric acid pool in the body can be calculated by administering the uric acid isotope (N^{15}). The normal value of miscible uric acid pool is 1200 mg and this value is greatly increased to 3000 mg or more in gout patients.

Treatment: Allopurinol is the drug used for the treatment of primary gout. Allopurinol competitively inhibits the *xanthine oxidase* enzyme because it is chemically a structural analog of hypoxanthine. In addition, alloxanthine is produced by allopurinol by simple oxidation in presence of *xanthine oxidase*. Alloxanthine is a more powerful *xanthine oxidase* inhibitor than allopurinol. This type of enzyme inhibition is known as suicide inhibition. Hypoxanthine and xanthine are accumulated in the body due to inhibition of *xanthine oxidase* by allopurinol. Compared to uric acid, hypoxanthine and xanthine are more soluble in water, hence, it is easily excreted in urine.

Restriction of dietary intake of purines and alcohol is also advised besides the drug therapy. In addition, drinking more water is also very useful.

In general, for the treatment of gouty arthritis, anti-inflammatory drug colchicine is used. Other anti-inflammatory drugs such as indomethacin, phenylbutazone, oxyphenbutazone and corticosteroids are also used for the treatment of gouty arthritis.

Pseudogout: It is similar to gout by clinical manifestation but it is caused by deposition of calcium pyrophosphate crystals in joints. In addition, serum uric acid level is normal in pseudogout.

Biosynthesis of Pyrimidine Nucleotides

Pyrimidine biosynthesis process is much simpler than that of the purine biosynthesis process. First, pyrimidine nitrogen base is synthesized and then sugar molecule i.e., ribose-5-phosphate is attached to the pyrimidine nitrogen base to synthesize pyrimidine nucleotide. In case of purine nucleotide synthesis purine nitrogen base is synthesized in a pre-existing ribose-5-phosphate. Pyrimidine rings of the nucleotides are contributed by many compounds which are presented in Figure 4.2. They are,

1. N_1, C_4, C_5 and C_6 of pyrimidine are derived from aspartate.
2. C_2 of pyrimidine is derived from carbon dioxide.
3. N_3 of pyrimidine is derived from the amide group of glutamine.

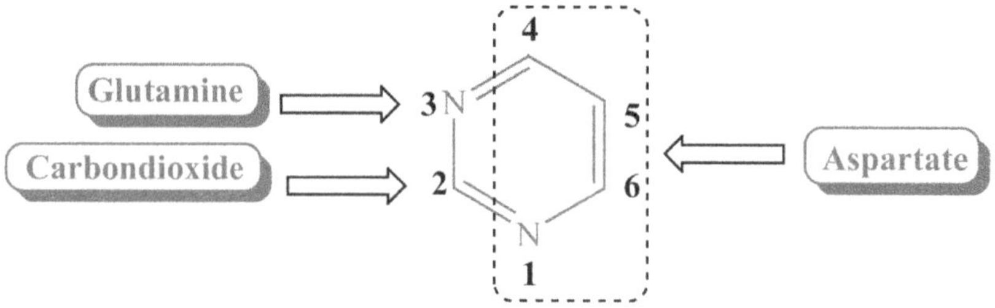

Figure 4.2 Sources of individual atoms in pyrimidine ring.

Pathway:

1. At first, carbondioxide reacts with glutamine and ATP to produce carbamoyl phosphate in presence of cytosomal enzyme *carbamoyl phosphate synthetase – II (CPS – II)* (The product formed is "carbamoyl phosphate" and the type of reaction involved is "synthesis") by simple condensation. In this reaction, energy needed by the reaction is provided by the breakdown of ATP and glutamate is liberated after donating the amine group of glutamines. Two ATP is used in this reaction. One for phosphorylation and the another one for energy purpose **(2 ATP is utilized)**.

   ATP and phosphoribosyl pyrophosphate (PRPP) activate *carbamoyl phosphate synthetase – II (CPS – II)*; whereas UTP inhibits *CPS – II*. In urea biosynthesis, carbamoyl phosphate is synthesized from ammonia and carbondioxide in presence of microsomal enzyme *carbamoyl phosphate synthetase – I (CPS – I)* which needs N-acetyl glutamate (NAG) for its activity. Only one *carbamoyl phosphate synthetase* is present in eukaryotes for the biosynthesis of pyrimidines and arginine.
2. In the next step, carbamoyl phosphate is reacted with aspartate by simple condensation and produces carbamoyl aspartate with a loss of inorganic phosphate in the presence of *aspartate transcarbamoylase* (The substrate is "aspartate" and the type of reaction involved is "transfer of carbamoyl group").
3. Later, in presence of *dihydroorotase* (The product formed is "dihydroorotate" and the type of reaction involved is "hydrolysis" in reverse manner), carbamoyl aspartate undergoes ring closure reaction with a loss of water molecule produces dihydroorotate. Enzymes such as *CPS – II, aspartate transcarbamoylase* and *dihydroorotase* are the functional units of the same protein. Hence, it is also a very good example for a **multi-functional enzyme**.
4. Orotate is synthesized from dihydroorotate by dehydrogenation i.e., oxidation reaction which are dependent on NAD^+ in presence of *dihydroorotate dehydrogenase* (In NAD^+ / $NADP^+$ / FAD involved reactions, the enzymes acted are "*dehydrogenase*" and the substrate is "dihydroorotate"). In this reaction one NAD^+ is converted to NADH + H^+. In ETC, one NADH + H^+ produces 3 ATP **(3 ATP is generated).**
5. In this step, phosphoribosyl pyrophosphate (PRPP) donates ribose-5-phosphate to orotate in order to synthesize orotidine monophosphate (OMP) with the liberation of pyrophosphate. This reaction is catalyzed by *orotate phospho ribosyl transferase* (The substrate is "orotate" and the type of reaction involved is "transfer of ribose-5-phosphate group"). This enzyme is usually compared with *hypoxanthine-guanine phosphoribosyl transferase (HGPRT)* in its function.
6. In the succeeding step, OMP loss its carboxyl group present in C-6 as carbondioxide by simple decarboxylation in presence of *OMP decarboxylase* (The substrate is "OMP" and the type of reaction involved is "decarboxylation") to produce uridine monophosphate (UMP). *Orotate phospho ribosyl transferase* and *OMP decarboxylase* is the functional unit of the same protein. Hence, it is also a very good example for a bifunctional enzyme and the deficiency of this bifunctional enzyme causes orotic aciduria.
7. Later, UMP is converted into uridine diphosphate (UDP) by simple phosphorylation reaction by reacting with ATP with liberation of ADP in the presence of *kinase* (In ATP / GTP involves reaction the enzyme acted are "*kinase*"). In this reaction, one ATP is converted to ADP **(1 ATP is utilized)**. UDP acts as a precursor for the synthesis of deoxyuridine diphosphate (*d*UDP), deoxyuridine monophosphate (*d*UMP), deoxythymidine monophosphate (*d*TMP), uridine triphosphate (UTP), and cytidine triphosphate (CTP).

8. UDP undergoes two different types of reactions. In first reaction, UDP reacts with the reduced form of thioredoxin (2 SH) to produce *d*UDP by simple reduction reaction in the presence of *ribonucleotide reductase* (The substrate is "UDP which is ribonucleotide" and the type of reaction involved is "reduction"). After the reaction, oxidized form of thioredoxin (S-S) is liberated. Later, *d*UDP

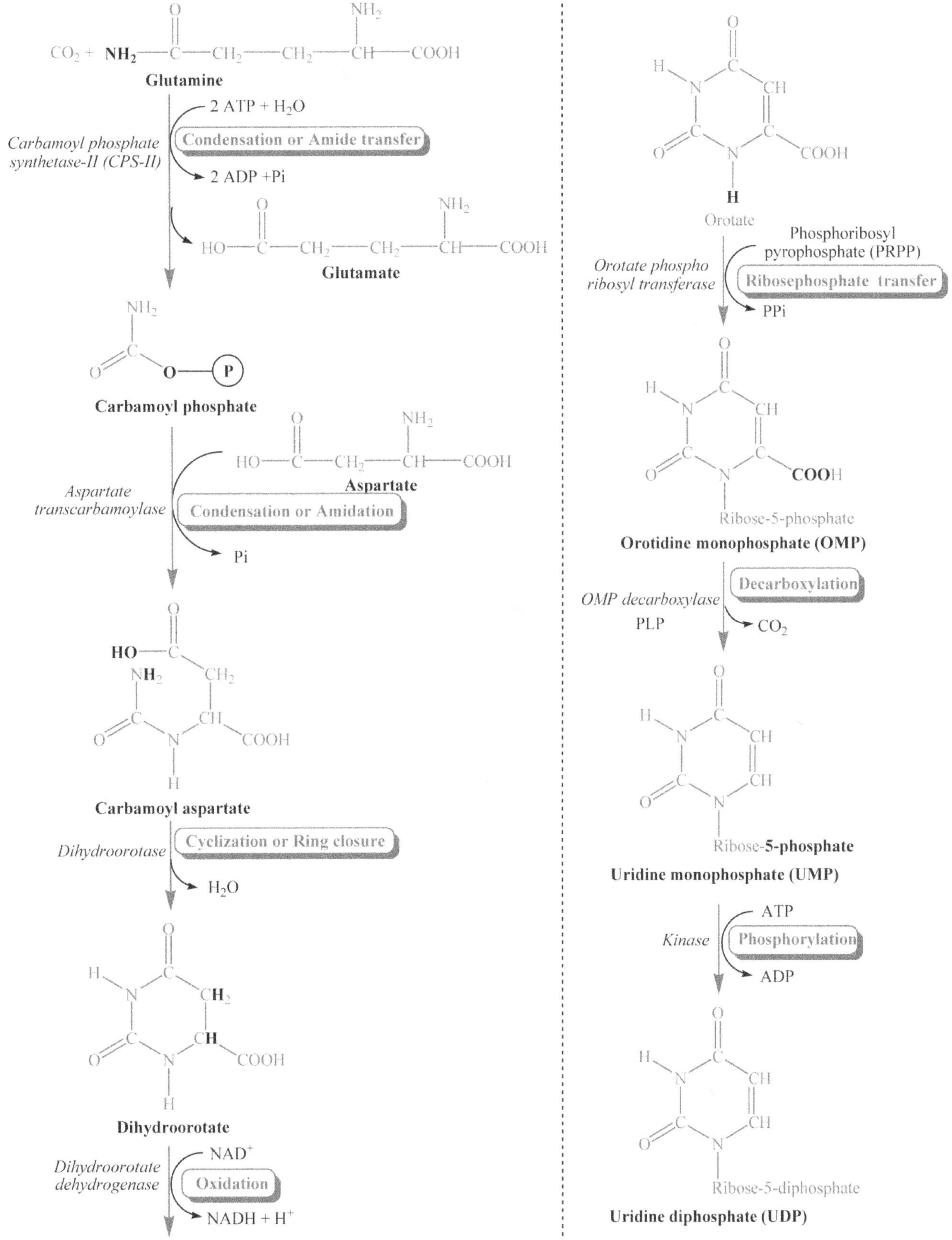

CO_2 + NH_2—C(=O)—CH_2—CH_2—CH(NH_2)—COOH

Glutamine

Carbamoyl phosphate synthetase-II (CPS-II) — 2 ATP + H_2O — **Condensation or Amide transfer** — 2 ADP + Pi

HO—C(=O)—CH_2—CH_2—CH(NH_2)—COOH

Glutamate

NH_2—C(=O)—O—(P)

Carbamoyl phosphate

Aspartate transcarbamoylase — HO—C(=O)—CH_2—CH(NH_2)—COOH **Aspartate** — **Condensation or Amidation** — Pi

Carbamoyl aspartate

Dihydroorotase — **Cyclization or Ring closure** — H_2O

Dihydroorotate

Dihydroorotate dehydrogenase — NAD^+ — **Oxidation** — $NADH + H^+$

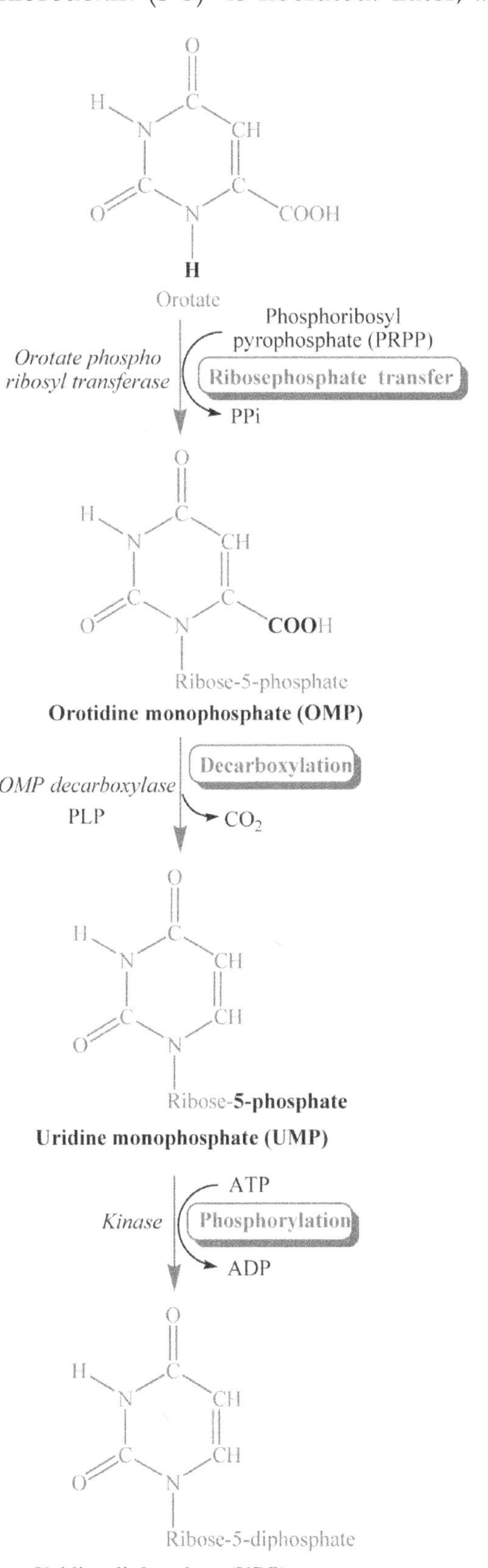

Ribose-5-diphosphate

Uridine diphosphate (UDP)

Ribonucleotide reductase

Thioredoxin (2 SH)

Reduction

Thioredoxin (-S-S-)

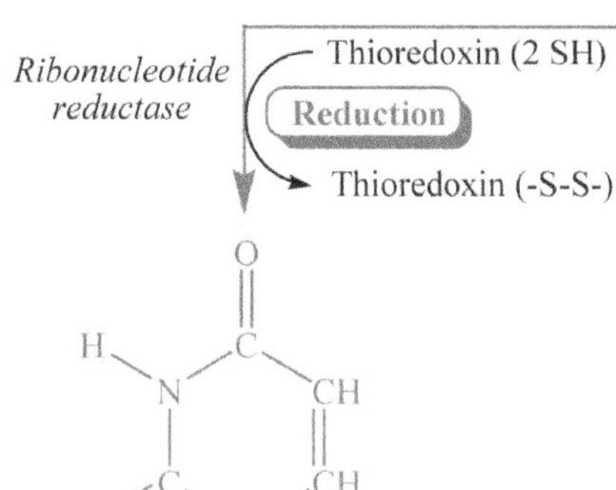

Deoxyribose-**5-diphosphate**

Deoxyuridine diphosphate (*d*UDP)

dUMP kinase

ADP

Dephosphorylation

ATP

Deoxyribose-5-phosphate

Deoxyuridine monophosphate (*d*UMP)

Thymidylate synthetase

N^5, N^{10}-Methylene THF

Methylation

THF

CH_3

Deoxyribose-5-phosphate

Deoxythymidine monophosphate (*d*TMP)

Kinase

ATP

Phosphorylation

ADP

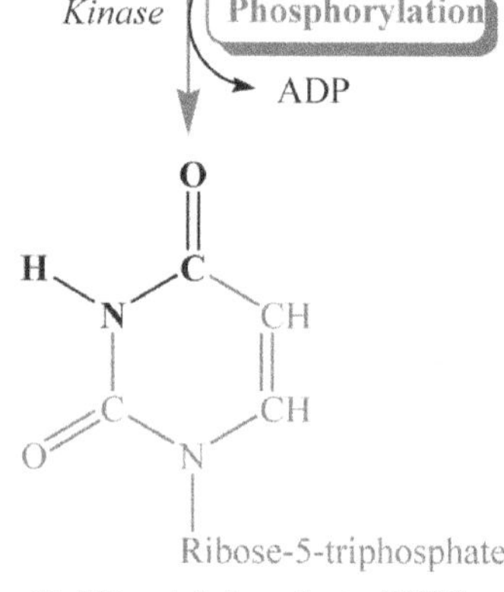

Ribose-5-triphosphate

Uridine triphosphate (UTP)
(Keto form)

Keto-enol tautomerism

Tautomerization

OH

Ribose-5-triphosphate

Uridine triphosphate (UTP)
(Enol form)

CTP synthetase

Glutamine + ATP + H_2O

Amination

Glutamate + ADP + Pi

NH_2

Ribose-5-triphosphate

Cytidine triphosphate (CTP)

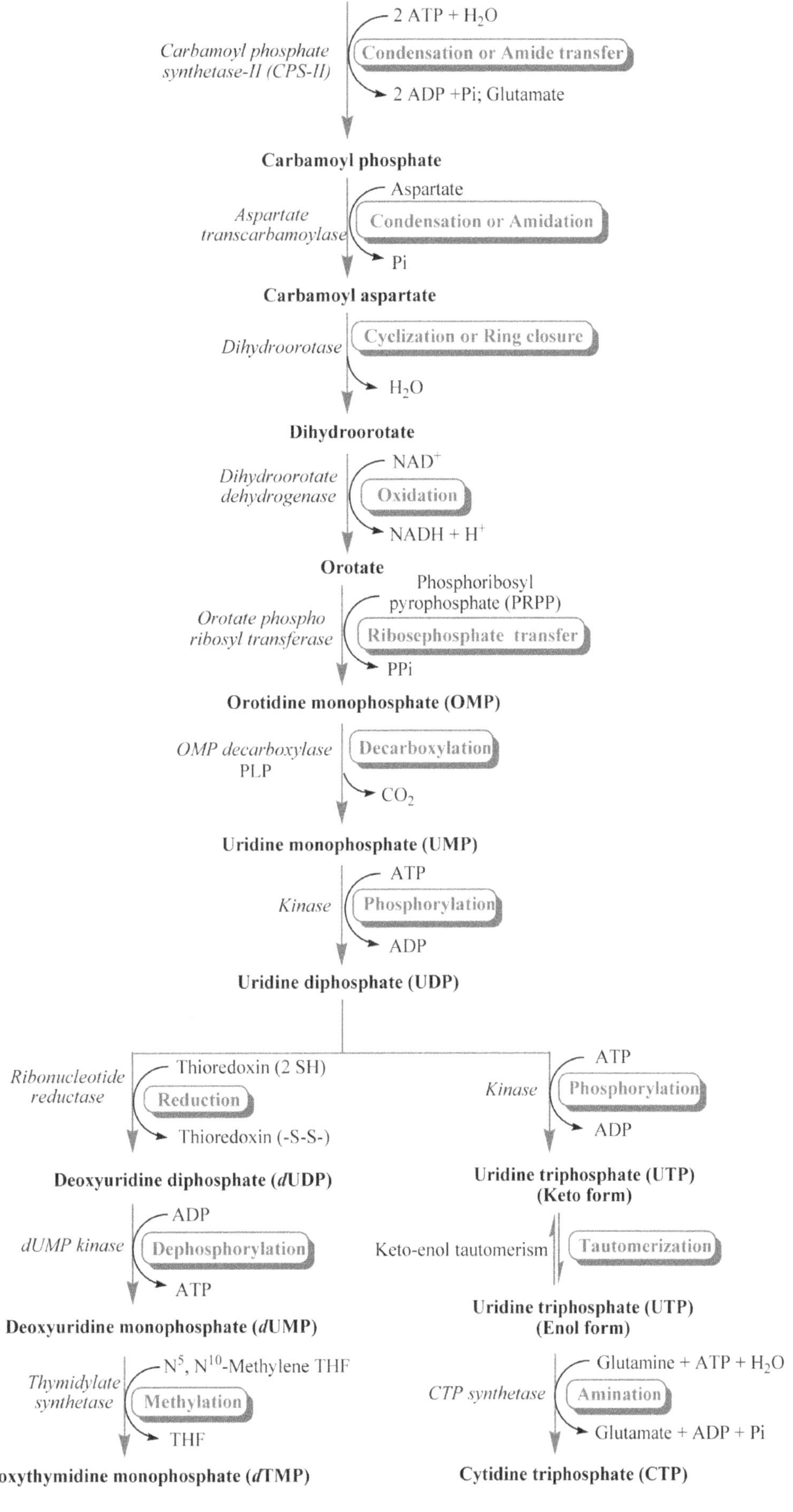
CO_2 + Glutamine
2 ATP + H_2O
Carbamoyl phosphate synthetase-II (CPS-II)
Condensation or Amide transfer
2 ADP +Pi; Glutamate
Carbamoyl phosphate
Aspartate
Aspartate transcarbamoylase
Condensation or Amidation
Pi
Carbamoyl aspartate
Dihydroorotase
Cyclization or Ring closure
H_2O
Dihydroorotate
NAD^+
Dihydroorotate dehydrogenase
Oxidation
$NADH + H^+$
Orotate
Phosphoribosyl pyrophosphate (PRPP)
Orotate phospho ribosyl transferase
Ribosephosphate transfer
PPi
Orotidine monophosphate (OMP)
OMP decarboxylase PLP
Decarboxylation
CO_2
Uridine monophosphate (UMP)
ATP
Kinase
Phosphorylation
ADP
Uridine diphosphate (UDP)
Thioredoxin (2 SH)
Ribonucleotide reductase
Reduction
Thioredoxin (-S-S-)
Deoxyuridine diphosphate (dUDP)
ADP
dUMP kinase
Dephosphorylation
ATP
Deoxyuridine monophosphate (dUMP)
N^5, N^{10}-Methylene THF
Thymidylate synthetase
Methylation
THF
Deoxythymidine monophosphate (dTMP)
ATP
Kinase
Phosphorylation
ADP
Uridine triphosphate (UTP) (Keto form)
Keto-enol tautomerism
Tautomerization
Uridine triphosphate (UTP) (Enol form)
Glutamine + ATP + H_2O
CTP synthetase
Amination
Glutamate + ADP + Pi
Cytidine triphosphate (CTP)

undergoes a dephosphorylation reaction to produce *d*UMP and the liberated inorganic phosphate is taken by ADP and converted to ATP. The reaction is catalyzed by *kinase* enzyme (In ATP / GTP involved reaction the enzyme acted are "*kinase*"). Finally, *d*UMP is converted to *d*TMP by the transfer of the methyl group from N^5, N^{10}-methylene THF in the presence of *thymidylate synthetase* (The product formed is "*d*TMP which is a thymidine analog" and the type of reaction involved is "synthesis") with the liberation of THF.

9. In another way, UDP is converted into uridine triphosphate (UTP) by simple phosphorylation reaction by reacting with ATP with the liberation of ADP in the presence of *kinase* (In ATP / GTP involved reaction the enzyme acted are "*kinase*"). In this reaction, one ATP is converted to ADP **(1 ATP is utilized)**. Later, in enol form, UTP reacts with glutamine and produces CTP with the liberation of glutamate after removing the amine group. This reaction is a simple amination reaction and is anabolic in nature. The energy is obtained from the breakdown of ATP into ADP. In this reaction, one ATP is converted to ADP **(1 ATP is utilized)**.

Structure of DNA

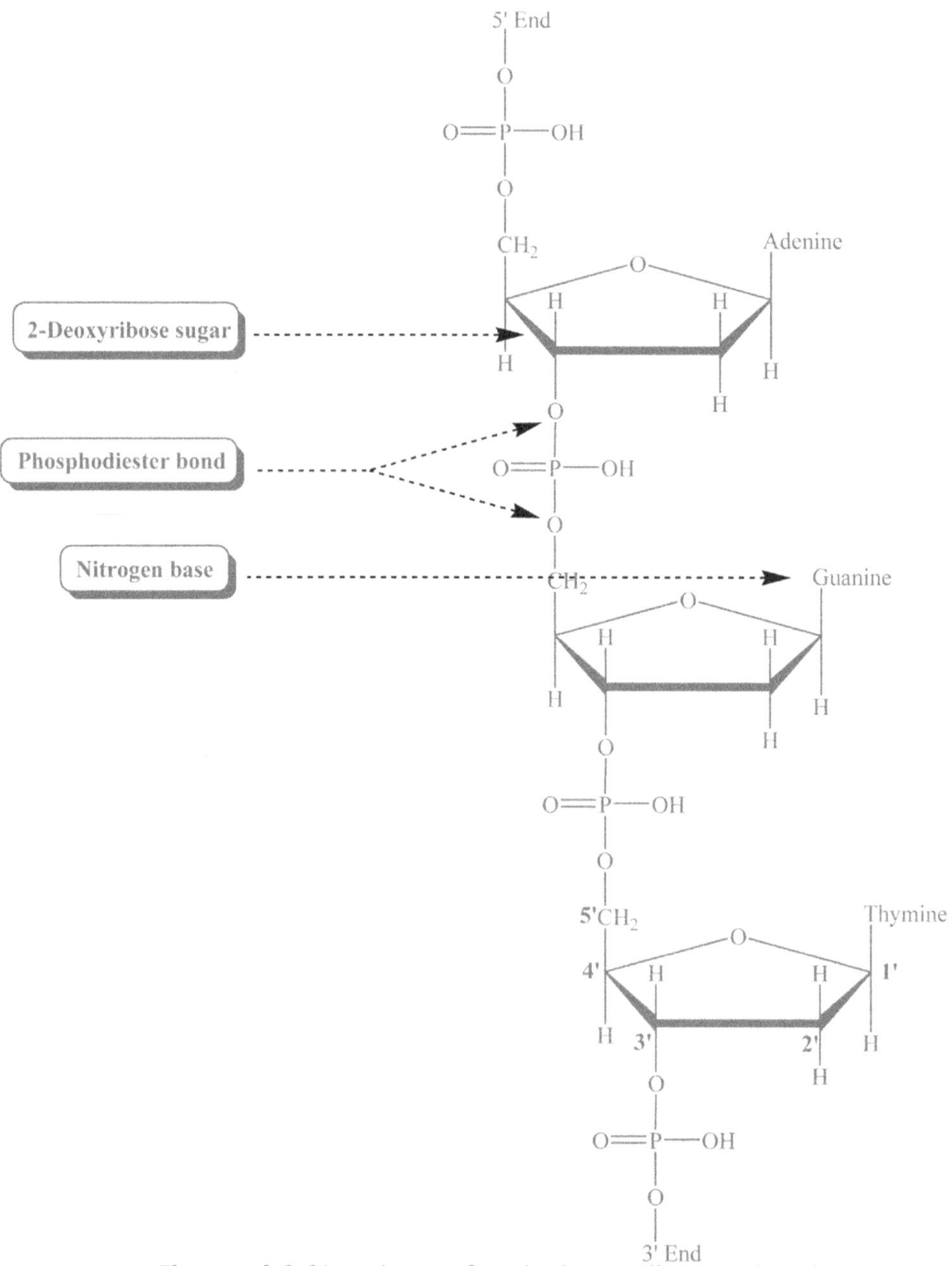

Figure 4.3 Structure of polydeoxyribonucleotide.

Composition:

DNA is a polymer of deoxyribonucleotides or simply deoxynucleotides Figure 4.3. The various monomeric units present in DNA are as follows,

1. Deoxyadenylate (*d*AMP)
2. Deoxyguanylate (*d*GMP)
3. Deoxycytidylate (*d*CMP) and
4. Deoxythymidylate (*d*TMP)

The DNA contains,

1. **Nitrogen base:** Purine (Adenine & guanine) and pyrimidine (Cytosine & thymine)
2. **Sugar:** 2-Deoxyribose and
3. Phosphate group.

Schematic representation:

In DNA, the monomeric deoxyribonucleotides are attached together by 3′,5′-phosphodiester bridges. It is often observed that the structure of nucleic acid such as DNA and RNA is represented by a shorthand form (Figure 4.4). The carbon chains of sugars are usually indicated by a horizontal line; the base attached at C-1 is represented at the right hand side corner of the horizontal line and the phosphate linkage is present between C-3 of one sugar which is mentioned near the middle of the horizontal line and the C-5 of another sugar which is mentioned in next horizontal line left hand side corner.

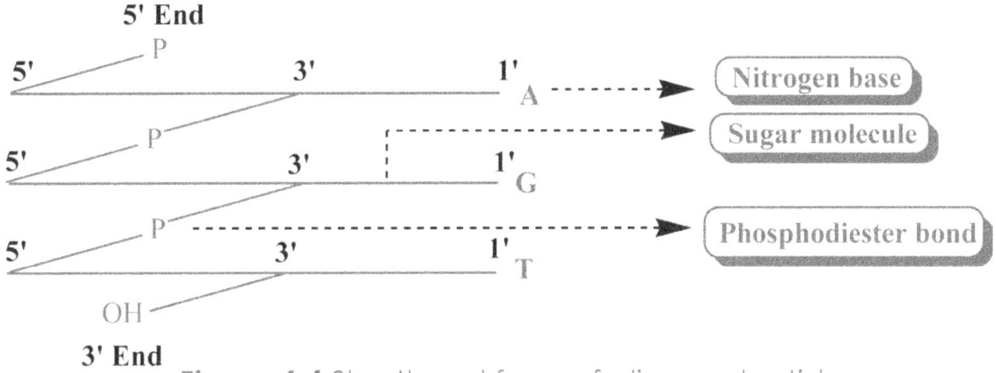

Figure 4.4 Shorthand form of oligonucleotides.

Chargaff's rule:

In the year 1940, from the different species, Erwin Chargaff quantitatively analyzed DNA hydrolysis and observed that in all the species the number of adenine and thymine residue (A = T) are equal in DNA and similarly, guanine and cytosine residue (G = C) are equal in the DNA. This concept is known as Chargaff's rule of molecular equivalence between the purines and pyrimidines in DNA structure. This rule gives

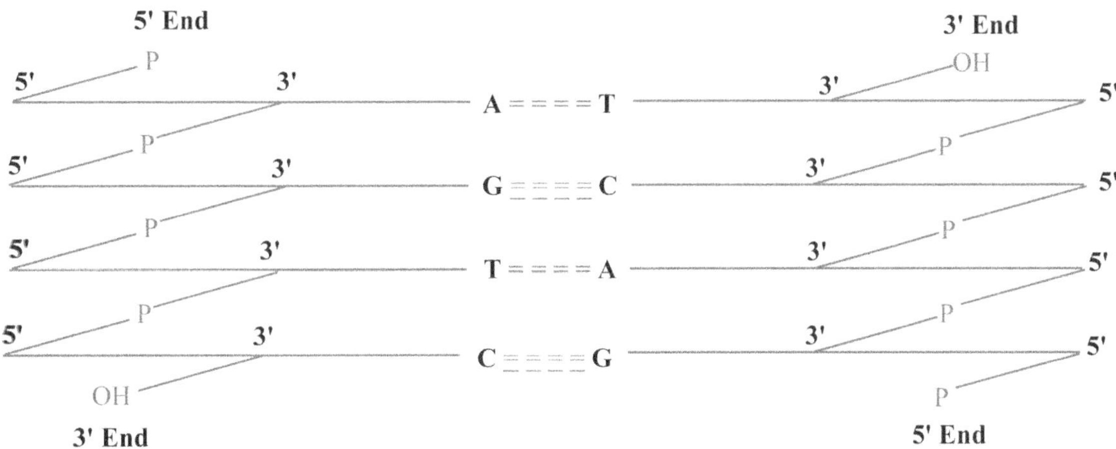

Figure 4.5 Complementary base pairing in DNA helix.

strength to the double helical structure of DNA. This Chargaff's rule is not obeyed by single stranded DNA and RNA (usually single stranded). In certain viruses, as a genetic material, RNA is present in a double stranded form which obeys the Chargaff's rule.

DNA double helix:

In the year 1953, James Watson and Francis Crick proposed the double helical structure of DNA. In modern biology, the DNA structure elucidation is considered as a milestone. Usually, the twisted ladder was used to compare the DNA double helix. Now, the Watson-Crick model of DNA is known as B-DNA and its various salient features are as follows.

1. DNA is the right-handed double helix composed of two strands i.e., polydeoxyribo nucleotide chains twisted around a common axis.
2. Out of these two strands, one strand runs in 5′ to 3′ direction; whereas the other strand runs in the opposite direction i.e., 3′ to 5′ direction. Hence, the two strands of DNA are antiparallel to each other and are usually compared with two parallel roads carrying traffic in opposite directions.
3. 20 A° or 2 nm is the width or diameter of the double helix.

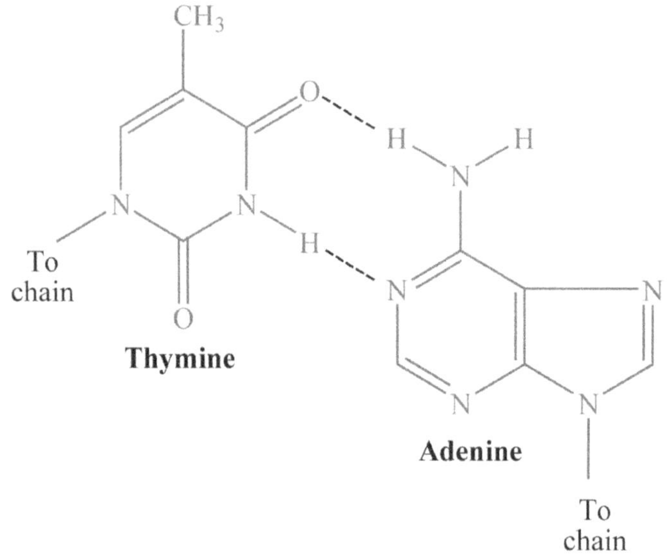

CH_3 H H N N N H N N To chain O N N **Thymine** **Adenine** To chain

(A) Thymine pairs with adenine by 2 hydrogen bonds

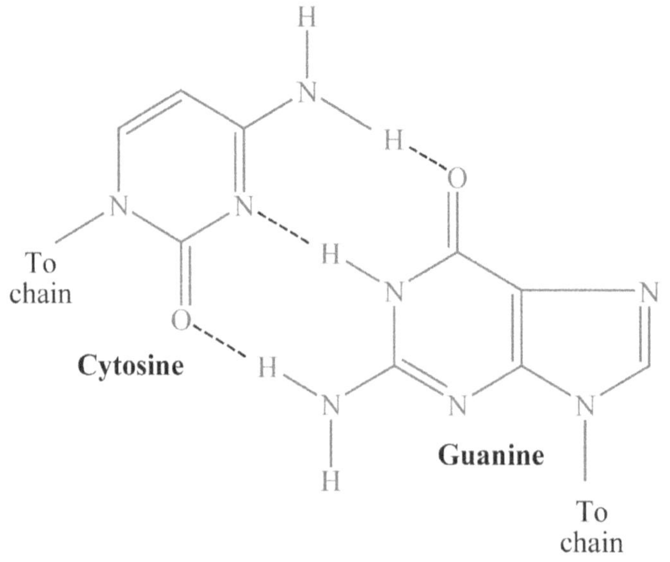

H N H O N N H N N To chain O N **Cytosine** H N N N H **Guanine** To chain

(B) Cytosine pairs with guanine by 3 hydrogen bonds

Figure 4.6 Complementary base pairing in DNA.

4. 34 A° or 3.4 nm is the size of each pitch or turn of the helix. Each turn contains ten pairs of nucleotides and each pair is placed at 3.4 A° or 0.34 nm distance.
5. The periphery or outside of each strand contains hydrophilic deoxyribose phosphate backbone (3′-5′ phosphodiester bonds) and inside or core the hydrophobic bases are stacked.
6. Due to base pairing, the two strands or polydeoxyribonucleotide chains of DNA are complementary to each other and are not identical.
7. Complementary base pairs (Figure 4.5 & 4.6) form hydrogen bonds which are used to hold together the two strands. Two hydrogen bonds are formed between adenine and thymine (A = T) and three hydrogen bonds are formed between guanine and cytosine (G ≡ C). In addition, guanine-cytosine hydrogen bond (G ≡ C) is 50 % stronger than adenine-thymine hydrogen bond (A = T).
8. In general, the hydrogen bond is formed between purine base with pyrimidine base only. If two purines are facing each other, it will not fit in the allowable space. Similarly, if two pyrimidine bases face each other it will be too far to form the hydrogen bonds. In DNA, only the following four base arrangements are possible due to spatial consideration. They are, A-T, G-C, T-A and C-G.
9. The Chargaff's rule is proved by the complementary base pairing in the DNA helix. In general, in the DNA, the content of adenine is equal to thymine and the content of guanine is equal to cytosine.
10. Out of two strands, the genetic information resides in only one strand which is known as the sense strand or the template strand. The other strand is known as the anti-sense strand. Along the phosphodiester backbone, the double helix has major groove (wide) and minor groove (narrow). In these grooves without disturbing the base pairs and double helix, proteins interact with DNA.

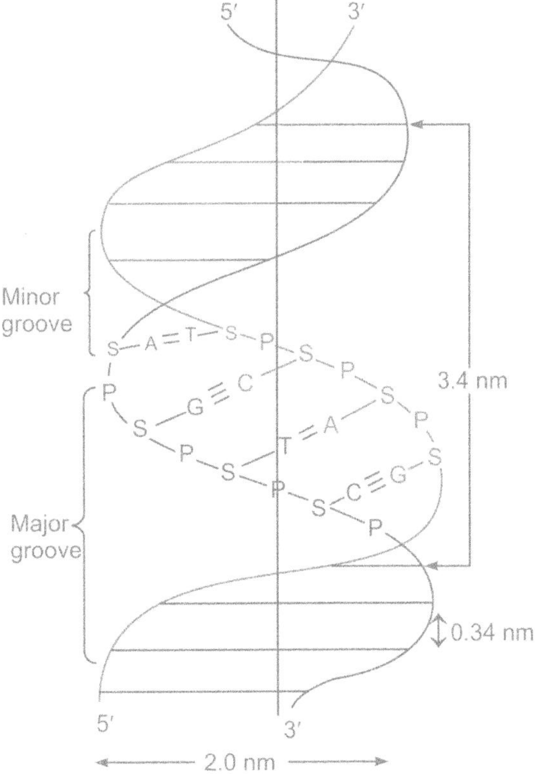

Figure 4.7 Right-handed double helical structure of DNA.

Conformations of DNA double helix: In nucleotides of DNA, the conformation variation is associated with conformational variants of DNA. At least six different forms of DNA double helical structures such as A to E and Z exist in nature. B, A and Z forms are important among these six forms. Under physiological conditions, the most predominant form is B-form of DNA double helix described by Watson and Crick model. The width of the B-form is 2 nm and ten base pairs are present in each turn, spanning a distance of 3.4 nm. The A-form is also a right-handed helix and it contains eleven base pairs in each turn. From the central axis the base pairs are tilted by 20 °C away. The Z-form is a left-handed helix and it contains twelve base pairs in each turn. In zig-zag fashion, the polynucleotide strands of DNA are moving; hence, this form is named as Z-form. In regulation of gene expression, the transition between different helical forms of DNA plays a significant role. The right-handed double helical structure of DNA is depicted in Figure 4.7.

Other types of DNA structure:

DNA also exists in other unusual structures. It is believed that for molecular recognition of DNA by proteins and enzymes, these structures are important. In addition, for DNA to exhibit its function in an appropriate manner, it needs these structures. The following are the various important unusual structures of DNA.

1. Bent DNA
2. Triple stranded DNA and
3. Four stranded DNA

Organization of Mammalian Genome or Organization of DNA in the Cell

In each chromosome, the length of double stranded DNA is thousand times of its diameter of the nucleus. In humans, 2 meter long DNA is packed in 10 μm diameter of the nucleus. It is possible inside the cell due to the excellent and compact organization and packing of DNA.

Organization of prokaryotic DNA:

In the form of a double stranded circle, DNA is organized in prokaryotic cells as a single chromosome. By interacting with proteins and certain cations like polyamines, in the form of nucleoids these bacterial enzymes are packed.

Organization of eukaryotic DNA:

Naked DNA double helix (**2 nm**)

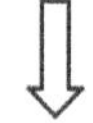

Beads on a string which is a form of chromatin (**10 nm**)

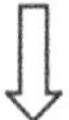

30 nm chromatin fiber composed of nucleosomes (**30 nm**)

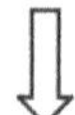

Chromosomes in an extended form (non-condensed loops; **300 nm**)

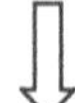

Condensed form of chromosome (**700 nm**)

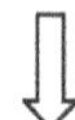

Metaphase chromosome (**1400 nm**)

In eukaryotic cells, to form chromatin the DNA is associated with various proteins. Later, chromatin is getting organized into compact structures known as chromosomes. The basic histones are the core proteins which wrapped the double helix of DNA. Two molecules of histones (H2A, H2B, H3 and H4) compose the core proteins. The basic unit of chromatin is nucleosome which wraps round each core with two turns of DNA (approximately with 150 base pairs). Spacer DNA separates the nucleosomes in which histones are attached. 10 nm fibers are the continuous string of nucleosomes representing beads on a string form of chromatin. This 10 nm fibers formation considerably reduces the length of DNA. Further, 30 nm fiber is formed from 10 nm fiber by coiling. 30 nm fibers have a solenoid structure with six nucleosomes in every turn. Further, by anchoring the fiber these 30 nm fibers are organized into loops at A/T rich regions namely scaffold associated regions (SARS) to a protein scaffold. The loops are further coiled and the chromosomes are condensed and become visible during the process of mitosis.

Structure of RNA

Composition:

RNA is a polymer of ribonucleotides and is linked by 3′,5′-phosphodiester bridges. The various monomeric units present in RNA are as follows,

1. Adenosine monophosphate (AMP)
2. Guanosine monophosphate (GMP)
3. Cytidine monophosphate (CMP) and
4. Uridine monophosphate (UMP)

The RNA contains,

1. **Nitrogen base:** Purine (Adenine & guanine) and pyrimidine (Cytosine &uracil)
2. **Sugar:** Ribose and
3. Phosphate group.

Comparison between DNA and RNA:

The following are the differences between RNA and DNA even though they have certain similarities.

1. **Pentose sugar:** Ribose is present in RNA in contrast to deoxyribose in DNA.
2. **Pyrimidine base:** In place of thymine in DNA, RNA contains uracil.
3. **Single strand:** In general RNA is single stranded polynucleotide whereas DNA is double stranded polynucleotide. Even though in RNA at certain places if complementary base pairs are in close proximity this single strand may fold to give a double stranded structure.
4. **Chargaff's rule:** In RNA there is no specific relationship between purine and pyrimidine contents due to the single stranded nature. That means content of cytosine is not equal to content of guanine (C # G).
5. **Alkali hydrolysis susceptibility:** Due to the presence of hydroxyl group at C-2 of ribose, RNA undergoes alkali hydrolysis and produces 2′,3′-cyclic diesters. Whereas DNA is not hydrolyzed by alkali due to lack of hydroxyl group at C-2 of sugar molecules.
6. **Orcinol color reaction:** RNA contains ribose in its structure, hence historically it gives orcinol color reactions; whereas DNA not due to lack of ribose sugar.

   The various similarities and differences between the DNA and RNA are summarized in the Table 4.1.

Table 4.1 Comparison between DNA and RNA.

S. No.	Parameter	DNA	RNA
Differences			
1	Nucleotide	Deoxyribonucleotide	Ribonucleotide
2	Pentose sugar	2-Deoxyribose	Ribose
3	Pyrimidine base	Cytosine & thymine	Cytosine & uracil
4	Structure	Double helix	Single strand
5	Chargaff's rule	Obey	Not obey
6	Alkali hydrolysis	Not susceptible	Susceptible
7	Orcinol color reaction	No characteristic reaction (Negative)	Characteristic reaction (Positive)
8	Types	No types	mRNA, tRNA, rRNA, hnRNA, snRNA, snoRNA, scRNA, tmRNA
9	Other forms	Bent DNA, triple stranded DNA and four stranded DNA	No other forms
10	Function	Hereditary function or genetic information	Biosynthesis of protein
11	Enzyme function	Not act as enzyme	Certain RNA like ribozymes act as enzyme
12	Biosynthesis	From parent DNA by replication	From DNA by transcription
Similarities			
13	Purine base	Adenine & guanine	Adenine & guanine
14	Linkage or bridges	3',5'-phosphodiester bridges	3',5'-phosphodiester bridges
15	Composition	Nitrogen base, sugar and phosphate	Nitrogen base, sugar and phosphate

Types of RNA:

RNAs are primarily involved in the process of protein biosynthesis and are synthesized from DNA. RNAs vary in their structure and functions. Based on the cellular composition there are many different types of RNAs that exist. Among them the first three types are major. They are,

1. **Messenger RNA (mRNA):** 5-10 % mRNA is present in total RNA. To synthesize proteins mRNA transfers genetic information from genes to ribosomes.
2. **Transfer RNA (tRNA):** 10-20 % tRNA is present in total RNA. For protein synthesis it transfers amino acids to mRNA.
3. **Ribosomal RNA (rRNA):** 50-80 % rRNA is present in total RNA. It provides a structural framework for ribosomes.
4. **Heterogenous nuclear RNA (hnRNA):** It serves as a precursor for the synthesis of all RNAs including mRNA.
5. **Small nuclear RNA (snRNA):** It is involved in the processing of mRNA.
6. **Small nucleolar RNA (snoRNA):** It plays a major role in processing of rRNA.
7. **Small cytoplasmic RNA (scRNA):** It is involved in the secretion of proteins for export.
8. **Transfer messenger RNA (tmRNA):** In bacteria it is mostly present and it facilitates the degradation of incorrectly synthesized proteins by adding short peptide tags to proteins.

Messenger RNA (mRNA):

In the nucleus of eukaryotes messenger RNA (mRNA) is synthesized as heterogenous nuclear RNA (hnRNA). The functional mRNA is liberated from hnRNA on processing and this functional mRNA enters into cytoplasm to participate in protein biosynthesis. The half-life of mRNA is short and it has high molecular weight. Compared to prokaryotes mRNA, eukaryotes mRNA is more stable and possess long half-life. 7-Methylguanosine triphosphate capped the 5′-terminal end of eukaryotic mRNA. Hydrolysis of mRNA is prevented by this cap form *5′-exonucleases*. In addition, for protein synthesis this cap is involved in recognition of mRNA. Poly (A) tail is the 3′-terminal ends of mRNA composed of 20 to 250 adenylate residues. This tail prevents mRNA from the attack of 3′-exonuclease and also provides stability to mRNA. Often in the internal structures of mRNA 6-methyl adenylates which are modified bases are present.

Transfer RNA (tRNA):

It is otherwise known as soluble RNA made up of mostly 75 (71 to 80) nucleotides with 25,000 molecular weight. Corresponding to 20 amino acids present in protein there are at least 20 different species of tRNAs present. Holley first elucidated the structure of tRNA for alanine. The structure of tRNA resembles clover leaf and contains four arms. Due to the existence of complementary base pairs in the arms of tRNA, the structure of tRNA is maintained. Base paired stem is present in each arm. Structure of tRNA is presented in (Figure 4.8). The following are the five arms of tRNA.

1. **The acceptor arm:** To the acceptor arm amino acid is attached and is capped in 5′ to 3′ direction with a sequence of CCA. Seven base pairs are present in this arm.
2. **The anticodon arm:** Triplet codon of mRNA is recognized by this anticodon arm only. Three specific nucleotide bases are present in this arm. The codon and anticodon are complementary to each other. In this arm five base pairs are present.
3. **The D-arm:** Dihydrouridine is present in this arm; hence, it is named as D-arm. Four base pairs are present in this arm.
4. **The TΨC-arm:** This arm contains a sequence of T, pseudo define (represented by psi, ø) and C. In this arm five base pairs are present.
5. **The variable arm:** In tRNA this arm is most variable. tRNAs are classified into two major categories based on this variability as follows,
   (a) **Class - I tRNA:** The length of this class tRNA is 3 to 5 base pair length and is the most predominant one with around 75 %.
   (b) **Class - II tRNA:** The length of this class tRNA is 13 to 20 base pair length and is less common with around 25 %.

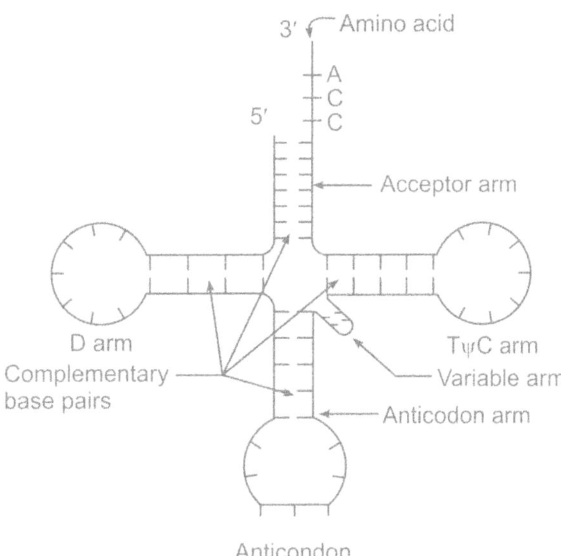

Figure 4.8 Structure of tRNA.

Ribosomal RNA (rRNA):

The protein synthesis factories are ribosomes. Two major nucleoprotein complexes such as 60S subunit and 80S subunit are present in eukaryotic ribosomes. 28S rRNA, 5S rRNA and 5.8S rRNA are present in 60S subunit and 18S rRNA is present in 40S subunit. In ribosomes the function of rRNA is not clearly known. It is believed that they play a significant role in the binding of mRNA to ribosomes and protein synthesis.

Ribozymes (Catalytic RNA):

Ribonucleoproteins (protein associated RNA) of RNA is catalytically active in certain instances and such RNAs are known as ribozymes. Just like proteins i.e., enzymes, RNA molecules adapt tertiary structures. The reason behind the biocatalyst functions of RNA is its specific conformation. During the course of evolution before the occurrence of protein enzymes, ribozymes were functioning as catalysts. The following are some important ribozymes.

(a) **rRNA:** In protein synthesis it is involved in peptide bond formation.
(b) ***Ribonuclease P (RNase P):*** It is a component of RNA and is a ribozyme containing protein. It is involved in cleavage of RNA particularly tRNA precursors to generate mature tRNA molecules. It is also involved in the ligation.
(c) **Self-splicing RNA:** It is involved in the cleavage of DNA.
(d) **RNAs of spliceosome:** It is involved in splicing of RNA.
(e) ***In vitro* selected RNAs:** It is involved in RNA polymerization, RNA aminoacylation, RNA phosphorylation, redox reactions, glycoside bond formation and disulfide exchange.

Recombinant ribozymes (rRibozymes): Any RNA can be cleaved by designing recombinant ribozymes. At present for curing diseases these recombinant ribozymes are considered as therapeutic agents. Theoretically in disease, recombinant ribozymes selectively degrades faulty RNAs such as mutated or inappropriately expressed RNAs. From the cells the specific RNAs can be eliminated by this way which will help to inhibit the disease process.

The Central Dogma of Life

The central dogma of life is flowing of biological information from DNA to RNA and from there to proteins. Through protein synthesis DNA ultimately controls every function of the cell.

In the cell as a carrier of genetic information, DNA must be replicated (duplicated), maintained and passed down accurately to the daughter cells. For this purpose, three Rs of DNA such as replication, recombination and repair are specifically designed. The following are the common features of these three Rs of DNA

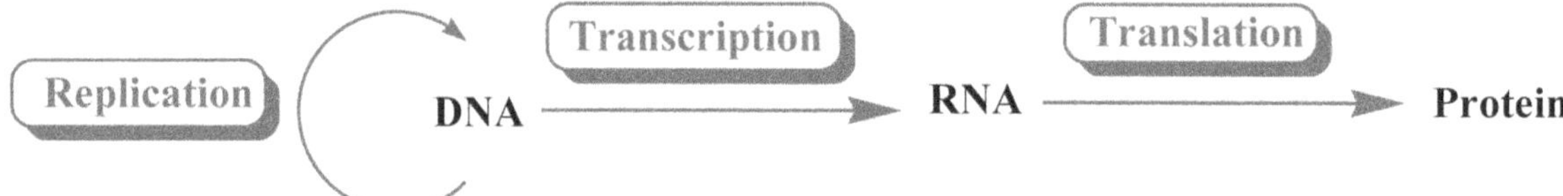

1. They act on DNA (Same substrate)
2. The backbone of DNA structure is phosphodiester bonds. These three Rs are primarily concerned with the making and breaking of these phosphodiester bonds.
3. In these three processes, the enzymes used are similar or comparable.

DNA Replication

Definition: From the parent cell, the daughter cells receive identical copies of genetic information when the cell divides. **The replication is defined as a process in which DNA copies itself to produce identical daughter molecules of DNA.** For the survival of species DNA is essential, hence, with high loyalty replication is carried out. Replication process is a complex one involving a series of steps.

Replication in prokaryotes:

Semi-conservative replication: Two strands which are complementary to each other are present in parent DNA. Two daughter molecules are produced by simultaneous replication of both two strands. In a newly synthesized DNA, one half is original i.e., one strand from parent DNA and the other half is duplicate i.e., another strand is newly synthesized or copied. Since, half of the original DNA is conserved in the daughter DNA this type of replication is called a semi-conservative model. In 1958, Meselson and Stahl provided the first experimental evidence for this semi-conservative DNA replication. In Figure 4.9, semi-conservative DNA replication is presented.

Initiation of replication: Origin of replication is the site for DNA synthesis initiation. There are multiple sites of origin in eukaryotes whereas in prokaryotes only a single site of origin. Mostly in these sites, a short sequence of A-T base pairs is present. For replication, dna A is a specific protein containing 20 to 50 monomers bound with the site of origin leads to separation of double stranded DNA.

Replication bubble: To form a replication bubble, at the site of replication two complementary strands of DNA are separated. For a rapid replication process in eukaryotic DNA, multiple replication bubbles are formed. Multiple replication bubbles formed in DNA replication is schematically presented in Figure 4.10.

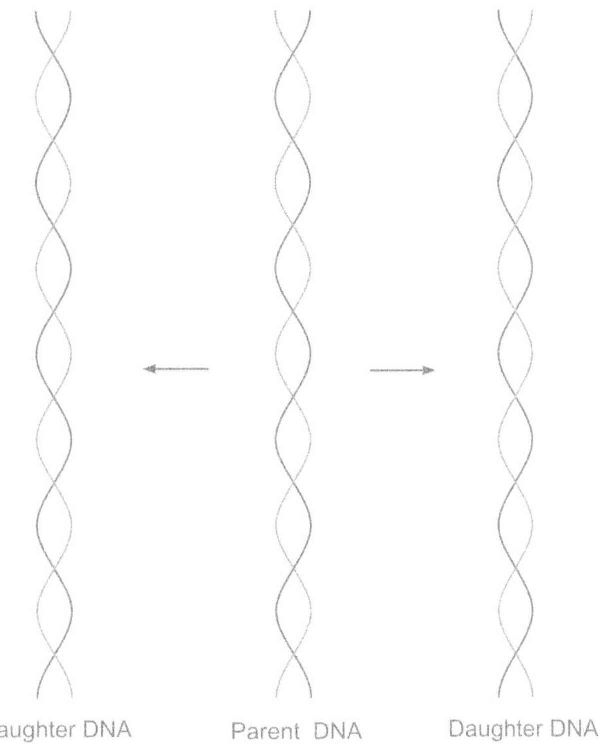

Figure 4.9 Semi-conservative DNA replication.

RNA primer: RNA primer is a short fragment of RNA (contains 5 to 50 nucleotides which is variable with species) needed for the synthesis of new DNA. Primosome is a complex formed by a specific *RNA polymerase* enzyme i.e., *primase* in association with single stranded DNA binding protein (SSBP). RNA primers are produced by *primase*. On the lagging strand of DNA, RNA primer synthesis and supply should occur constantly. In the case of leading strands, almost a single RNA primer is occurring.

Semi discontinuous and bidirectional synthesis of DNA: On both strands of DNA, replication simultaneously occurs in 5′ to 3′ direction. The DNA synthesis is continuous in one strand and that strand

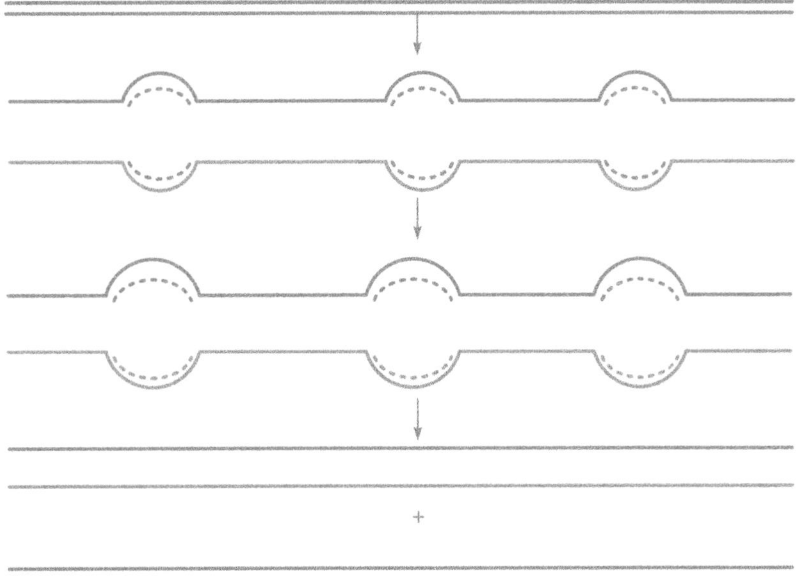

Figure 4.10 Multiple replication bubbles in DNA replication (Schematic representation).

is called a leading or continuous or forward strand. In the other strand, DNA synthesis is discontinuous and that strand is known as lagging or discontinuous or retrograde strand. In the latter strand i.e., lagging strand, short pieces of DNA possessing 15 to 250 nucleotides are produced. From the point of origin of replication bubble, DNA synthesis occurs in both the directions.

Replication fork: Replication fork is formed as a result of separation of two strands of parent DNA. In this region, only active synthesis of DNA takes place. As the daughter DNA molecules are synthesized, the replication fork moves along the parent DNA.

***DNA helicase*:** At the replication fork the enzyme *DNA helicase* binds to both DNA strands. Two strands of DNA are separated when a *DNA helicase* moves along the DNA helix. The function of *DNA helicase* is usually compared with a zip opener and is dependent on ATP for supply of energy.

Single stranded DNA binding protein (SSBP): DNA helix destabilizing protein is the other name of single stranded DNA binding protein (SSBP). Only to a single stranded DNA separated by *DNA helicase*, single stranded DNA binding protein (SSBP) bounds and keep the two strands separate. The template for new DNA synthesis is provided by single stranded DNA binding protein (SSBP). In addition, degradation of single stranded DNA by *nuclease* is also protected by a single stranded DNA binding protein (SSBP).

***DNA polymerase - III*:** In 5′ to 3′ direction new strands of DNA is synthesized and this reaction is catalyzed by *DNA polymerase - III*. To the parent template DNA strand this synthesis is antiparallel. The essential prerequisite for the replication is the presence of all four deoxyribonucleotide such as *d*ATP, *d*GTP, *d*CTP and *d*TTP. Simultaneously two new DNA strands are synthesized but in the opposite direction (One is in 5′ to 3′ direction which is continuous towards the replication fork and another one in 3′ to 5′ direction which is discontinuous away from the replication fork). To the 3′ end of the growing DNA chain one after another the incoming deoxyribonucleotides are added. For addition of each nucleotide one mole of pyrophosphate is removed. The base sequence of the newly synthesized complementary DNA is determined by the parent template DNA strand.

Polarity problem: By sequential addition of new nucleotides, the DNA leading strand with its 3′ end oriented towards the fork can be elongated. In case of DNA lagging strand with 5′ end present some problem due to lack of *DNA polymerase* enzyme which catalyze the addition of nucleotide to the 5′ end i.e., 3′ to 5′ direction of the growing chain. A series of small fragments are synthesized in these strands to solve this problem. In this small fragment synthesis takes place in a normal 5′ to 3′ direction and later joined together. Overview of DNA replication is presented in Figure 4.11.

Okazaki fragments: The small fragments of the discontinuously synthesized DNA are known as Okazaki fragments or pieces. In the parent DNA Okazaki fragments are produced on the lagging DNA strand and are later joined together to form a continuous strand of DNA in presence of *DNA polymerase - I* and *DNA ligase*.

***DNA polymerase - III*:** For the very existence of an organism, fidelity of replication is most important. *DNA polymerase - III* also performs proof reading activity along with 5′to 3′ directed catalytic activity. To the growing DNA strand, it allows only the correct complementary base by checking the incoming nucleotides. In addition, it removes the wrongly placed nucleotide base and edits its mistakes, if any.

RNA primer replacement: Till close proximity to RNA primer, the synthesis of DNA strand continues. *DNA polymerase - I* takes its position by removing the RNA primer. Generally, RNA primer is replaced by a small fragment of DNA synthesized in 5′ to 3′ direction catalyzed by *DNA polymerase - I*.

***DNA ligase*:** DNA synthesized by *DNA polymerase - III* and the small fragment of DNA synthesized by *DNA polymerase - I* are linked by phosphodiester linkage in which the reaction is catalyzed by *DNA ligase*. This process is called nick sealing and it needs energy which is provided by the breakdown of ATP into AMP and pyrophosphate.

***DNA polymerase - II*:** In the DNA repair process, this enzyme participates.

***DNA topoisomerase*:** From one side DNA double helix separates and on the other side, the replication proceeds and super coils form. One end tied two twisted ropes are generally used for the comparison of

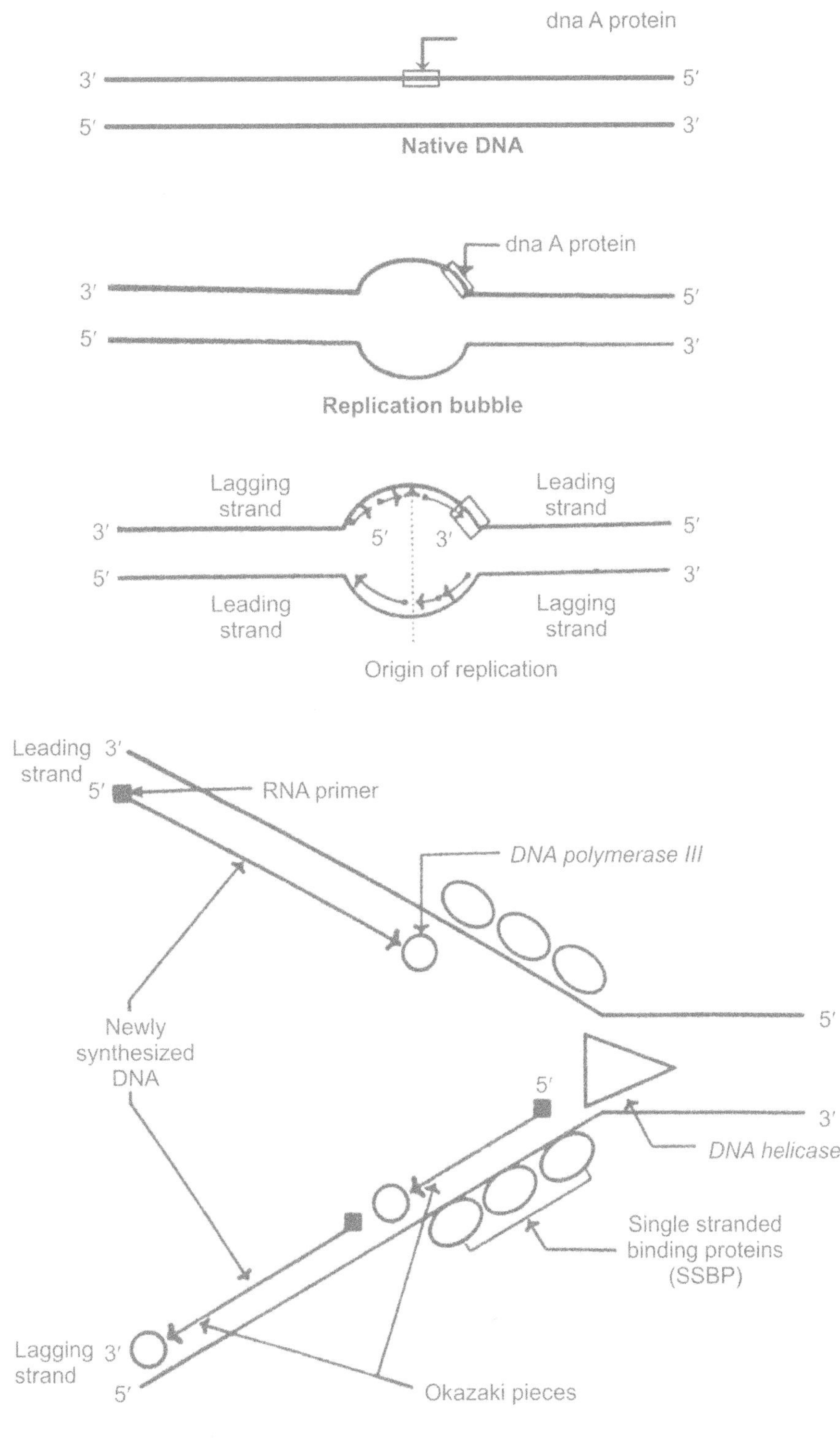

Figure 4.11 Overview of DNA replication.

DNA helix to understand the formation of super coils. The formation of the super coil is clearly observed by holding the rope at the tied end in a fixed position and letting your friend pulls the ropes apart from the other side. There are two *DNA topoisomerase i.e., DNA topoisomerase – I* and *DNA topoisomerase –II*. Among these two, *DNA topoisomerase – I* exhibited *nuclease* activity to overcome the super coils problem by cutting the single DNA strand and then resealed by *DNA ligase*. *DNA topoisomerase – II* is otherwise known as

DNA gyrase which cuts both strands and reseals them to overcome the super coil problem. In the cancer treatment many drugs target *DNA topoisomerases* only. **Example**: Camptothecin targets *DNA topoisomerase -I* and amsacrine and etoposide targets *DNA topoisomerase - II*.

Inhibitors of DNA replication:

DNA topoisomerase - II is otherwise known as *DNA gyrase* is a specific enzyme present in bacteria which cuts and reseals the circular DNA of bacteria to overcome the super coil problem. Antibiotics such as ciprofloxacin, novobiocin and nalidixic acid exhibit its activity by inhibiting this *DNA gyrase* enzyme. These antibiotics effectively block the DNA replication and multiplication of cells; hence they are widely used as antibacterial agents. On human enzymes, these antibiotics have almost no effect.

Anticancer agents such as etoposide, and doxorubicin inhibit human *topoisomerase*. In addition, nucleotide derivatives such as 6-mercptopurine and 5-fluorouracil which inhibit DNA replication are also used as anticancer agents.

Transcription

Definition:

The process of synthesizing ribonucleic acid (RNA) from deoxyribonucleic acid (DNA) is known as transcription. The functional unit of the DNA that can be transcribed is called a gene. Hence, through RNA, DNA expresses the genetic information stored in it. The working copies of RNA molecules produced from antisense or non-coding or template strand which is one of the two strands of DNA. Another one strand is represented as a sense or coding or non-template strand which does not participate in the process of transcription.

Transcription is selective because the entire molecule of DNA is not expressed in transcription. In some selected regions of DNA only RNA is synthesized. In other regions of DNA, there is no transcription at all. In DNA molecules, some inbuilt signals are present which may be responsible for this selectiveness but the exact reasons not known. The primary RNA transcript is the product formed in the transcription and is generally inactive. The functionally active RNA is produced from the primary RNA transcript by some alterations such as splicing, terminal addition, base modification, etc. Some differences are observed between prokaryotes transcription and eukaryotes transcription.

Transcription in Prokaryotes

In prokaryotes, *RNA polymerase* or *DNA dependent RNA polymerase* is the single enzyme involved in the synthesis of all RNAs. Five polypeptide units (Molecular weight: 465 kDa) such as two α, one β, one β' and one σ is present in the *RNA polymerase* which is a complex holoenzyme of *Escherichia Coli (E. coli)*. *RNA polymerase* of *E. coli* & overview of transcription is presented in Figure 4.12 & Figure 4.13, respectively. Without sigma factor or subunits, the enzyme is referred as core enzyme i.e., $\alpha_2\beta\beta'$. Three different stages are involved in the transcription. They are,

1. Stage - 1 or Initiation stage
2. Stage - 2 or Elongation stage
3. Stage - 3 or Termination stage

Stage - 1 or Initiation stage:

For the starting of transcription, the prerequisite needed is the binding of *RNA polymerase* to DNA. Promoter region is the specific region of the DNA where the enzyme binds. The transcription initiation is recognized by *RNA polymerase* through two base sequences present on the coding strand. The two base sequences are,

1. **TATA box or Pribnow box:** In the promoter region of DNA this is the first recognition site. From the starting point of transcription, the TATA box is located about 10 bases away (upstream) on the left side and consists of six nucleotide bases such as TATAAT.

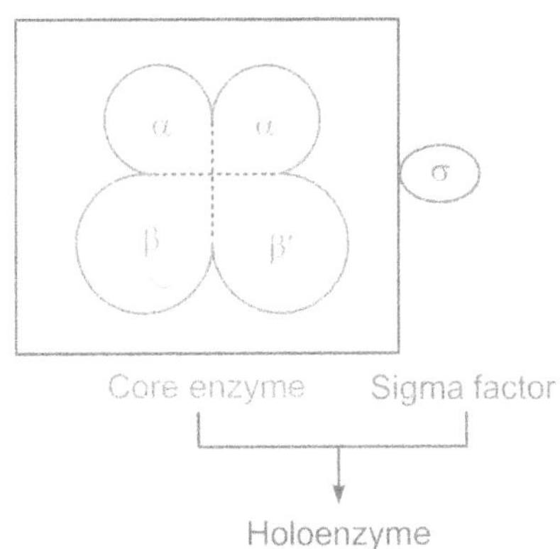

Figure 4.12 *RNA polymerase of E. coli.*

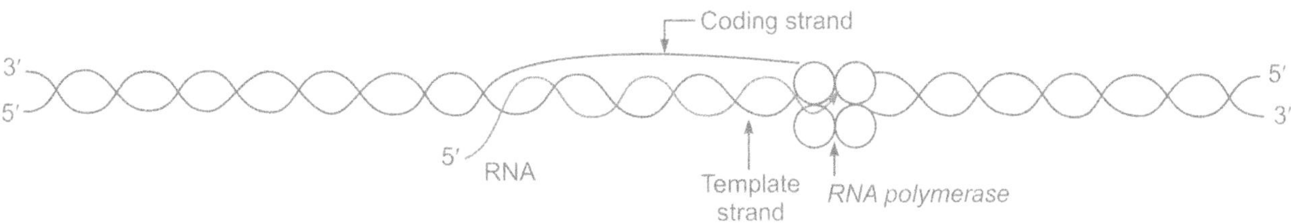

Figure 4.13 Overview of transcription.

2. **The -35 sequence:** In the promoter region of DNA, this is the second recognition site. From the starting point of transcription, the -35 sequence is located about 35 bases away (upstream) on the left side and consists of six nucleotide bases such as TTGACA.

Stage - 2 or Elongation stage:

The sigma factor is released and the transcription proceeds when the *RNA polymerase* recognizes the promoter region as holoenzyme. To the DNA template, RNA is synthesized antiparallelly i.e., 5′ end to 3′ end. RNA is formed using ribonucleotide triphosphate such as ATP, GTP, CTP and UTP by *RNA polymerase.* A pyrophosphate moiety is released for addition of each nucleotide to the growing chain. In mRNA, nucleotide base sequence is complementary to the template DNA strand. However, it is identical to that of

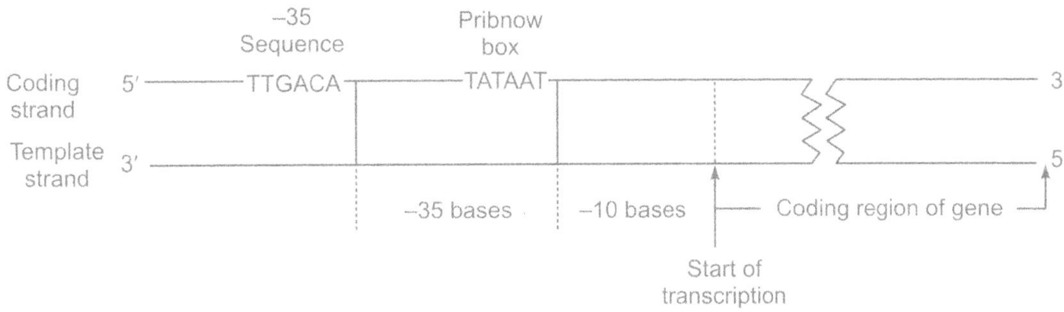

Figure 4.14 Promoter regions of DNA in prokaryotes.

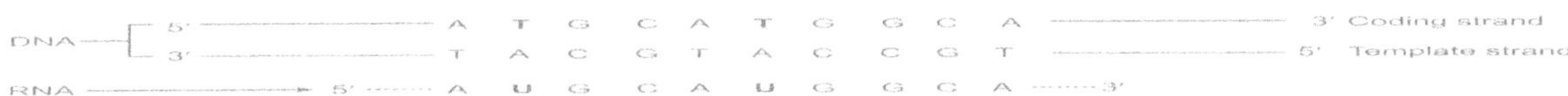

Figure 4.15 Complementary base pair relationship in transcription.

coding strand except that RNA contains U in place of T in DNA. In two aspects *RNA polymerase* is differ from *DNA polymerase*. They are,

1. *RNA polymerase* does not require primer for its activity, whereas *DNA polymerase* requires primer for its activity.
2. *RNA polymerase* does not possess *endonuclease* and *exonuclease* activity whereas *DNA polymerase* possesses *endonuclease* and *exonuclease* activity.

Mistakes in the synthesized RNA cannot be repaired i.e., proofreading activity by *RNA polymerase* due to lack of *endonuclease* and *exonuclease* activity. In the case of DNA, the replication process is carried out with high fidelity; even though mistakes in RNA synthesis are less dangerous because it is not transmitted to the daughter cells. In addition, super coiling problems in DNA replication due to double helical structure of DNA is overcome by *topoisomerase*.

Stage - 3 or Termination stage:

Termination signals stop the process of transcription. Two different terminations are identified. They are,

1. **Rho (ρ) dependent termination:** To the growing RNA (not to *RNA polymerase*) or weakly to DNA, a specific protein namely ρ factor is bound. This ρ factor terminates transcription and releases RNA by acting as *ATPase* in bound state. In addition, for dissociation of *RNA polymerase* from DNA, this ρ factor is also responsible.
2. **Rho (ρ) independent termination:** In this case, termination is brought by hairpins formation in the newly synthesized RNA due to palindromes presence. Palindrome is a word that reads alike forward and backward (**Example:** Madam and rotor). The termination region is known by the presence of palindromes (same when read in opposite directions also) in the base sequence of DNA template. Hence, hairpins are formed by the newly synthesized RNA by folding due to complementary base pairing. This may lead to termination of transcription. The various stages involved in the process of prokaryotes transcription is presented in Figure 4.16.

Inhibitors of transcription:

Certain toxins and antibiotics inhibit the synthesis of RNA.

1. **α-Amanitin:** *Amanita phalloide* is a delicious mushroom in taste but it produces a toxin called α-amanitin. This α-amanitin inhibits transcription by binding with *RNA polymerase – II* of eukaryotes. Hence, *Amanita phalloide* mushroom is a poisonous one.
2. **Actinomycin-D or Dactinomycin:** *Streptomyces* species synthesize dactinomycin. It blocks the movement of *RNA polymerase* by binding with DNA template strand. For the treatment of cancer this was the very first antibiotic used.
3. **Rifampin:** For the treatment of tuberculosis and leprosy, the antibiotic rifampin is widely used. It inhibits the activity of prokaryotic *RNA polymerase* by binding with their β-subunit.

Genetic code

Genetic code is simply known as codons. Genetic code is constituted by triplet (three nucleotides) base sequences in mRNA that act as code words for amino acids in protein. In protein the sequence of amino acids is determined by genetic code and this genetic code is considered as a dictionary of nucleotide bases (A, G, C and U). Generally, codons consist of four nucleotide bases such as purine bases [adenine (A) and guanine (G)] and pyrimidine base [cytosine (C) and uracil (U)]. 64 (4^3) combinations of three base codons are produced by these four bases. In mRNA, from 5′ to 3′ direction, the nucleotide sequence of codons is written. For the twenty different amino acids in protein sixty-one codons are available. The remaining three codons such as UAA, UAG and UGA do not code for amino acids. In protein synthesis, these three codons stop the signals, hence they are termed as termination codons or non-sense codons. The codons UAA, UAG and UGA are often referred to as ochre, amber and opal codons, respectively. In addition, codons AUG and sometimes GUG act as initiating codons. The Various genetic codes are summarized in Table 4.2.

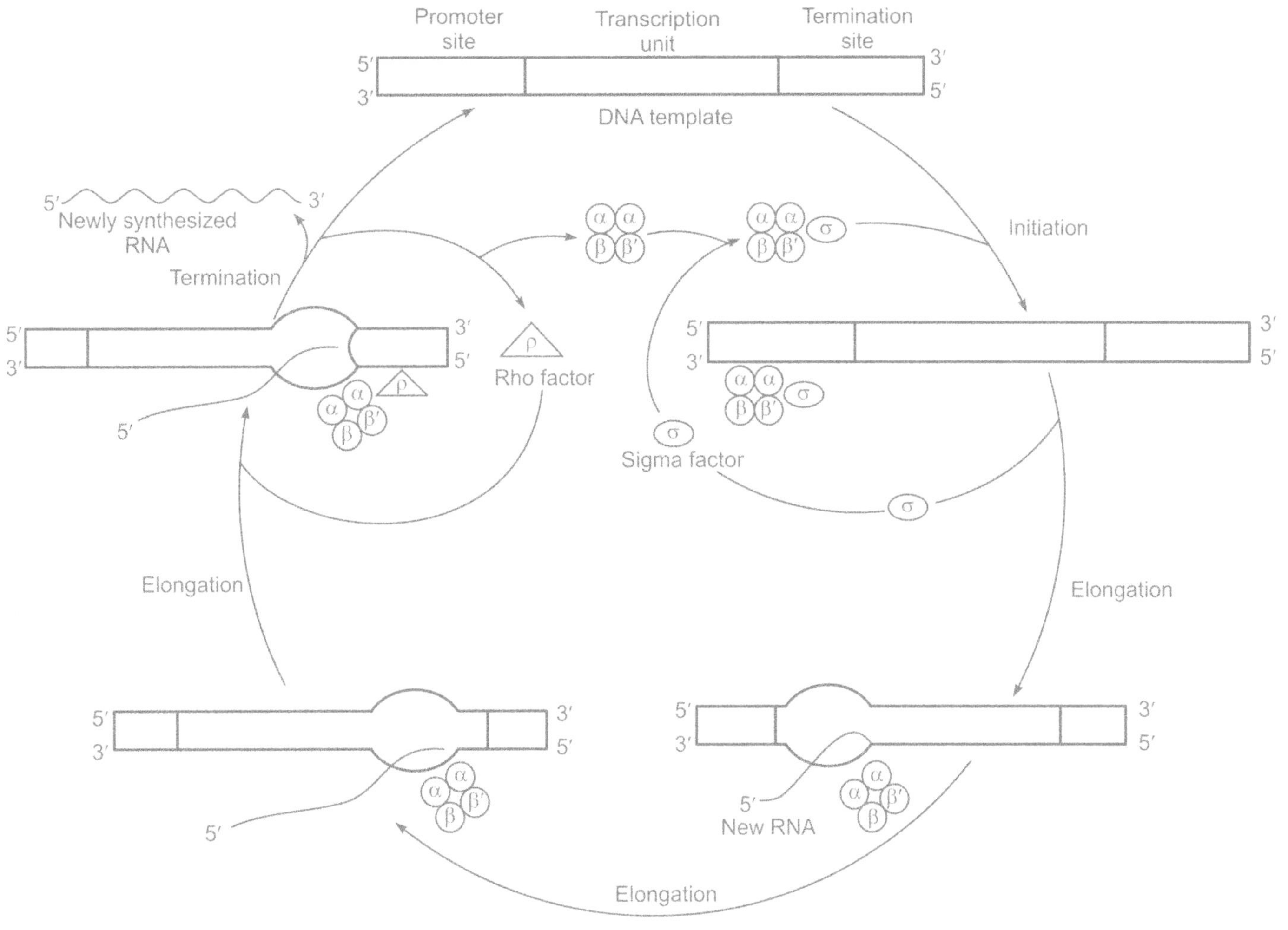

Figure 4.16 Stages involved in prokaryotes transcription.

The following are some other characteristics of genetic code.

1. **Universal:** In all the living organisms, for the same amino acids, same codons are used. Thus, during the course of evolution, the genetic code has been conserved. Hence, the genetic code is regarded as universal, approximately. Even though there are few exceptions. **Example:** In mitochondria for methionine the codon is AUA, whereas in cytoplasm the same codon codes for isoleucine. Therefore, the genetic code is universal with some exceptions.
2. **Specific:** Same amino acid is always coded by a particular codon only. Hence, genetic code is highly specific or unambiguous. **Example:** For tryptophan the codon is UGG.
3. **Non overlapping:** As a continuous base sequence the genetic code is read from a fixed point. It is usually non overlapping, comma less and without any punctuations. **Example:** UUUCUUAGAGGG is read as UUU / CUU / AGA / GGG. In mRNA the message sequence is radically changed due to addition or deletion of one or two bases. Such mRNA will produce protein which is totally different. This is encountered in the frame shift mutations which cause an alteration in the reading frame of mRNA.
4. **Degenerate:** More than one codon is available for most of the amino acids. For twenty amino acids there are sixty-one codons available, hence, the codon is redundant or degenerate. **Example:** Four codons available for glycine. The codons that designate the same amino acids are called synonyms and differ only in the third base (3′ end) of the codon.

The various genetic code along with their respective amino acids are tabulated in Table 4.2.

Table 4.2 Genetic code along with respective amino acids.

First base 5' end	Second base (Middle one)				Third base 3' end
	U	C	A	G	
U	UUU Phe UUC UUA Leu UUG	UCU UCC Ser UCA UCG	UAU Try UAC UAA Stop UAG Stop	UGU Cys UGC UGA Stop UGG Trp	U C A G
C	CUU CUC Leu CUA CUG	CCU CCC Pro CCA CCG	CAU His CAC CAA Gin CAG	CGU CGC Arg CGA CGG	U C A G
A	AUU AUC Ile AUA AUG Met (initiation)	ACU ACC Thr ACA ACG	AAU Asn AAC AAA Lys AAG	AGU Ser AGC AGA Arg AGG	U C A G
G	GUU GUC Val GUA GUG	GCU GCC Ala GCA GCG	GAU Asp GAC GAA Glu GAG	GGU GGC Gly GGA GGG	U C A G

Protein Biosynthesis

The following are the five different stages involved in the synthesis of proteins which involves the translation of nucleotide base sequence of mRNA into the language of amino acid sequences.

1. Components requirement
2. Amino acids activation
3. Proper protein synthesis
4. Chaperones and protein folding
5. Post-translational modifications of proteins

1. Components requirement:

Protein synthesis needs many components such as amino acids, ribosomes, messenger RNA (mRNA), transfer RNA (tRNA), energy sources like ATP and GTP and protein factors.

Amino acids: Proteins are the polymer of amino acids. Hence, amino acid presence is the primary requirement for protein synthesis. Protein present in nature only twenty amino acids are repeatedly present. Among these, the body is able to synthesize ten amino acids which are known as non-essential amino acids and hence these amino acids are not necessary to take through dietary sources. The remaining ten amino acids are not synthesized in the body which are known as essential amino acids and hence, these amino acids are necessary to be taken through dietary sources. When all the amino acids needed for the synthesis of protein are available, then only the protein synthesis takes place. Even deficiency of one essential amino acid in dietary sources leads to stopping of translation. Hence, the dietary source must contain all essential amino acids in sufficient quantities to maintain protein synthesis as amino acids are pre-requisite for synthesis of proteins. In case of prokaryotes from inorganic components, all twenty amino acids are synthesized, hence, no amino acid is required.

Ribosomes: The center or factories for protein synthesis are ribosomes. In translation, ribosomes are considered as workbenches. Ribosomes are the huge complex structure (70S for prokaryotes and 80S for eukaryotes) of proteins and ribosomal RNAs. One big and one small sub units are present in each ribosome. A-site and P-site are the two sites of functional ribosomes. Both the sub units are covered by each site. During the course of translation, A-site is considered as acceptor site and aminoacyl tRNA binds in it; whereas P-site is considered as donor site and peptidyl tRNA binds in it. In case of eukaryotes, a third site is present which is commonly known as E-site or exit site. In the cytosomal fraction of the cell, ribosomes are present.

In general, ribosomes are found in association with rough endoplasmic reticulum (RER) to form RER-ribosomes in which synthesis of protein takes place. On a single mRNA, if many ribosomes simultaneously translate then the ribosome is known as polysome or polyribosome.

Messenger RNA (mRNA): For the synthesis of a given protein, the specific information required is present on the mRNA. In the form of codons, the genetic information is passed from DNA to mRNA to translate into a protein sequence.

Transfer RNA (tRNA): To the growing polypeptide chain, the amino acids are carried and handed over by tRNA. At 3′-end amino acids are covalently bonded to tRNA. Anticodon is the three-nucleotide base sequence present in each tRNA which is responsible to recognize the codon (complementary bases) of mRNA for protein synthesis. In a bacteria, forty different tRNAs and in a man fifty different tRNAs are found. Amino acids with multiple codons have more than one tRNA.

Energy sources: During protein synthesis, energy is supplied by both ATP and GTP. In general, energy is obtained by the breakdown of ATP and GTP into AMP and GMP, respectively with liberation of pyrophosphate. Two high energy phosphates equivalent to two ATP is consumed by each one of these reactions.

Protein factors: There are a number of protein factors involved in the process of translation. In the translation process, these protein factors are needed for initiation, elongation and termination. Compared to prokaryotes, the protein factors are complex in eukaryotes.

2. **Amino acids activation:**

   In a two-step reaction, the amino acids are activated and attached to tRNAs. *Aminoacyl tRNA synthetases* are a group of enzymes needed for this process. For the amino acids and their corresponding tRNAs these enzymes are highly specific. First, to the enzyme utilizing ATP, amino acids are attached to form enzyme-AMP-amino acid complex. Later, to form aminoacyl tRNA, the amino acid is transferred to the 3′ end of the tRNA.

3. **Proper protein synthesis:**

   Rather polyribosomes, the polypeptide or protein synthesis is occurring on ribosomes only. The polypeptide synthesis proceeds from N-terminal end to C-terminal end by mRNA reading in the 5′ to 3′ direction. Translation is directional and collinear with mRNA. Eukaryotic mRNA codes for a single polypeptide, hence termed as monocistronic and in contrast prokaryotic mRNA codes for a multiple polypeptide due to presence of many coding regions in mRNA, hence termed as polycistronic.

   In prokaryotes, both transcription and translation take place simultaneously because before transcription of gene is completed translation commences. In case eukaryotes, it is not possible because in nucleus transcription occurs and in cytosol translation occurs. In addition, to generate functional mRNA, the hnRNA (primary transcript synthesized from DNA) undergoes several modifications. Compared to eukaryotes in prokaryotes, the protein synthesis is comparatively simple. Earlier in eukaryotic translation, many steps were not understood but now it is better understood due to advancement in molecular biology.

   Eukaryotic translation is divided into three different stages as initiation, elongation and termination.

   (a) **Initiation:**

   In eukaryotes, at least ten different eukaryotic initiation factors (eIFs) are involved in initiation of translation, hence it is complex. Multiple (3 to 8) sub-units are present in some of eIFs. Four steps are involved in the initiation process. They are,

   1. Dissociation of ribosomes

2. 43S pre-initiation complex formation
3. 48S initiation complex formation
4. 80S initiation complex formation

1. **Dissociation of ribosomes:** 40S and 60S subunits are formed by dissociation of 80S ribosomes. To the newly formed 40S subunit eIF-1A and eIF-3 are binds and blocks the re-association of eIF-1A and eIF-3 with 60S subunit. Hence these initiating factors are also known as anti-association factors.
2. **43S pre-initiation complex formation:** 43S pre-initiation complex is formed by attaching GTP bound a ternary complex possessing met-rRNA′ (Superscript ′ is used in met-tRNA because it is specifically involved in binding to the initiation codon AUGs) and elf-2 to 40S ribosomal subunit. This complex is stabilized by the presence of elf-3 and elf-1A.
3. **48S initiation complex formation:** This complex is formed by binding of mRNA to 43S pre-initiation complex through the intermediate 43S initiation complex. In this interaction between elFs and activation of mRNA is involved.
4. **80S initiation complex formation:** This complex is formed by binding of 48S initiation complex with 60S ribosomal subunit. Hydrolysis of elF bound GTP is involved in the binding. elF-5 is involved in the facilitation of this step.

   Recognition and regulation of initiation: The initiation codon is 5′-AUG and the specific nucleotides surrounding it facilitates its recognition. Identification of AUG by this marker sequence is known as Kozak consensus sequences. In case of prokaryotes, Shine - Dalgarno sequence recognizes initiation codon sequence. The initiation and thus translation are controlled by elF-4F complex formation by the assembly of three initiation factors. The rate limiting step in the translation is recognition of mRNA cap by the elF-4F complex in which elF-4E is the primary component involved in this. To some extent, protein synthesis is also controlled by elF-2 involved in the formation of 43S pre-initiation complex.

   Initiation of translation in prokaryotes: Compared to eukaryotes the initiation of translation in prokaryotes is a simple process and less complicated. IF-3 is bound to the 30S ribosomal subunit and attached to the ternary complex of IF-2, formyl met-tRNA and GTP. In the formation of pre-initiation complex IF-1 also participates. Shine - Dalgarno sequence recognizes initiation codon AUG sequence. In prokaryotes 70S initiation complex is produced by binding of a 50S ribosome unit with 30S unit.

(b) Elongation:

Polypeptide chain is elongated by ribosomes through a sequential addition of amino acids. In the specific mRNA the order of codons determines the amino acid sequence. Certain elongation factor is involved in the cyclic process of elongation. This cyclic process involves three steps as follows,

1. Binding of aminoacyl tRNA to A-site
2. Formation of peptide bond
3. Translocation

Binding of aminoacyl tRNA to A-site: A-site is free and in the P-site met-tRNA′ is present in the 80S initiation complex. In the A-site another aminoacyl tRNA is placed. Energy supply by CTP, involvement of EF-1a (elongation factor 1a) and mRNA proper codon recognition is required for this process. Another aminoacyl tRNA is brought by recycled EF-1a and GDP because in the A-site, aminoacyl tRNA is placed.

Formation of peptide bond: Peptide bond formation is catalyzed by the enzyme *peptidyl transferase*. On 28S RNA of 60S ribosomal subunit the activity of *peptidyl transferase* lies. Hence, the peptide bond formation is catalyzed by rRNA (and not protein) referred to as ribozyme. For peptide bond formation there is no need for additional energy because in the aminoacyl tRNA, amino acid is already activated. In the A-site, a growing peptide chain is attached as the net result of peptide bond formation.

Translocation: Towards 3′-end, ribosomes are moved to the next codon of the mRNA as the peptide bond formation occurs. In the basic process of translocation from A-site growing peptide chain is moved to P-site. EF-2 and CTP are required for translocation and the energy for mRNA movement is provided by the hydrolysis of GTP. For translocation EF-2 and GTP complex recycles. In eukaryotes recently E-site i.e., exit site is identified. Into the E-site the deacylated tRNA moves from where it leaves the ribosome. The elongation factors are different in case of prokaryotes and they are, EF-Tu and EF-Ts in place of EF-1a and EF-G in place of EF-2.

In eukaryotes during the course of translocation, per second about six amino acids are incorporated; whereas in prokaryotes it is twenty amino acids. Hence with a great speed and accuracy in translation the protein or polypeptide synthesis occurs.

(c) **Termination:**

Compared to initiation and elongation, the process of termination is simple. The growing polypeptide chain is terminated by one of the termination codons i.e., UAA, UAG and UCA after the several cycles of elongation. No specific tRNA is available to bind for the termination codons. A-site of the ribosome is occupied by termination codon and the stop signal is recognized by the release factor namely eRF. In the P-site the peptide bond formed between the polypeptide and tRNA is cleaved by eRF-GTP complex in association with enzyme *peptidyl transferase*. Instead of amino acid, water molecules are added in this step. From the P-site, protein and tRNA is released by this hydrolysis. 40S and 60S subunits (obtained from dissociation of 80S ribosome) are recycled and the mRNA is also released.

4. **Chaperones and protein folding:**

Chaperones are the heat shock proteins which facilitate and favor the interactions on the polypeptide surfaces to finally give the specific conformation of a protein. One major function of chaperones is to prevent both newly synthesized polypeptide chains and assembled subunits from aggregating into nonfunctional structures. Chaperones are found mainly in the endoplasmic reticulum (ER), since protein synthesis often occurs in this area. Human chaperones are broadly classified into four major types. They are,

1. General chaperones: GRP78/BiP, GRP94, GRP170
2. Lectin chaperones: Calnexin and calreticulin
3. Non-classical molecular chaperones: HSP47 and ERp29
4. Folding chaperones: *Protein disulfide isomerase (PDI), Peptidyl prolyl cis-trans-isomerase (PPI),* ERp57

5. **Post-translational modifications of proteins:**

As such the protein synthesized in the translation is not functional. In the polypeptides many changes are takes place after initiation of protein synthesis or mostly after the completion of protein synthesis. The following processes are collectively known as post-translational modifications. They are,

1. Protein folding
2. Trimming by proteolytic degradation
3. Intern splicing
4. Covalent changes

Inhibitors of Protein Synthesis

The favorite target for antibiotics is translation only. In general antibiotics are the compounds produced by bacteria or fungi which inhibit the growth of other organisms. Most of the antibiotics are harmless to the higher organism and it only interferes with the protein synthesis of bacteria because eukaryotes and prokaryotes are sufficiently different in their translation process. The following are the various inhibitors of protein synthesis.

1. **Streptomycin:** It inhibits the initiation of protein synthesis by causing misreading of mRNA and interfering with the normal pairing between codons and anticodons.

2. **Tetracycline:** Binding of aminoacyl tRNA to ribosomal complex is inhibited by tetracycline. Eukaryotic protein synthesis can also be blocked by tetracycline but eukaryotic cell membrane is not permeable to tetracycline; hence it does not happen.
3. **Puromycin:** It is structurally related to aminoacyl tRNA. Into the growing polypeptide chain puromycin is incorporated by entering into the A-site. In both eukaryotes and prokaryotes, protein synthesis is prevented by puromycin.
4. **Chloramphenicol:** It is a competitive inhibitor of *peptidyl transferase*. Hence, it interferes with peptide chain elongation.
5. **Erythromycin:** It binds with 50S subunit of bacterial ribosome and inhibits translocation.
6. **Diphtheria toxin:** It inactivates the elongation factor eEF_2. Hence, eukaryotes prevent translocation in protein synthesis.

PROBABLE QUESTIONS

PART - A: Multiple Choice Questions

1. Which of the following compound is not involved in the synthesis of pyrimidine?
   (a) Glutamine (b) Aspartate
   (c) N^{10}-formyl THF (d) CO_2
2. Numbering of pyrimidine follows which pattern?
   (a) Anti-clockwise (b) Clockwise
   (c) Either (a) or (b) (d) Both (a) and (b)
3. Which is the rate limiting enzyme of purine biosynthesis?
   (a) *PRPP glutamyl ketotransferase* (b) *PRPP glutamyl methyltransferase*
   (c) *RPP glutamyl aminotransferase* (d) *PRPP glutamyl sulphotranaferase*
4. What is the end product of purine metabolism?
   (a) Xanthine (b) Uric acid
   (c) Hypoxanthine (d) IMP
5. What is the end product of pyrimidine metabolism?
   (a) Acetyl CoA (b) Uric acid
   (c) Ammonia (d) Xanthine
6. Reye's syndrome is a metabolic disorder of ______________.
   (a) Purine (b) Cholesterol
   (c) Bile acids (d) Pyrimidine
7. Synthesis of protein from RNA is known as______________?
   (a) Replication (b) Transcription
   (c) Translation (d) All of them
8. DNA synthesis is continuous in which strand?
   (a) Lagging (b) Leading
   (c) Either (a) or (b) (d) Both (a) and (b)
9. Which performs proof reading activity?
   (a) *DNA polymerase-I* (b) *DNA polymerase-II*
   (c) *DNA polymerase-III* (d) *DNA polymerase-IV*

10. Which enzyme separates the strands of DNA?
    (a) *DNA ligase* (b) *DNA polymerase*
    (c) *DNA gyrase* (d) *DNA helicase*
11. Which is the promoter region of transcription?
    (a) TATA box (b) CAAT box
    (c) Either (a) or (b) (d) Both (a) and (b)
12. Which is the initiating codon?
    (a) AUG (b) UAA
    (c) UAG (d) UGA
13. An amino group donated by glutamine is attached at C-1 of PRPP, this results in ___________
    (a) 5-Phosphoribosylamine (b) 4-Phosphoribosylamine
    (c) 3-Phosphoribosylamine (d) 2-Phosphoribosylamine
14. The first intermediate with a complete purine ring is ___________
    (a) Inosinate (b) Formate
    (c) Aspartate (d) Glycine
15. Which of the following is an important precursor in the purine pathway?
    (a) Glycine (b) Aspartate
    (c) Glutamine (d) Leucine
16. Which of the following is an important precursor in pyrimidine pathway?
    (a) Glycine (b) Aspartate
    (c) Glutamine (d) Leucine
17. In the first committed step of pyrimidine biosynthesis, the reaction is catalyzed by ___________.
    (a) *Adenylate kinase* (b) *Aspartate transcarbamoylase*
    (c) *Dihyhroorotase* (d) *Cytidylate synthase*
18. The phenomenon of twisting around itself by a molecule to relieve helical stress is ___________
    (a) Supercoiling (b) Coiling
    (c) Elongation (d) Compression
19. When there is no net bending of the DNA axis upon itself, the DNA is said to be in a ___________
    (a) Elongated state (b) Compressed state
    (c) Relaxed state (d) Denatured state
20. Over-twisting of a molecule results in ___________
    (a) Negative supercoiling (b) Positive supercoiling
    (c) Elongation (d) Compression
21. Changing twist from the relaxed state requires adding energy and increases the ___________
    (a) Forces in molecule (b) Stress along molecule
    (c) Strain over molecule (d) None of the above
22. The enzyme responsible for the removal of supercoiling in replicating DNA ahead of the replication fork is ___________
    (a) *Topoisomerase* (b) *Primase*
    (c) *DNA polymerase* (d) *Helicase*
23. Which type of *topoisomerases* generally relaxes DNA by removing negative supercoiling?
    (a) Type-I (b) Type-II
    (c) Type-III (d) Type-IV

24. The type of *topoisomerases* that can introduce negative supercoils is ___________
    (a) Type-I (b) Type-II
    (c) Type-III (d) Type-IV
25. Chromatin is composed of ___________
    (a) DNA (b) DNA and proteins
    (c) DNA, RNA and proteins (d) None of the above
26. What is DNA replication?
    (a) Conservative (b) Non-conservative
    (c) Semi-conservative (d) None of the above
27. Eukaryotes differ from prokaryote in mechanism of DNA replication due to ___________
    (a) Use of DNA primer rather than RNA primer
    (b) Different enzyme for synthesis of lagging and leading strand
    (c) Discontinuous rather than semi-discontinuous replication
    (d) Unidirectional rather than semi-discontinuous replication
28. Which of the following is true about *DNA polymerase*?
    (a) It can synthesize DNA in the 5′ to 3′ direction
    (b) It can synthesize DNA in the 3′ to 5′ direction
    (c) It can synthesize mRNA in the 3′ to 5′ direction
    (d) It can synthesize mRNA in the 5′ to 3′ direction
29. What is the reaction in DNA replication catalyzed by *DNA ligase*?
    (a) Addition of new nucleotides to the leading strand
    (b) Addition of new nucleotide to the lagging strand
    (c) Formation of a phosphodiester bond between the 3′-OH of one Okazaki fragment and the 5′-phosphate of the next on the lagging strand
    (d) Base pairing of the template and the newly formed DNA strand
30. Which of the following reactions is required for proof reading during DNA replication by *DNA polymerase-III*?
    (a) 5′ to 3′ *exonuclease* activity (b) 3′ to 5′ *exonuclease* activity
    (c) 3′ to 5′ *endonuclease* activity (d) 5′ to 3′ *endonuclease* activity
31. Which of the following enzyme remove supercoiling in replicating DNA ahead of the replication fork?
    (a) *DNA polymerase* (b) *Helicase*
    (c) *Primase* (d) *Topoisomerase*
32. DNA unwinding is done by ___________
    (a) *Ligase* (b) *Helicase*
    (c) *Topoisomerase* (d) *Hexonuclease*
33. Which of the following enzymes is the principal replication enzyme in *E. coli*?
    (a) *DNA polymerase-I* (b) *DNA polymerase-II*
    (c) *DNA polymerase-III* (d) None of the above
34. Which enzyme is used to join bits of DNA?
    (a) *DNA polymerase* (b) *DNA ligase*
    (c) *Endonuclease* (d) *Primase*

35. Which of the following has the self-repairing mechanisms?
    (a) DNA and RNA
    (b) DNA, RNA and protein
    (c) Only DNA
    (d) DNA and protein
36. Which of the following involves remarkable capacity of a short segment of DNA to move from one place to another?
    (a) DNA transposition
    (b) DNA replication
    (c) Translation
    (d) Transcription
37. Which of the following process occurs between DNA molecules of very similar sequences?
    (a) Homologous genetic recombination
    (b) Site specific recombination
    (c) Non-homologous recombination
    (d) Replicative recombination
38. Transcription is catalyzed by ___________
    (a) DNA-dependent *RNA polymerase*
    (b) RNA-dependent *DNA polymerase*
    (c) *Reverse transcriptase*
    (d) *DNA ligase*
39. Where does *RNA polymerase* bind DNA?
    (a) Promoter
    (b) Operator
    (c) Enhancer
    (d) None of the above
40. Which of the following is true about RNA synthesis?
    (a) Synthesis of RNA is always in the 5′ to 3′ direction
    (b) *RNA polymerase* requires a primer for initiating transcription
    (c) "U" is inserted opposite "T" in transcription
    (d) New nucleotides are added on the 2′-OH of the ribose sugar
41. What is the role of sigma factor in bacterial *RNA polymerase*?
    (a) Catalyzing RNA synthesis
    (b) Positioning *RNA polymerase* correctly on the DNA template
    (c) Terminating RNA synthesis
    (d) Unwinding DNA template
42. TBP stands for?
    (a) *TATA box polymerase*
    (b) TATA box binding protein
    (c) Transcription associated factor
    (d) Transcription factor binding protein
43. Actinomycin-D is an inhibitor of ___________
    (a) Transcription
    (b) Translation
    (c) Replication
    (d) None of the above
44. Number of hydrogen bonds that form between "U" and "A" in a Watson-Crick base pair interactions?
    (a) 0
    (b) 1
    (c) 2
    (d) 3
45. Repressors bind to ___________
    (a) Promoter
    (b) Enhancer
    (c) Operator
    (d) Hormone response element
46. RNA primer is removed from the Okazaki fragment by ___________
    (a) *DNA polymerase-I*
    (b) *DNA polymerase-II*
    (c) *DNA polymerase-III*
    (d) *RNA polymerase*

47. Binding of the prokaryotic DNA dependent *RNA polymerase* to promoter site is inhibited by ___________

(a) Rifampicin (b) Tetracycline
(c) Puromycin (d) Streptomycin

48. Which of the following is an incorrect statement about m-RNA?

(a) Cap is added to the 5′ end
(b) Introns are removed and exons are spliced together
(c) Histone mRNAs lack 5′ cap
(d) Poly-A tail is added to the 3′ end

Key for Multiple Choice Questions

1. (c)	2. (b)	3. (c)	4. (b)	5. (a)
6. (d)	7. (c)	8. (b)	9. (c)	10. (d)
11. (c)	12. (a)	13. (a)	14. (a)	15. (a)
16. (b)	17. (b)	18. (a)	19. (c)	20. (b)
21. (b)	22. (a)	23. (a)	24. (b)	25. (c)
26. (c)	27. (c)	28. (a)	29. (c)	30. (b)
31. (d)	32. (b)	33. (c)	34. (b)	35. (c)
36. (a)	37. (a)	38. (a)	39. (a)	40. (a)
41. (b)	42. (b)	43. (a)	44. (c)	45. (c)
46. (a)	47. (a)	48. (b)		

PART - B: Short Answers

1. How AMP & GMP is synthesized from IMP?
2. Note on Salvage pathway for purine nucleotide synthesis.
3. How deoxyribonucleotides are synthesized from ribonucleotides?
4. What is genetic code? Write characteristic features of genetic code.
5. Explain the role of various *DNA polymerases* in prokaryotic replication process.
6. Write the mechanism of inhibition of protein synthesis by chloramphenicol.
7. Name the enzymes involved in DNA replication.
8. Write a note on inhibitors of protein synthesis.
9. What is semi-conservative DNA replication?
10. Outline the role of ribosomes in protein synthesis.
11. What is hyperuricemia & uricosuria?
12. Write a note on gout.
13. Explain Chargaff's rule.
14. Write a note on denaturation of DNA strands.
15. What is central dogma of life?
16. Explain Okazaki fragments.
17. Write a note on Wobble hypothesis.

PART - C: Long Answers

1. How purine nucleotides are degraded?
2. Enumerate the biosynthesis and degradation of uric acid?
3. Explain the structure of DNA.
4. Write a detailed note on structure of RNA?
5. Explain various metabolic disorders of purine metabolism.
6. Write a detailed note on organization of mammalian genome.
7. Write in detail prokaryotic translation process.
8. Explain in detail DNA replication process in prokaryotes.
9. Outline various steps involved in eukaryotic protein synthesis.
10. Write about various steps involved in protein synthesis.
11. Write about metabolic diseases associated with defective nucleic acid metabolism.
12. Write about DNA replication mechanism. Discuss about the different types of DNA replication and repair mechanisms.
13. Explain the mechanism and function of DNA replication.
14. Write about catabolism of purine nucleotides.
15. Write a note on transcription & translation.
16. Explain replication in detail.
17. Explain the biosynthesis of purines.
18. Sketch the biosynthesis of pyrimidines.
19. Enumerate the salient features of DNA replication & its regulation.
20. Explain the transcription taking place in eukaryotes
21. Write about catabolism of pyrimidine nucleotides.

UNIT 5

Enzymes

Enzymes are the bio-chemicals synthesized by living cells which increases the rate of the biochemical reaction without undergoing any changes itself. They are protein in nature (except RNA acting as *ribozyme*), colloidal (does not form true solution in water due to huge size), thermolabile (affected by heat) and specific in their action. They are huge in size with a small active site.

In biochemical lab, enzymes are highly used for diagnosis of various diseases. For example, in laboratory condition a couple of days are needed for hydrolysis of proteins even at 100 °C in presence of strong acid like hydrochloric acid, etc.; whereas the same reaction in a biological system is completed within 2 hours at body temperature itself in presence of GIT enzymes. This reaction shows the efficiency of enzymes.

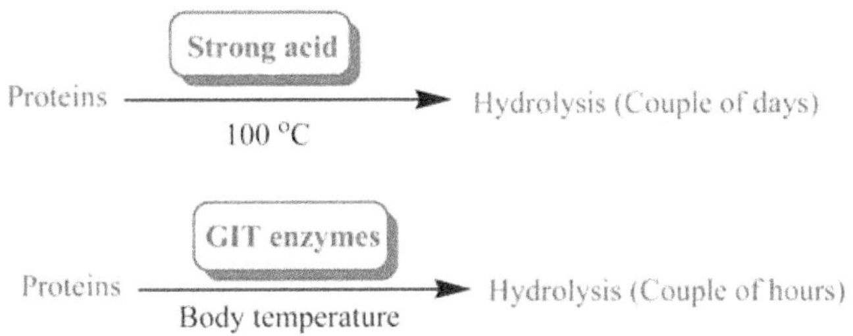

Properties of Enzymes

1. All enzymes are proteins except RNA as a *ribozyme*.
2. Holo-enzyme is the functional unit of enzyme and it is composed of two major parts namely apo-enzyme and co-enzyme. The Protein part of enzyme is called as apo-enzyme and the non-protein part of enzyme is called as co-enzyme.

Holoenzyme (Active enzyme) ⟶ **Apoenzyme** (Protein part) + **Co-enzyme** (Non-protein part)

3. Generally, co-enzymes are loosely bounded to apo-enzyme, hence can be easily separated by the process called dialysis. If the non-protein parts are tightly (covalently) bonded to the apo-enzyme then it is known as "prosthetic group" and it cannot be separated by dialysis.
4. Generally, enzymes are soluble in water but it does not form true solution instead it forms a colloidal solution. This property of an enzyme is due to its huge size.
5. The molecular weight of enzymes varies which depends upon the proteins present in enzymes.
6. Enzymes are varied in shape. It may be globular, oval, fibrous or elongated, etc.
7. Isoelectric pH (p^I) is defined as the pH at which proteins exists as zwitterion or dipolar ion. These dipolar or zwitterion are electrically neutral, hence in the electric field they do not migrate. Generally, at isoelectric pH the solubility is minimum, the precipitability is maximum and the buffering capacity is least.

8. Enzymes are big in size when compared to relatively smaller substrates. Only a smaller portion of the huge enzyme is directly involved in the substrate binding and catalysis. Active site or center of an enzyme represents the smaller region at which the substrate binds and participates in catalysis.
9. Enzymes contain a small active site and substrates bind with these active sites through weak non-covalent bonds.
10. The existence of an active site is due to the tertiary structure of protein resulting in three dimensional native confirmations. The amino acid present in the active site is responsible for the activity and specific action of the enzymes.
11. The active site is made up of amino acids which are far from each other in the linear sequences of amino acids (For example, the *lysozyme* is composed of 129 amino acids in which 35, 52, 62, 63 and 101 amino acids are present in the active site).
12. Active sites are not rigid in structure and are regarded as clefts or cervices or pockets occupying a small region in a big enzyme molecule. Serine is the most frequently found amino acid in active site.
13. Substrate binding site and catalytic binding sites are present in the active site of enzymes. The first one is for substrate and the second one is for catalyst for specific reactions. The co-enzymes or cofactors or prosthetic groups bind in the catalytic site only.
14. In general, enzyme binds with substrate and forms enzyme-substrate complex. This step is a reversible one. Later enzyme-substrate complex produces a product and regenerates enzymes for other fresh reaction.

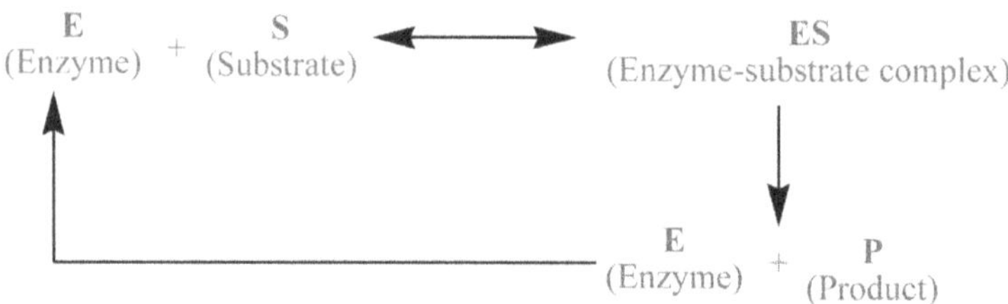

Nomenclature of Enzymes

Enzymes are named in three different ways a) Arbitrary manner, b) Tribal name, c) Enzyme commission name.

1. **Arbitrary Manner:** In olden days,the enzymes are named based on the discoveries. This system of naming doesn't convey any information like nature of the substrate on which it acts, the function of enzyme, etc. **Example:** *Pepsin, trypsin* and *chymotrypsin*.
2. **Tribal Name:** In this type of nomenclature the suffix "ase" is added to the substrate for giving a name to enzymes. This system also fails to provide complete information of enzyme catalyzed reaction such as type of reaction, cofactors required, etc. **Example:** *Lipase* acts on lipids, *nuclease* acts on nucleic acid, *protease* acts on protein, *lactase* acts on lactose. But this naming does not indicate about the type of reaction.
3. **IUB Name:** Enzyme commission allotted a four-digit enzyme commission (EC) number to every enzyme. This number is known as IUB (International union of biochemistry) name of enzymes. Each digit indicates certain information. The first digit of EC number indicates class of enzyme, the second digit indicates sub-class of enzyme, the third digit indicates sub-sub-class of enzyme and the fourth digit indicates individual enzyme name. This system provides all information related to biochemical reactions such as type of substrate, type of reaction catalyzed by the enzymes, co-enzyme required if any, etc. IUB names are not accepted for general use because they are complex and difficult to remember even though they are specific and unambiguous. Hence, usually tribal names along with EC numbers as and when needed are commonly used and are widely accepted.

Classification of Enzymes

Enzymes are classified in different ways as follows, a) IUB classification, b) Classification based on place or site of action, c) Classification based on the number of polypeptide chain, d) Classification based on the number of enzymes.

(a) IUB classification: In the year 1961, enzyme commission classified enzymes into six major categories according to the type of reactions catalyzed by enzyme. In general, the word **"OTHLIL"** may be memorized to remember six major categories of enzymes in correct order. All six classes of enzymes are summarized in Table 5.1 with type of reaction catalyzing, general reaction, example and biochemical reaction example.

Table 5.1 IUB classification of enzymes.

S. No.	Class of Enzyme	Type of reaction catalyzing	General Reaction	Example	Biochemical Reaction Example
1.	*Oxidoreductases*	It catalyzes oxidation reduction (redox) reaction	$AH_2 + B$ → (Oxidation-Reduction) → $A + BH_2$	*Alcohol dehydrogenase, cytochrome oxidase, L-amino acid oxidase, D-amino acid oxidase*	$CH_3CH_2OH + NAD^+$ Ethanol → (*Alcohol dehydrogenase*; Oxidation-Reduction) → $CH_3CHO + NADH + H^+$ Acetaldehyde
2.	*Transferases*	It catalyzes the transfer of functional group other than hydrogen from one compound to another compound	$AX + B$ → (Functional group transfer other than hydrogen) → $A + BX$	*Choline acetyl transferase, transaminase, transmethylase, phoshorylase, hexokinase*	$CH_3COSCoA$ + Choline (Acetyl CoA) → (*Choline acetyl transferase*; Transfer of acetyl group) → CH_3CO-Choline + CoASH (Acetyl choline)
3.	*Hydrolases*	It catalyzes hydrolysis reactions	$AB + H_2O$ → (Hydrolysis) → $AH + BOH$	*Cholinesterase, lipase, urease, pepsin, acid phosphatase, alkaline phosphatase*	CH_3CO-Choline + H_2O (Acetyl choline) → (*Choline esterase*; Hydrolysis) → CH_3COOH + Choline (Acetic acid)
4.	*Lyases*	It catalyzes addition or removal of water, ammonia, carbon dioxide, etc. and results in the formation of double bond	A—X + B—Y → (Addition - Elimination) → AX—BY	*Aldolase, fumarase, Histidase*	Glyceraldehyde-3-phosphate + Dihydroxy acetone phosphate → (*Aldolase*; Addition - Elimination) → Fructose-1,6-bisphosphate
5.	*Isomerases*	It catalyzes isomerization reaction	A ⇅ (Interconversion of isomers) A'	*Phospho triose isomerase, Phosphohexose isomerase, retinol isomerase*	Glyceraldehyde-3-phosphate ⇅ (*Phospho triose isomerase*; Isomerization) Dihydroxy acetone phosphate
6.	*Ligases* or *synthetases*or *synthases*	It catalyzes synthetic reaction (In Greek "ligate" means to bind where two molecules joined together).It needs ATP	A + B → (Condensation usually depends on ATP; ATP → ADP + Pi) → A—B	*Glutamine synthase, succinate thiokinase, fatty acid synthase, acetyl CoA carboxylase*	Glutamic acid + NH_3 → (*Glutamine synthase*; Condensation; ATP → ADP + Pi) → Glutamine

(b) Classification based on place of action: Enzymes are classified into 2 major types according to the place where it exhibits action.

1. **Intracellular enzyme:** In Greek "intra" means "within". These enzymes exhibit activity within the cell where they are synthesized. **Example:** *Hexokinase (HK), aldolase,* etc.
2. **Extracellular enzymes:** These enzymes exhibit activity outside the cell where they are not synthesized and not within the cell. **Example:** All digestive enzymes.

(c) Classification based upon the number of polypeptide chains: Based on the number of peptide chains present in enzyme it was classified into two major categories.

1. **Monomeric enzyme:** In Greek "mono" means "single". This enzyme is composed of single peptide chains. **Example:** *Trypsin.*
2. **Oligomeric enzyme:** In Greek "oligo" means "few". These enzymes are made up of a few peptide chains. **Example:** *Lactate dehydrogenase* **(LDH).**

(d) Classification based upon the number of enzymes: Enzymes are classified into two major categories according to the number of enzymes present in it.

1. **Mono-enzymes:** These enzymes are composed of single enzyme molecule only and are not depends on any enzyme for its activity. **Example:** Almost all enzymes like *hexokinase (HK), aldolase,* etc.
2. **Multi enzyme complex:** These are enzyme complexes made up of many enzyme molecules. The activity of enzymes depends on the activity of other enzymes present in complex. If any one enzyme is removed or inactivated the whole enzyme system becomes inactive. **Example:** *Lactate dehydrogenase (LDH), pyruvate dehydrogenase (PDH), fatty acid synthase (FAS)* complex.

Mechanism of Enzyme Action

Enzyme Decreases Activation Energy

Enzymes are powerful catalyst and catalysis is the prime functions of the enzyme. Similar to non-biological catalysis, it takes place in biological system also. The reactant must be changed to an activated state or transition state for any chemical reaction to take place. For this, the substances (reactants) needs some energy. The energy required by the reactants to undergo a chemical reaction is called activation energy. When heated the reactants attain this activation energy. The catalyst (enzyme in biological systems) brings down the activation energy hence the reactions takes place at lower temperature itself. Generally, equilibrium constants are not altered by enzymes and it only increases the velocity of reactions.

The role of enzyme or catalyst is usually compared with a tunnel made in the mountain to reduce the barrier as illustrated in Figure 5.1. Enzymes make the reaction go faster because it lowers the energy barriers of reactants. Enzyme made possible that all biochemical reaction occurs at body temperature itself (below 40 °C) by reducing activation energy of reactants as follows-.

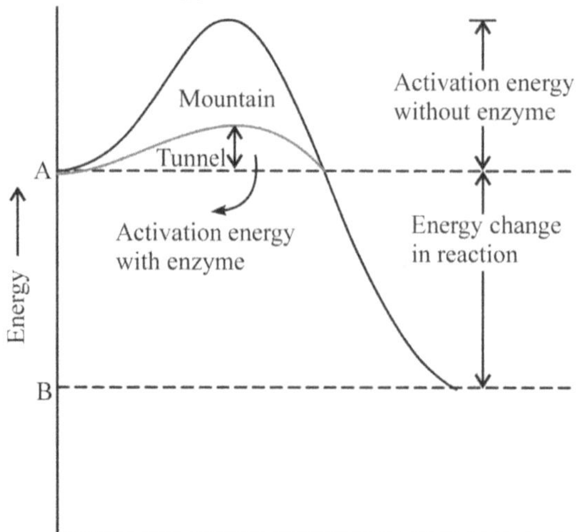

Figure 5.1 Effect of enzyme on activation energy of a reaction; A is substrate; B is product.

Formation of Enzyme-Substrate Complex

The primary basic in enzyme catalysis is binding of the substrate (S) with enzyme (E) on active site of enzyme and forms enzyme-substrate complex (ES). Finally, the product (P) is formed from enzyme-substrate complex (ES) with the regeneration of enzyme (E). This enzyme-substrate complex is otherwise called as a "Michaelis" complex.

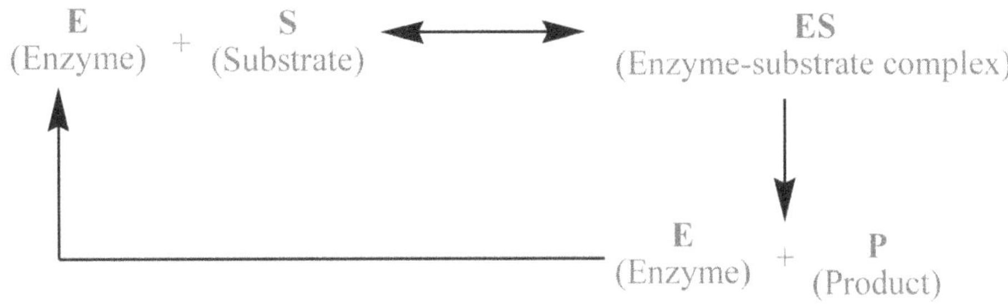

The above mechanism of enzyme-substrate complex formation is explained by the following theories like 1) Lock and key model or Fischer's template theory, 2) Induced fit theory or Koshland's model, 3) Substrate strain theory.

1. **Lock and key model or Fischer's template theory**

   The first theory to explain the mechanism of enzyme catalyzed reaction was proposed by German biochemist "Emil Fischer". According to this theory, the structure or conformation of enzymes is rigid in nature. Hence a particular substrate only fit into the enzymes just like a key fitted into a proper lock or hand in to the proper gloves. Hence the active site of an enzyme is pre-shaped and rigid where only specific substrate can bind and forms enzyme-substrate complex. But this theory not explains the flexible nature of enzymes, hence this theory fails to explain many facts of enzyme-catalyzed reactions particularly allosteric modulators. According to this theory, both enzyme and substrate are rigid in structure.

2. **Induced fit theory or Koshland's model**

   For enzyme-substrate complex formation, Koshland proposed more realistic and accepted model in 1958. According to this theory, the active sites of enzymes are not rigid and pre-shaped in structure. In nascent active site, the essential features of the substrate binding sites are present. When the enzyme is approached by a substrate, the enzyme undergoes some conformational changes which lead to the formation of strong substrate binding site. In addition, the active site is formed by the repositioning of appropriate amino acids due to induced fit and brings about the catalysis. As the substrate induces enzyme for binding it is known as induced fit theory. This theory explains the allosteric modulators and competitive enzyme inhibition on enzyme. There is enough evidence from X-ray diffraction studies for this model. According to this theory, enzyme is flexible in nature whereas substrate is rigid in structure.

3. **Substrate strain theory**

   This is another important theory which explains the mechanism of enzyme-substrate complex formation. In this model, the substrate is strained due to the induced conformation change in the enzyme. It is also possible that the enzyme induces a strain to the substrate when a substrate binds to the pre-formed active site. Product is formed from the strained substrate. According to this theory, both substrate and enzymes are flexible and not rigid in structure. In the enzymatic action, combination of induced fit theory or Koshland's model and substrate strain theory is operative. All three theories are represented in simple form in Figure 5.2 and Table 5.2

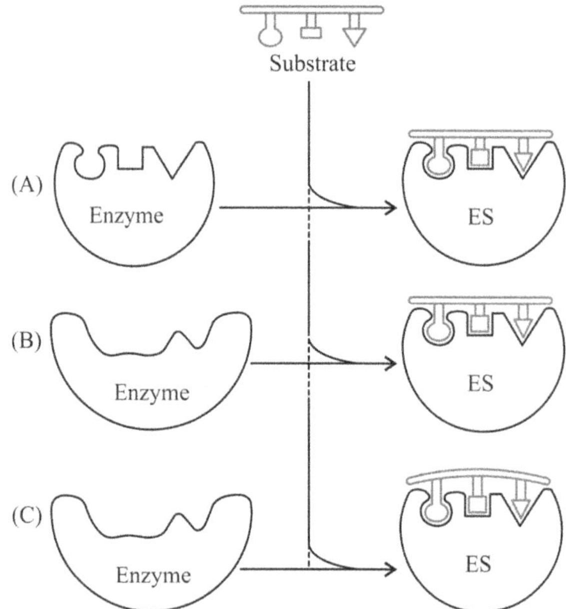

Figure 5.2 Theories of enzyme-substrate complex formation; A) Lock and key model or Fischer's template theory; B) Induced fit theory or Koshland's model; C) Substrate strain theory.

Table 5.2 Theories of enzyme substrate complex formation.

S. No.	Theory name	Structure or conformation	
		Enzyme	**Substrate**
1	Lock and key model or Fischer's template theory	Rigid	Rigid
2	Induced fit theory or Koshland's model	Flexible	Rigid
3	Substrate strain theory	Flexible	Flexible

Enzyme Kinetics

Initially, the increase in substrate concentration gradually increases the velocity of enzyme-catalyzed reactions within the limited range of substrate levels. After that concentration, a large change in substrate concentration produces a small change in velocity. Further increased concentration of substrate does not produce any change in velocity of reaction. The relationship between substrate concentration and velocity is explained by drawing a plot (graph) taking substrate concentration on X-axis and velocity on Y-axis. Generally, the graph for effect of concentration of substrate will be rectangular hyperbola (Figure 5.3).

In this graph three phases of reactions are observed. 1) Linear (A), 2) Curve (B), 3) Almost unchanged (C). Two different plots are used to explain the effect of substrate concentration in enzyme catalyzed reactions. They are a) Michaelis plot, and b) Lineweaver - Burk double reciprocal plot.

(a) Michaelis plot:

K_m value or Michaelis-Menten constant is defined as the substrate concentration (in moles) required to produce half maximum velocity ($\frac{1}{2} V_{max}$) in an enzyme-catalyzed reactions. It is also known as **Brig's and Haldane's constant.** It indicates that when the substrate concentration is equal to K_m value, about 50 % of enzyme molecules are bonded with the substrate molecules. K_m value is not dependent on the concentration of enzymes. In K_m "K" stands for constant and "m" stands for Michaelis.

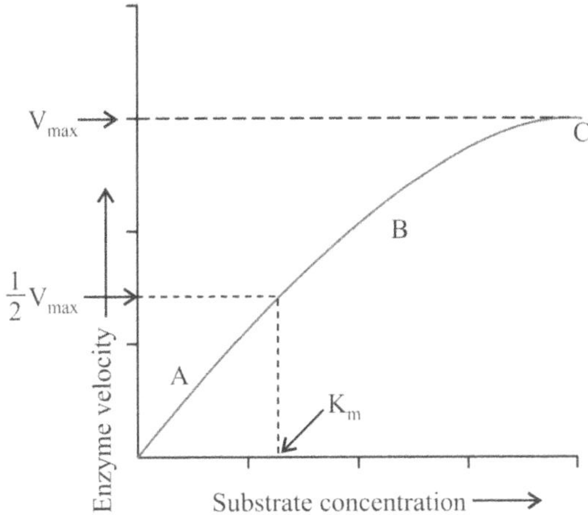

Figure 5.3 Effect of concentration of substrate on velocity of enzyme; A is linear; B is curve; C is almost unchanged.

In an enzyme catalyzed reaction, low K_m value indicates the strong affinity between enzyme and substrate; whereas high K_m value indicates the weak affinity between substrate and enzyme. Generally, the K_m value of most of the enzymes is in the ranges between 10^{-5} to 10^{-2} moles. When a substrate concentration is less than K_m value then the rate of reaction follows first order kinetics for substrate concentration; whereas when the substrate concentration is much greater than K_m value then it follows zero order kinetics in which the rate of reaction is independent of substrate concentration.

$$\underset{\text{(Enzyme)}}{E} + \underset{\text{(Substrate)}}{S} \underset{K_2}{\overset{K_1}{\rightleftharpoons}} \underset{\text{(Enzyme-substrate complex)}}{ES} \xrightarrow{K_3} \underset{\text{(Enzyme)}}{E} + \underset{\text{(Product)}}{P}$$

Where, K_1, K_2 and K_3 are velocity constants for respective reactions.

$$K_m = \frac{K_2 + K_3}{K_1}$$

After suitable modification of algebra,

$$V = \frac{V_{max}[s]}{K_m + [s]}$$

Where,

V = Measured velocity

V_{max} = Maximum velocity

[S] = Substrate concentration

K_m = Michaelis-Menten constant

If the measured velocity is equal to half maximum velocity *i.e.*, ($V = \frac{1}{2}V_{max}$) and substituting this in above equation results in,

$$\frac{1}{2}V_{max} = \frac{V_{max}[S]}{K_m + [S]}$$

$$K_m + [S] = \frac{2\,V_{max}[S]}{V_{max}}$$

$$K_m + [S] = 2\,[S]$$

$$K_m + 2[S] - [S]$$
$$K_m = [S]$$

(b) Lineweaver–Burk double reciprocal plot:

Lineweaver–Burk double reciprocal plot is used to understand the effect of various inhibitors. For K_m value determination substrate saturation curve i.e., Michaelis plot is not very accurate. Lineweaver–Burk double reciprocal plot is very easier to calculate the K_m value.

$$V = \frac{V_{max}[S]}{k_m + [S]}$$

Therefore,
$$\frac{1}{V} = \frac{K_m + [S]}{V_{max}[S]}$$

$$\frac{1}{V} = \frac{K_m}{V_{max}} \times \frac{1}{[S]} + \frac{[S]}{V_{max}[S]}$$

$$\frac{1}{V} = \frac{K_m}{V_{max}} \times \frac{1}{[S]} + \frac{1}{V_{max}}$$

$$y = ax + b$$

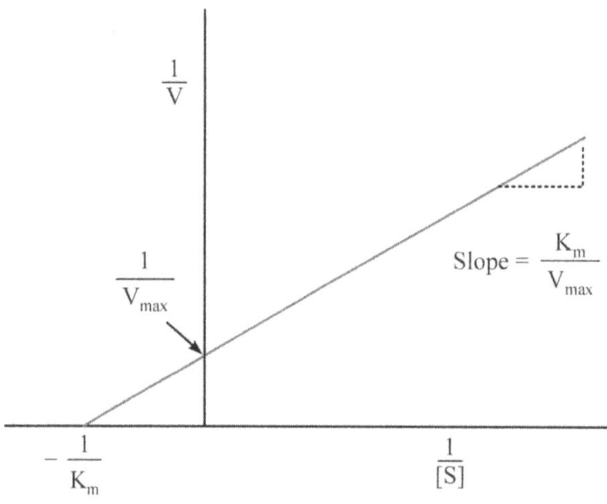

Figure 5.4 Lineweaver–Burk double reciprocal plot.

Where "a" is slope & "b" is the intercept. While drawing a graph by taking reciprocal of velocity ($\frac{1}{V}$) in "X" axis and reciprocal of substrate concentration ($\frac{1}{[S]}$) in "Y" axis, respectively it gives a straight line (Figure 5.4). Here the slope "a" is $\frac{K_m}{V_{max}}$ and the intercept "b" is $\frac{1}{V_{max}}$. It is very easy to calculate the K_m value from the intercept on "X" axis which is $\frac{-1}{K_m}$.

Enzyme Inhibition

Enzyme inhibitor is defined as the substance which binds with the enzyme and decreases the enzyme catalytic activity. The process by which the enzyme activity is decreased is known as enzyme inhibition. Enzyme inhibition is broadly classified into three major types.

1. Reversible enzyme inhibition
2. Irreversible enzyme inhibition
3. Allosteric enzyme inhibition

1. Reversible enzyme inhibition (REI):

As the name indicates this type of enzyme inhibition is reversible in nature. In this type inhibitor binds with the enzyme by a weak non-covalent bond. Hence, the reactions can be reversed if the inhibitor is removed. Reversible enzyme inhibition is further sub-classified into two categories as a) Competitive enzyme inhibition (CEI), b) Non-competitive enzyme inhibition (NCEI).

(a) Competitive enzyme inhibition: There is a competition between substrate and inhibitor for binding to the active site of enzyme. The competition is due to structural similarities between real substrate (S) and the inhibitors (I). Hence, these inhibitors are regarded as analogue of substrate. Once the inhibitor (I) is bonded with enzyme (E) it forms enzyme inhibitor complex (EI) which leads to unavailability of enzyme for binding with substrate. During the reaction enzyme substrate complex (ES) are also formed.

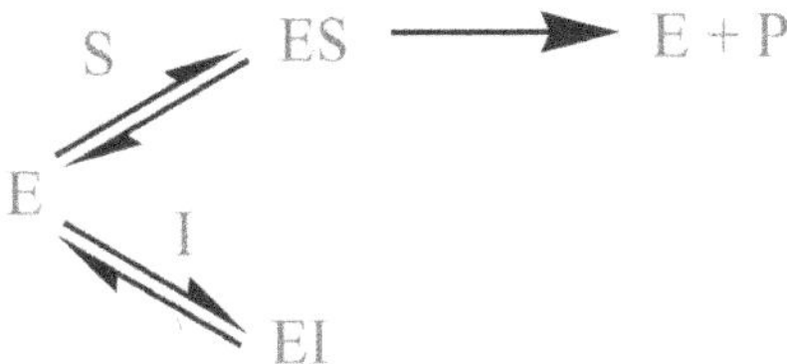

Followings are the two major factors which influence the competitive enzyme inhibition. They are i) Concentration of substrate and inhibitor, ii) Affinity of substrate and inhibitor with the enzyme. In general, high substrate concentration overcomes the competitive enzyme inhibition. K_m value is increasing and V_{max} is unchanged in competitive enzyme inhibition. A diagrammatic representation of competitive enzyme inhibition is presented in Figure 5.5 (A)and effect of competitive inhibitor on velocity of enzyme is presented in Figure 5.6.

Example 1: Enzyme: *Succinate dehydrogenase* (SDH), **Substrate:** Succinic acid, **Inhibitor:** Oxalic acid, malonic acid and glutaric acid. Here the structural similarities between substrate and inhibitors are presence of dicarboxylic group. Hence the inhibitors oxalic acid, malonic acid and glutaric acid competes with succinic acid for the active site of enzyme "*succinate dehydrogenase (SDH)*".

Succinic acid	Oxalic acid	Malonic acid	Glutaric acid
CH_2COOH – CH_2COOH	COOH – COOH	COOH – CH_2 – COOH	CH_2COOH – CH_2 – CH_2COOH

Example 2: Enzyme: *Alcohol dehydrogenase*(ADH), **Substrate:** Methanol (CH_3OH), **Inhibitor:** Ethanol (CH_3CH_2OH). In this example the structural similarities between substrate and inhibitors are presence of primary alcohol group. Hence the inhibitor ethanol competes with methanol for active site of enzyme "*alcohol dehydrogenase (ADH)*". For this reason, ethanol may be used

in the treatment of methanol poisoning. Some more clinical and pharmacological significances of competitive enzyme inhibitors are listed in Table 5.3.

Example 3: Antimetabolites are the chemical substances which block the metabolic reaction due to its competitive enzyme inhibition with enzymes. Generally, they are used in the treatment of cancer. Examples are mentioned in Table. 5.3. The term antivitamins are used for the antimetabolites which block the biochemical actions of vitamins and leads to deficiencies of corresponding vitamins. **Example:** Sulphanilamide and dicoumarol.

Table 5.3 Clinical and pharmacological significances of competitive enzyme inhibitors.

S. No	Name of enzyme	Substrate name	Inhibitor name	Significance of inhibitors
1	*MAO (Monoamine oxidase)*	Nor-epinephrine, epinephrine	Ephedrine, amphetamine	Catecholamine elevators
2	*Xanthine oxidase*	Hypoxanthine, Xanthine	Allopurinol	Treatment of gout
3	*Dihydropteroate synthase*	PABA (*p*-Amino benzoic acid)	Sulfanilamide	Antibacterial agent
4	*Acetylcholine esterase*	Acetylcholine	Succinylcholine	In anesthetized patient used for muscle relaxation in surgery
5	*HMG CoA reductase*	HMG CoA	Lovastatin, Pravastatin	Antihyperlipidemic agent
6	*Dihydrofolate reductase*	Dihydrofolic acid	Methotrexate, Trimetrexate, Aminopterin	Treatment of leukemia and other cancers
7	*Vitamin K epoxide reductase*	Vitamin K	Dicoumarol	Anticoagulant

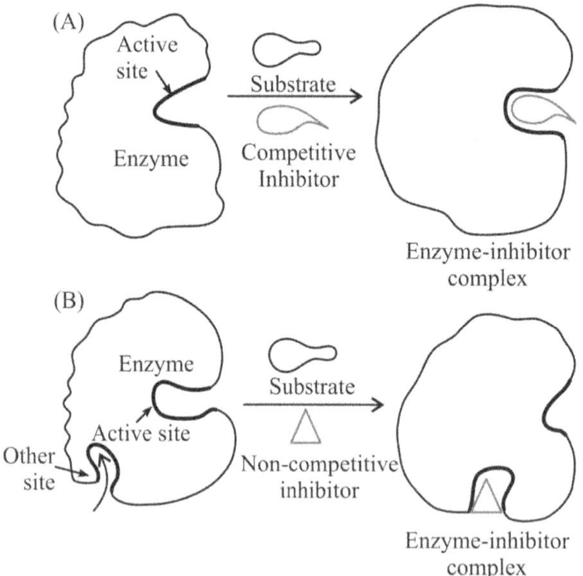

Figure 5.5 (A) Competitive enzyme inhibition; (B) Non-competitive enzyme inhibition.

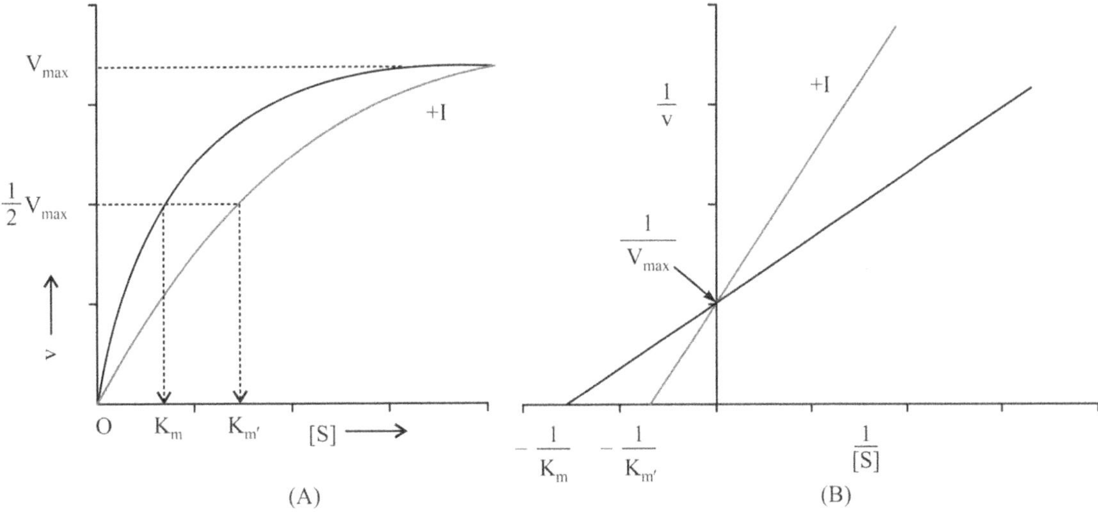

Figure 5.6 Effect of competitive inhibitor on velocity of enzyme; A) Velocity Vs Substrate; B) Lineweaver-Burk plot (Red line with inhibitor).

(b) Non-competitive enzyme inhibition (NCEI): In this type there is no competition between substrate and inhibitor for active site of enzyme because inhibitor bind with other sites on the enzyme surface and decreases the activity of enzyme. There are no structural similarities between substrate and inhibitors. Even though inhibitors exhibit strong affinities to bind in the second site of enzyme and it does not interfere with enzyme-substrate binding. The catalysis prevention may be due to enzyme conformation distortion. In this type, the inhibitor may bind with enzyme and enzyme-substrate complex as well . K_m value is unchanged and V_{max} is decreasing in non-competitive enzyme inhibition. A diagrammatic representation of non-competitive enzyme inhibition is presented in Figure 5.5 (B) and effect of non-competitive inhibitor on velocity of enzyme is presented in Figure 5.7.

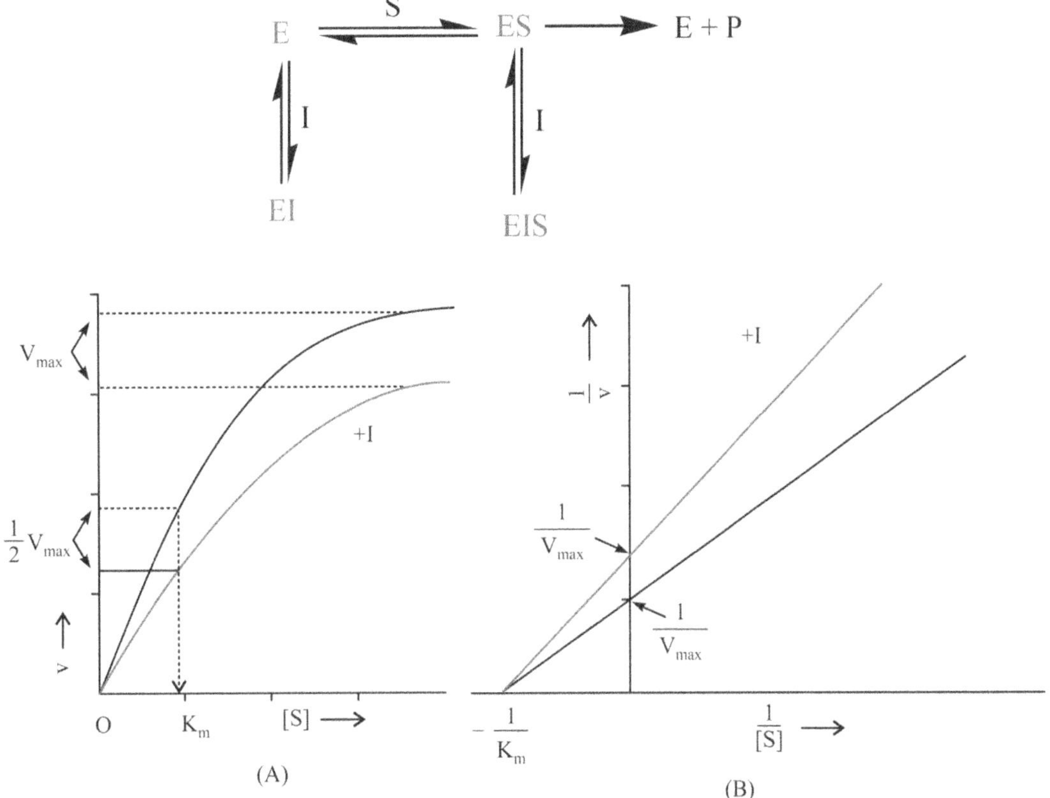

Figure 5.7 Effect of non-competitive inhibitor on velocity of enzyme; A) Velocity Vs Substrate; B) Lineweaver-Burk plot (Red line with inhibitor).

Example: Heavy metal ions like Hg^{2+}, Pb^{2+}, Ag^{+}, etc. binds with cysteinyl sulfhydryl group of enzymes non-competitively. Heavy metals also lead to formation of covalent bonds with carboxyl group and histidine often resulting in irreversible inhibition.

$$E—SH + Hg^{2+} \rightleftharpoons E—S{-}{-}{-}{-}Hg^{2+} + H^{+}$$

2. **Irreversible enzyme inhibition:**
In this type of enzyme inhibition substrate binds to the enzyme by a covalent bond which is very strong in nature. Hence, the bond cannot be broken easily. This leads to an irreversible reaction. Generally, these irreversible inhibitors are toxic substances which poisons the enzymes. The following reaction represents irreversible enzyme inhibition. The characteristics of various irreversible enzyme inhibitors are listed in Table 5.4.

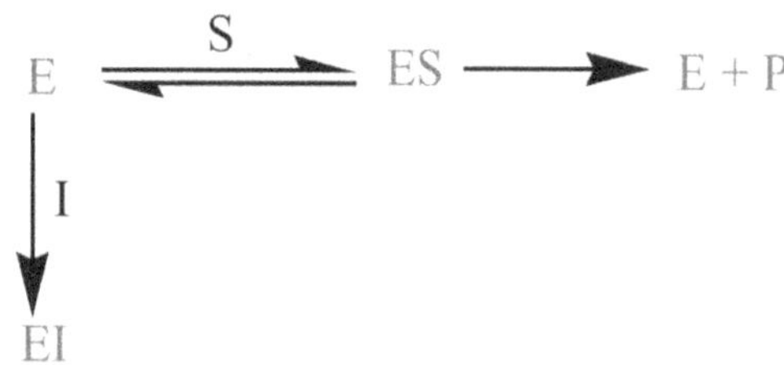

Table 5.4 Irreversible enzyme inhibitors.

S. No	Name of the enzyme	Inhibitor name	Characteristics
1	*Papain, and glyceraldehyde-3-phosphate*	Iodoacetate	Iodoacetate combine with –SH group of these enzyme and make them inactive
2	*Aldehyde dehydrogenase (ADH)*	Disulfiram	Treatment of alcoholism due to accumulation of acetaldehyde
3	Serine containing enzymes	Penicillin	Blocks the synthesis of bacterial cell wall.
4	*Serine protease, acetylcholine esterase (AchE)*	Diisopropyl fluorophosphates (DFP)	DFP is a nerve gas used in second world war by German.
5	*Acetylcholine esterase (AchE)*	Organophosphorus insecticides like parathion and malathion	Produces paralysis of vital body functions due to block of nerve conduction.

Suicide inhibition is a specialized form of irreversible inhibition. In this case, the actual or the original inhibitor is converted to a more potent form of inhibitor by the same enzyme itself. The actual or original inhibitor binds with enzyme reversibly (Mostly structural analogue or competitive inhibitor), whereas the newly formed inhibitor binds with enzyme irreversibly. Examples of various suicidal inhibitors and its uses are listed in Table 5.5.

Table 5.5 Suicide inhibitors.

S. No	Name of the enzyme	Original inhibitor name	Newly formed inhibitor	Uses
1	*Xanthine oxidase*	Allopurinol	Alloxanthine	Treatment of gout
2	*Thymidylate synthase*	5-Fluorouracil	Fluorodeoxy uridylate	Treatment of cancer

3. **Allosteric enzyme inhibition:**
In Greek, "allo" means "other". Few of the enzymes possess additional sites known as allosteric site along with the active site. These enzymes are known as allosteric enzymes. In the enzyme molecules, these allosteric sites are unique places. Generally, allosteric enzymes exist in two conformation state in the concerted model as a) T-state (Tense or taut), b) R-state (Relaxed). The T and R states are in equilibrium. If enzymes are present in relaxed form the activity will be more whereas if the enzymes

are present in tense form the activity will be less. In general, allosteric activators favors R-state of enzyme and allosteric inhibitors favor T-state. **Example:** Glucose-6-phosphate for *hexokinase(HK)*, ATP for *phosphofructokinase (PFK)* and *isocitrate dehydrogenase (ICDH)*, AMP for *fructose-1,6-bisphosphatase (F1,6BPase)*, and palmitate for *acetyl CoA carboxylase.* Various form of allosteric enzyme and its activator and inhibitor is diagrammatically represented in Figure 5.8.

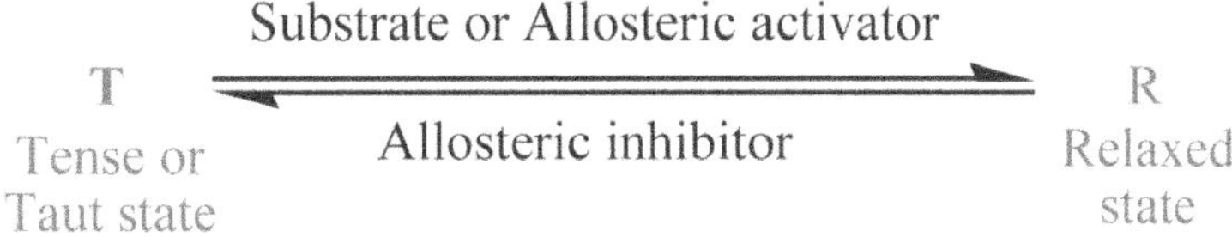

Enzyme Regulation

Enzyme regulation occurs in biological system in different stages in order to achieve cellular economy. Cellular metabolism is a molecular economy that is functionally organized into supply and demand blocks linked by metabolic products and co-factor cycles. The various ways of enzyme regulation are as follows.

1. Allosteric regulation
2. Latent enzyme activation
3. Metabolic pathways compartmentation
4. Enzyme synthesis control
5. Enzyme degradation
6. Iso-enzyme

1. Allosteric regulation:

The unique places of allosteric enzymes are alloesteric site which is additional site beside active site of enzyme. In these allosteric sites the allosteric modulators (modifiers or effectors) binds and regulate the activity of enzyme. In the allosteric site, binding of a positive allosteric modifiers results in increased enzyme activity and the allosteric site is known as activator site. Similarly, Binding of a negative allosteric modifier results in decreased enzyme activity and the allosteric site is known as inhibitor site.

Allosteric enzymes are the enzymes which are regulated by allosteric mechanism. Based on the effect of allosteric modifiers or effectors on K_m and V_{max} the allosteric enzymes are broadly classified into two types.

(a) K-class allosteric enzymes: In this class, allosteric effectors change the K_m and not the V_{max} value. Similar to competitive enzyme inhibition double reciprocal plots are obtained for this class of allosteric enzymes. **Example:** *Phosphofructokinase (PFK).*

(b) V-class allosteric enzymes: In this class, allosteric effectors change the V_{max} and not the K_m value. Similar to non-competitive enzyme inhibition double reciprocal plots are obtained for this class of allosteric enzymes. **Example:** *Acetyl CoA carboxylase.*

The sub-units of the oligomeric allosteric enzyme may be different or identical. In the active site of the enzyme conformational changes are taking place due to the reversible non-covalent binding of allosteric effectors that results in increased or decreased catalytic activity of enzyme. Generally, allosteric enzymes exist in two conformation state in the concerted model as a) T-state (Tense or taut), b) R-state (Relaxed). Normally allosteric activators favors R-state of enzyme and allosteric inhibitors favors T-state. Substrate will bind only to the R-state of the enzyme, hence increased substrate concentration increases R-state of the enzyme molecule. Hence, allosteric enzyme and substrate binding is said to be co-operative. Sigmoidal curve is obtained instead of rectangular hyperbola for allosteric enzymes when the graph is plotted between velocity and substrate concentration.

If the effects of allosteric modulator promote the binding of substrate to the enzyme which results in positive effect always is known as homotrophic effect. Incase if the effects of allosteric modulator promote the binding of substrate to the enzyme which results in either positive or negative effect is known as heterotrophic effect. The various examples for allosteric enzymes are listed in Table 5.6.

Table 5.6 Allosteric enzyme & their effectors.

S. No	Metabolic pathway name	Enzyme name	Allosteric activator	Allosteric inhibitor
1	Glycolysis	*Hexokinase (HK)*	-------	Glucose-6-phosphate
2	Glycolysis	*Phosphofructokinase (PFK)*	AMP, ADP	ATP
3	TCA cycle	*Isocitrate dehydrogenase (ICDH)*	ADP, NAD^+	ATP
4	Gluconeogenesis	*Pyruvate carboxylase (PC)*	Acetyl CoA	-------
5	Gluconeogenesis	*Fructose-1,6-bisphosphatase (F1,6-BPase)*	-------	AMP
6	Urea cycle	*Carbamoyl phosphate synthase – I (CPS – I)*	N-Acetyl glutamate (NAG)	-------
7	Tryptophan metabolism	*Tryptophan oxygenase (TO)*	L-Tryptophan	-------
8	Fatty acid synthesis	*Acetyl CoA carboxylase (ACC)*	Isocitrate	Palmitate

Feedback regulation: Feedback regulation is defined as the process in which first step of the series of enzyme catalyzed reaction is inhibited by the final product of that reaction. For example, product "E" is synthesized from substrate "A" in the following series of reaction.

$$A \xrightarrow[E]{e_1} B \xrightarrow{e_2} C \xrightarrow{e_3} D \xrightarrow{e_4} E$$

Where, A = Initial substrate

B, C and D = Intermediate compounds

E = End product

e_1, e_2, e_3 and e_4 = Enzymes

For regulating the pathway of above reactions, very first step (A to B by enzyme e_1) is the most effective by the final product E. This type of regulation is known as negative feedback regulation because increased final product concentration itself decreased its synthesis by inhibiting enzyme e_1. It will save the cellular economy by blocking the wasteful expenditure utilized for the synthesis of already existing compound. End product inhibition or feedback inhibition is the special type of allosteric enzyme inhibition used to control metabolic pathways for efficient cellular functions.

Example: *Aspartate transcarbamoylase (ATC)* is inhibited by CTP (cytidine triphosphate) in biosynthesis of pyrimidine.

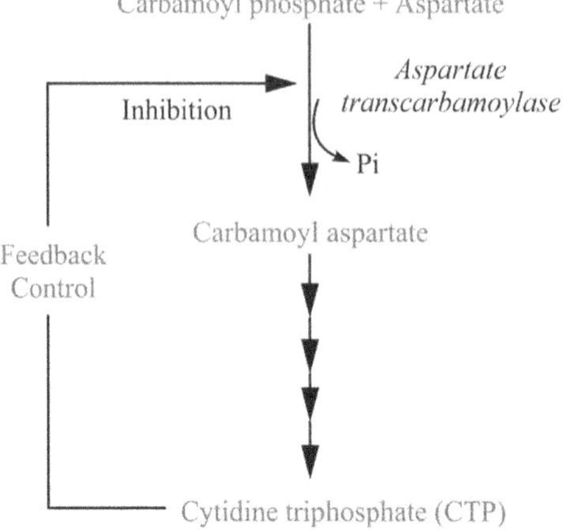

In general, feedback regulation represents a phenomenon while feedback inhibition involves the mechanism of regulation. For instance, through feedback regulation hepatic cholesterol synthesis is decreased by dietary cholesterol. Dietary cholesterol does not directly inhibit the regulatory enzyme *HMG CoA reductase*, hence feedback inhibition is not involved in this process. However, cholesterol reduces (repression) the activity of gene encoding this enzyme.

2. **Latent enzyme activation:**

As such latent enzymes are inactive. Latent enzymes whose activity only becomes manifest when the conditions are changed. The term "latent enzyme" is used especially of a particulate enzyme that becomes active when the particles are disrupted. Some of the enzymes are synthesized as zymogens or pro-enzymes which undergoes irreversible covalent activation by breakdown of one or more peptide bonds. Conversion of pro-enzymes *chymotrypsinogen, pepsinogen* and *plasminogen* into active enzymes *chymotrypsin, pepsin* and *plasmin*, respectively are very good examples.

Depending on the needs of biological systems some of the enzymes exist in both active and inactive forms which are inter convertible. Reversible covalent modifications such as oxidation and reduction of disulfide bonds and phosphorylation and dephosphorylation brings the above inter conversion.

Example 1: To provide energy, the muscle enzyme *glycogen phosphorylase* breaks glycogen. This enzyme possesses two identical subunits (homodimer) and exists in two inter convertible forms. The inactive form of enzyme is *phosphorylase-b* (dephospho enzyme) which is phosphorylated at serine residues and converted into active form *phosphorylase-a*. The inactive form *phosphorylase-b* is produced from active form by dephosphorylation reaction.

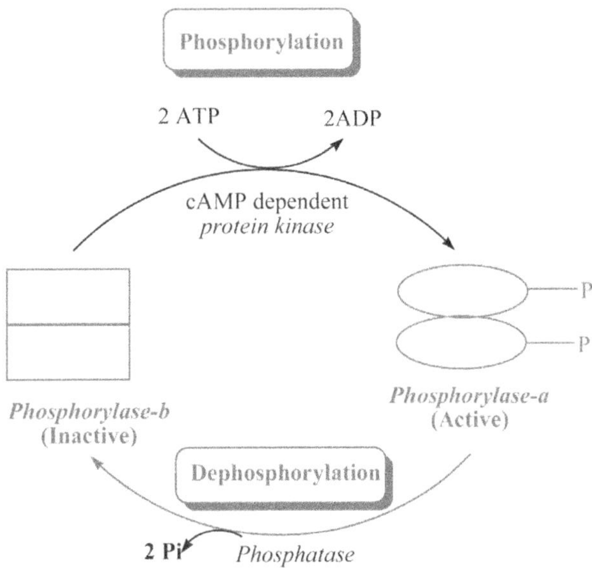

Citrate lyase and *fructose-2,6-bisphosphatase* are the other examples for phosphorylated active enzymes. Some enzymes are active in dephosphorylated form and converted into inactive form by phosphorylation. *Acetyl CoA carboxylase, glycogen synthase* and *HMG CoA reductase* are examples for dephosphorylated active enzymes.

Sulfhydryl (-SH) group is necessary for the activity of some enzymes. Stability of these enzymes is brought by reducing substances like glutathione.

E—S—S—E → E—SH + E—SH

Oxidized form of enzyme (Inactive) → **Reduced form of enzyme (Active)**

2G—SH → GS—SG

Glutathione **(Reduced form)** → Glutathione **(Oxidized form)**

3. **Metabolic pathways compartmentation:**

In biological systems, both synthesis and degradations are occurring for some substances like fatty acid and glycogen. Simultaneous occurrences of both the pathways are not possible. To achieve maximum cellular economy anabolic (synthetic) and catabolic (breakdown) pathways are taking place in different cellular organelles. For example, fatty acid oxidation occurs in mitochondria whereas fatty acid synthesis occurs in cytosol. Intracellular locations of certain enzymes are presented in Table 5.7.

Table 5.7 Intracellular locations of certain enzymes.

S. No	Intracellular organelle	Enzymes or metabolic pathways
1	Nucleus	Replication and transcription
2	Mitochondria	Krebs cycle, amino acid oxidation, urea cycle, fatty acid oxidation, oxidative phosphorylation and ETC
3	Microsomes (Endoplasmic reticulum)	Protein synthesis, triacylglycerol and phospholipid synthesis, steroid synthesis and reduction, *esterase* and *cytochrome* P_{450}
4	Golgi apparatus	*Glucose-6-phosphatase, glucosyl* and *galactosyl transferases* and *5-nucleotidase*
5	Lysosomes	*Proteases, lipases, nucleases, phosphatases, phospholipases, hydrolases* and *lysozyme*
6	Peroxisomes	*D-Amino acid oxidase*, long chain fatty acid oxidation, *urate oxidase* and *catalase*
7	Cytoplasm	Glycolysis, HMP shunt pathway, fatty acid synthesis, purine and pyrimidine catabolism, and *aminotransferases*

4. **Enzyme synthesis control:**

Many enzymes importantly regulating enzymes are present in very low concentration. The velocity of enzyme catalyzed reactions is directly controlled by number of enzymes. Enzyme levels are efficiently regulated because the half lives of many rate limiting enzymes are very short. Based on the level of enzymes present in biological systems, the enzymes are broadly classified into two classes namely a) Constitutive enzymes, b) Adaptive enzyme.

(a) **Constitutive enzymes:** The levels of these enzymes are fairly constant and are not controlled. It is otherwise known as housekeeping enzymes.

(b) **Adaptive enzymes:** The levels of these enzymes are not constant and are decreased or increased based on the body demands. Hence, these enzymes are well regulated by the genes. The enzyme levels may increase or decrease by increasing the synthesis of enzyme (Induction) or decreasing the synthesis of enzyme (Repression). At the gene level the enzyme concentrations are determined by induction or repression through the mediation of hormones or other substances.

Induction: Increased synthesis of enzyme is represented by the term "induction". **Example:** The synthesis of *glucokinase (GK), phosphofructokinase (PFK), pyruvate kinase (PK)* and *glycogen synthase (GS)* are induced by the hormone insulin. All these enzymes are involved in utilization of glucose. Similarly, the synthesis of *pyruvate carboxylase (PC), tryptophan oxygenase (TO)* and *tyrosine aminotransferase (TAT)* is induced by the hormone cortisol.

Repression: Decreased synthesis of enzyme is represented by the term "repression". Substrate can repress the enzyme synthesis in many instances. **Example:** The synthesis of *pyruvate carboxylase(PC)* is repressed by substrate glucose.

5. **Enzyme degradation:**

Generally, enzymes are not immortal because it creates many problems. Half-life of the individual enzymes varies a lot. Half-life of some enzymes are in days while for others in hours or in minutes (**Example:** LDH_4: 5 to 6 days, LDH_1: 8 to 12 hours, *Amylase*: 3 to 5 hours). The regulatory and key enzymes are most rapidly degraded. When there is no need it rapidly disappears and as when required it synthesized immediately. In majority cases long half-life possessing enzymes are sluggish in catalytic activity.

6. **Iso-enzymes:**

   Iso-enzymes are defined as the different form of the same enzyme [differ in amino acid sequence] exhibits similar activity. These iso-enzymes also help in regulation of enzyme activity. Many iso-enzymes are tissue specific. Iso-enzymes catalyze the same reaction of a given enzyme. But iso-enzymes differ in many properties such as K_m value, V_{max}, Isoelectric pH, electrophoretic mobility, optimum temperature, optimum pH, effect on heat, quantities present, etc.

Co-enzymes

Protein parts of the enzymes are not sufficient always to bring about the catalytic activity. Majority of the enzymes for its catalysis activity additionally need small non-protein factors collectively known as co-factors. In nature these co-factors may be either organic or inorganic.

Co-enzymes are defined as the non-protein, organic, low molecular weight and easily dialyzable substances associated with the functions of enzymes. If the organic non-protein substances are tightly bounded to protein part of enzyme then the term prosthetic group is used. Inorganic co-factors such as Ca^{2+}, Mg^{2+}, Mn^{2+}, etc. which are necessary to increase the activity of enzyme are called activators.. However, three terms such as co-enzyme, prosthetic group and activator are used interchangeably.

Holo-enzyme is the functional unit of enzyme and it is composed of two major parts namely apo-enzyme and co-enzyme. The protein part of enzyme is called as apo-enzyme and the non-protein part of enzyme is called as co-enzymes. Co-enzymes do not decide the specificity of enzyme. The specificity of enzyme is mostly depending on the apo-enzyme only.

Holoenzyme (Active enzyme) ⟶ Apo-enzyme (Protein part) + Co-enzyme (Non-protein part)

Usually co-enzymes are considered as co-substrate or second substrate because it also possess affinity with enzyme comparable with that of the substrates. During the enzymatic reactions co-enzymes undergoes modification but later regenerated, whereas substrate is converted to the product. Co-enzymes play a crucial role in functions of enzyme. In general co-enzymes are participated in several reactions involving transfer of atoms or groups like hydrogen, aldehydes, keto, amino, acyl, methyl, carbon dioxide, etc.

Types of co-enzymes:

There are four different types of co-enzymes as 1) Vitamin co-enzymes, 2) Non-vitamin co-enzymes, 3) Nucleotide co-enzymes, 4) Protein co-enzymes.

1. **Vitamin co-enzymes:** It is otherwise known as co-enzymes from vitamin B-complex because most of the co-enzymes are the derivatives of water-soluble B-complex vitamins. The B-complex vitamin exhibits its biological function through its respective co-enzymes only and the details are presented in Table 5.8.
2. **Non-vitamin co-enzymes:** Not all co-enzymes are vitamin derivatives. There are several other organic substances which have no relation with vitamins but act as co-enzymes. These organic substances are known as non-vitamin co-enzymes and various non-vitamin co-enzymes are listed in Table 5.9.

Table 5.8 Vitamin co-enzymes.

S. No	Vitamin name	Co-enzyme name	Chemical structure of co-enzyme	Important structural features of co-enzyme	Deficiency / Disorder	Atom or group transferred	Example of dependent enzyme
1	Vitamin-B_1 (Thiamine)	TPP (Thiamine pyrophosphate)	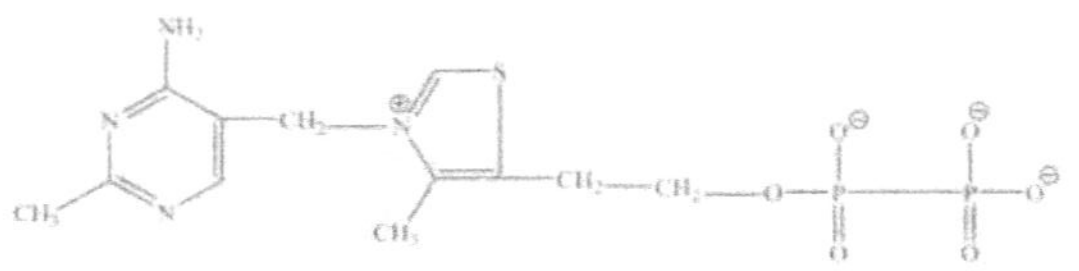	Pyrimidine, thiazole and methylene bridge	Beri-beri (dry or wet or mixed or infantile), peripheral neuropathy and Wernicke-Korsakoff syndrome	Aldehyde or keto	*Transketolase*
2	Vitamin B_2 (Riboflavin)	FMN (Flavin mono nucleotide)	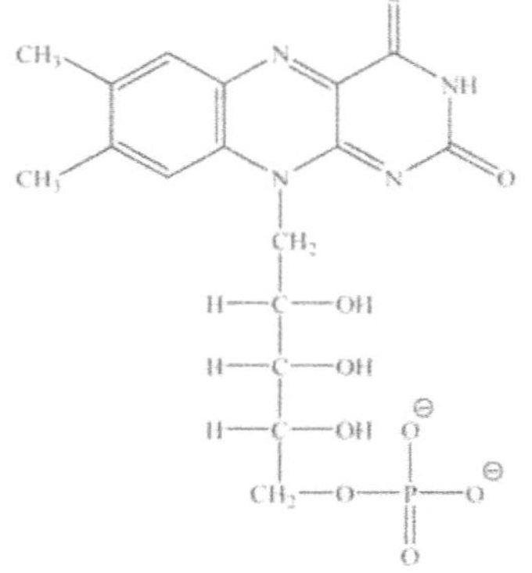	Isoalloxazine ring and ribitol	Cheilosis, glossitis and dermatitis	Hydrogen and electron	*L-Amino acid oxidase*
3		FAD (Flavin adenine dinucleotide)	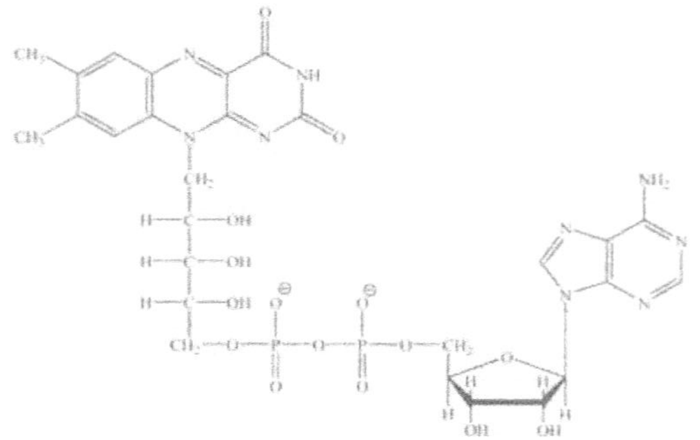	Isoalloxazine ring, ribitol, adenine and ribose	Cheilosis, glossitis and dermatitis	Hydrogen and electron	*D-Amino acid oxidase*

Table 5.8 Contd...

S. No	Vitamin name	Co-enzyme name	Chemical structure of co-enzyme	Important structural features of co-enzyme	Deficiency / Disorder	Atom or group transferred	Example of dependent enzyme
4	Vitamin-B_3 (Niacin)	NAD^+ (Nicotinamide adenine dinucleotide)	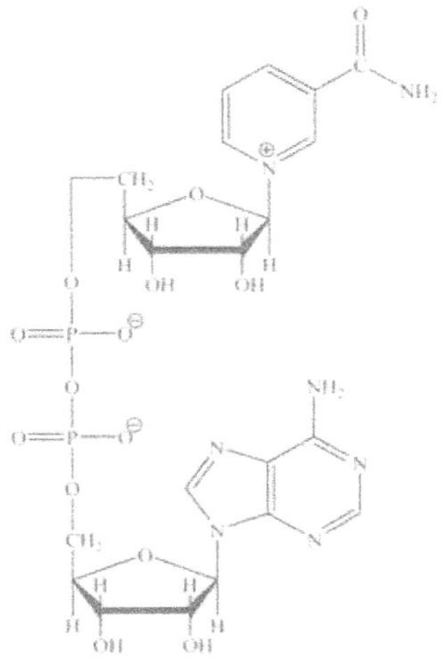	Pyridine, adenine and ribose	Pellagra (Dermatitis, diarrhea and dementia)	Hydrogen and electron	*Lactate dehydrogenase (LDH)*
5		$NADPH^+$ (Nicotinamide adenine dinucleotide phosphate)	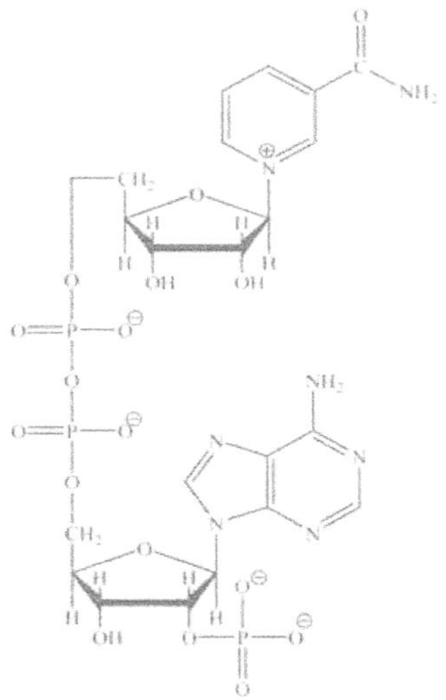	Pyridine, adenine and ribose	Pellagra (Dermatitis, diarrhea and dementia)	Hydrogen and electron	*Glucose-6-phosphate dehydrogenase (G6PD)*

Table 5.8 *Contd...*

S. No	Vitamin name	Co-enzyme name	Chemical structure of co-enzyme	Important structural features of co-enzyme	Deficiency / Disorder	Atom or group transferred	Example of dependent enzyme
6	Lipoic acid or Thioctic acid or 6,8-dithiooctanoic acid	Lipoic acid	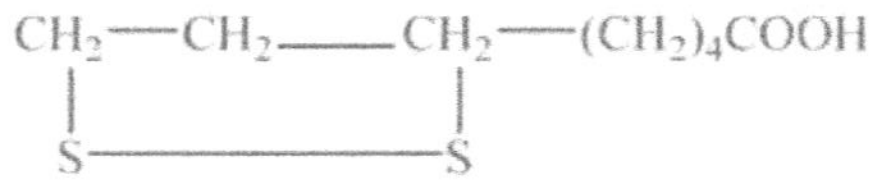 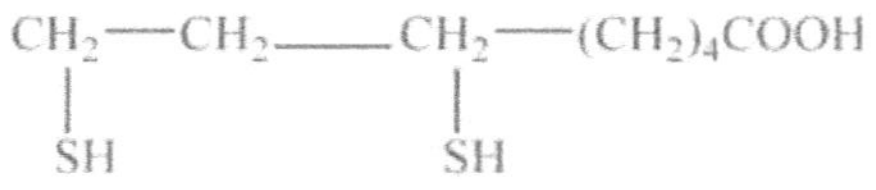 $CH_2—CH_2—CH_2—(CH_2)_4COOH$ (S—S bridge) **Oxidized form** $CH_2—CH_2—CH_2—(CH_2)_4COOH$ (SH, SH) **Reduced form**	Octanoic acid and thio group	Therapeutically used as antioxidant to prevent stroke, myocardial infarction, etc.	Hydrogen and electron	*Pyruvate dehydrogenase (PDH)*
7	Vitamin-B_5 (Pantothenic acid)	CoA (Co-enzyme-A)	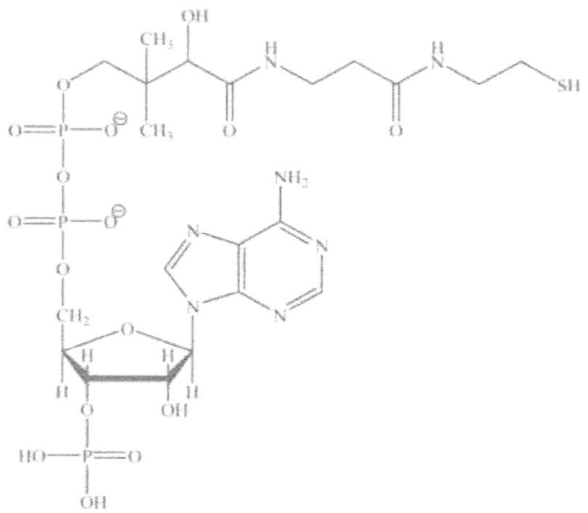	Pantoic acid, β-alanine, adenine and ribose	Burning feet syndrome (Pain and numbness in the toes, sleeplessness, fatigue, etc.). In animal (Anemia, fatty liver, decreased steroid synthesis)	Acyl group	*Thiokinase (TK)*
8	Vitamin-B_6 (Pyridoxine)	PLP (Pyridoxal phosphate)	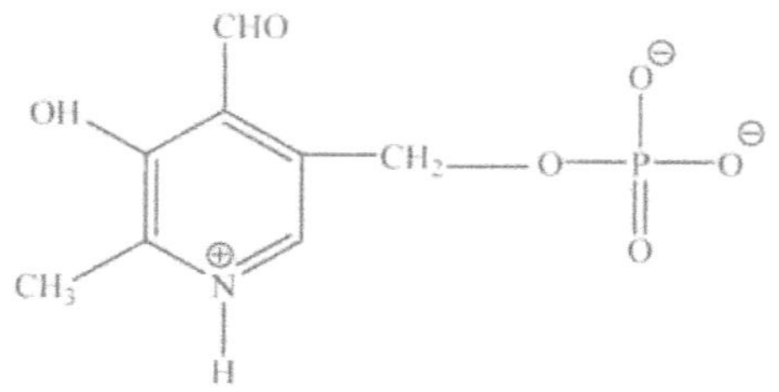	Pyridine	Neurological symptoms like depression, irritability, nervousness and mental confusion.	Amino or keto group	*Alanine transaminase (ATA)*

Table 5.8 *Contd...*

S. No	Vitamin name	Co-enzyme name	Chemical structure of co-enzyme	Important structural features of co-enzyme	Deficiency / Disorder	Atom or group transferred	Example of dependent enzyme
9	Vitamin-B_7 (Biotin)	Biocytin	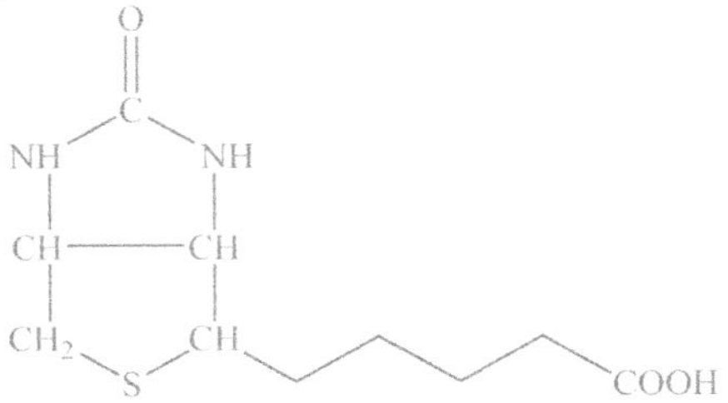 O, C, NH, NH, CH, CH, CH_2, S, CH, COOH	Imidazole and thiophene ring	Anemia, loss of appetite, nausea, dermatitis, glossitis, depression, hallucination and muscle pain.	Carbon dioxide	*Pyruvate carboxylase*
10	Vitamin-B_9 (Folic acid)	FH_4 or THF (Tetrahydro folic acid)	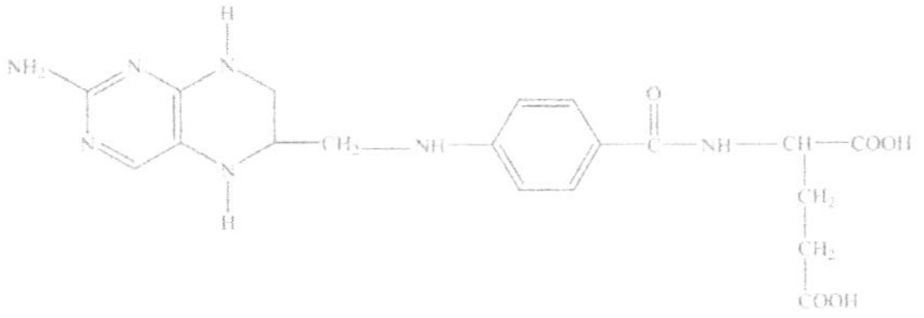 NH_2, N, H, CH_2, NH, O, C, NH, CH, COOH, CH_2, CH_2, COOH	Pteridine, PABA (*p*-amino benzoic acid) and glutamate	Macrocytic anemia and neural defects in fetus. Formiminoglutamate (FIGLU) accumulates and excretes in urine	Formyl, methyl, etc. (One carbon)	*Formyl transferase*
11	Vitamin-B_{12} (Cyanocobalamin)	Methyl cobalamin, S-Deoxy adenosyl cobalamin		Porphyrin ring, pyrrole ring, amino isopropanol, dimethyl benzimidazole and cobalt atom	Pernicious anemia, neuronal degeneration and demyelination of nervous system	Methyl or isomerization	*Methyl malonyl CoA mutase*

Table 5.9 Non-vitamin co-enzymes.

S. No.	Name	Abbreviation	Structure	Biochemical functions
1	Adenosine triphosphate	ATP	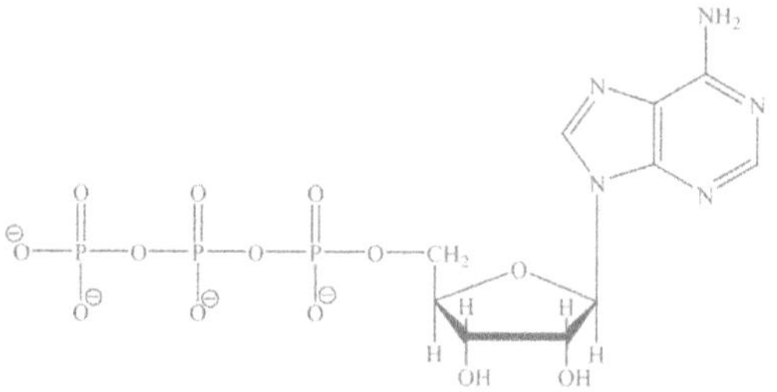	Donates phosphate, adenosine and AMP (adenosine monophosphate) moieties in biosynthetic reaction.
2	Uridine diphosphate	UDP	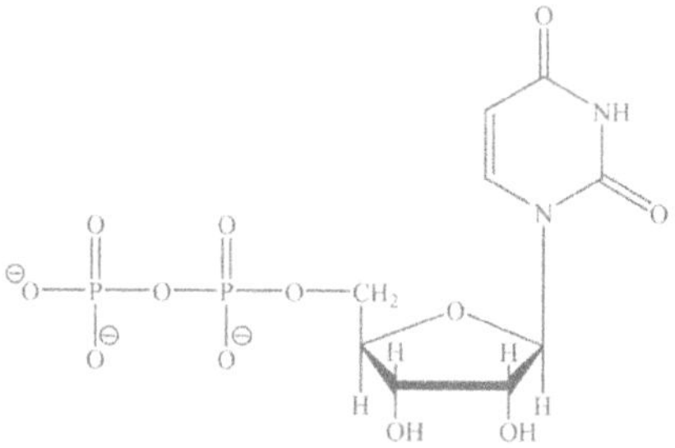	Carries molecule of mono saccharides like glucose and galactose for glycogen synthesis.
3	Cytidine diphosphate	CDP	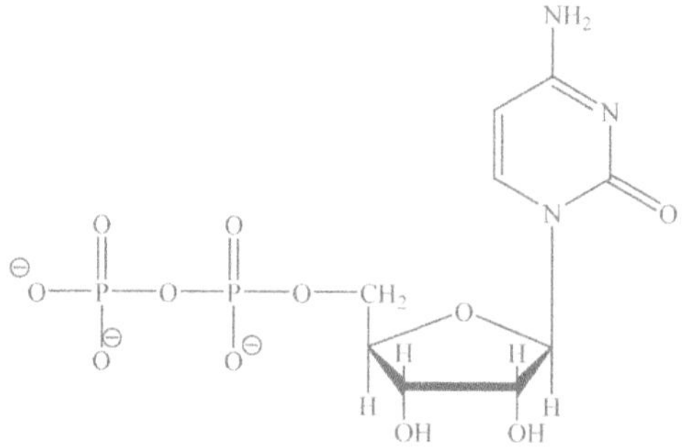	Carrier molecule of ethanolamine and choline for phospholipid synthesis.
4	S-Adenosyl methionine	SAM	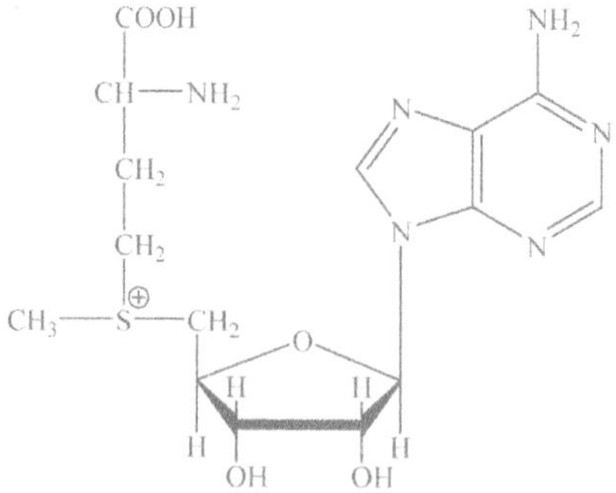	Donates methyl group in biosynthetic reaction.
5	Phosphoadenosine-phosphosulphate	PAPS	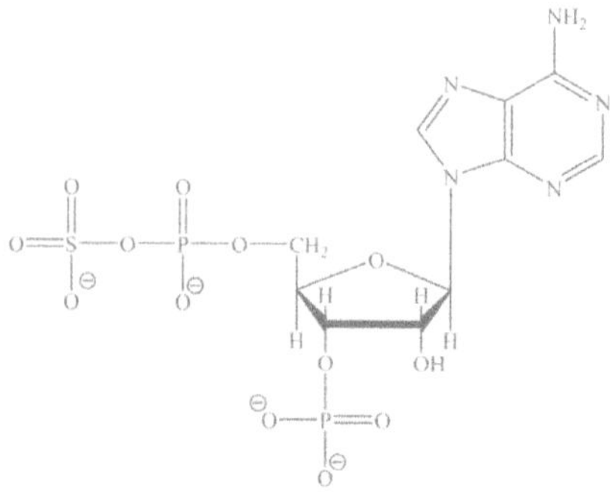	Donates sulphate groups for synthesis of muco ploy saccharides.

3. **Nucleotide co-enzymes:** The co-enzymes which are composed of nitrogen base, sugar and phosphate moieties are known as nucleotide co-enzymes. **Example:** FMN, FAD, NAD^+, $NADP^+$, Co-enzyme A, etc.
4. **Protein co-enzymes:** Some of the protein may serve as a co-enzyme for few enzymes. **Example:** Thioredoxin for *ribonucleotide reductase.*

Iso-enzymes

Iso-enzyme is defined as the multiple forms of an enzyme catalyzing the same reactions. They differ in their physical and chemical properties. The presences of iso-enzymes are confirmed from the following facts.

1. From the different genes iso-enzymes are synthesized. **Example:** *Malate dehydrogenase (MDH)* present in mitochondria is different from that found in cytosol.
2. Oligomeric enzymes are made up of more than one sub-units. **Example:** *Lactate dehydrogenase (LDH)* and *creatinine phosphokinase (CPK).*
3. As a monomer or oligomer, the enzymes may be active. **Example:** *Glutamate dehydrogenase (GDH).*
4. Difference in carbohydrate content in glycoprotein may be responsible for iso-enzymes. **Example:** *Alkaline phosphatase (AP).*

Therapeutic and Diagnostic Applications of Isoenzyme:

The following are the therapeutic and diagnostic applications of various iso-enzymes.

Example 1 (*Lactate dehydrogenase* or *LDH*):

$$CH_3-CH(OH)-COOH \xrightleftharpoons[\text{Lactate dehydrogenase (LDH)}]{\text{Oxidation};\ NAD^+ \rightarrow NADH + H^+} CH_3-C(=O)-COOH$$

Lactic acid **Pyruvic acid**

The enzyme commission number of *LDH* is 1.1.1.27. The systemic name of *LDH* is *L-lactate-NAD⁺ oxidoreductase* and it catalyzes the interconversion of lactate and pyruvate.

There are five different *LDH* iso-enzymes namely LDH_1, LDH_2, LDH_3, LDH_4 and LDH_5. It is an oligomeric (tetrameric) enzyme made up of four polypeptide sub units. Different genes produce two type of sub units namely "M" for muscle (Basic) and "H" for heart (Acidic). One or both the sub-units are present in the iso-enzymes LDH_1 to LDH_5.

Example 2 (*Creatinine phosphokinase* or *CPK*):

It is otherwise known as *creatine kinase* or *CK*. It catalyzes the interconversion of creatine phosphate or phosphocreatine into creatine.

$$\text{Creatine phosphate or Phosphocreatine} \xrightleftharpoons[\text{Creatine phosphokinase (CPK) or Creatine kinase (CK)}]{\text{Dephosphorylation};\ ADP \rightarrow ATP} \text{Creatine}$$

There are three different *CPK* iso-enzymes namely CPK_1, CPK_2 and CPK_3. It is an oligomeric (dimeric) enzyme made up of two polypeptide sub-units. Different genes produce two type of sub-units namely "M" for muscle and "B" for brain. The sub-unit of CPK_1, CPK_2 and CPK_3 are BB, MB and MM, respectively. CPK_1, CPK_2 and CPK_3 are mainly present in brain, heart and skeletal muscle, respectively. The normal serum level of CPK_{2-} is very less (less than 2 % of total *CPK*). Within first 6 to 18 hours after myocardial infarction serum level of CPK_{2-} increases to as high as 20 %. Hence, estimation of serum level of CPK_{2-} is the earliest reliable indication of myocardial infarction. In skeletal muscle disorder serum level of CPK_{2-} is not elevated.

Example 3 (*Alkaline phosphatase* or *ALP*):

It is otherwise known as *basic phosphatase*. It catalyzes the hydrolysis of phosphate monoesters at basic pH values.

There are six different *ALPs* iso-enzymes namely *α_1-ALP, α_2-heat labile ALP, α_2-heat stable ALP, pre-β-ALP, γ-ALP*, etc. It is a monomeric enzyme and the iso-enzymes are due to the difference in carbohydrate content (Sialic acid residues). Hepatitis is diagnosed by increased concentration of *α_2-heat labile ALP* and bone diseases are diagnosed from increased serum *pre-β-ALP*.

Example 4 (*Alcohol dehydrogenase* or *ADH*)

It catalyzes the interconversion of alcohol into aldehyde.

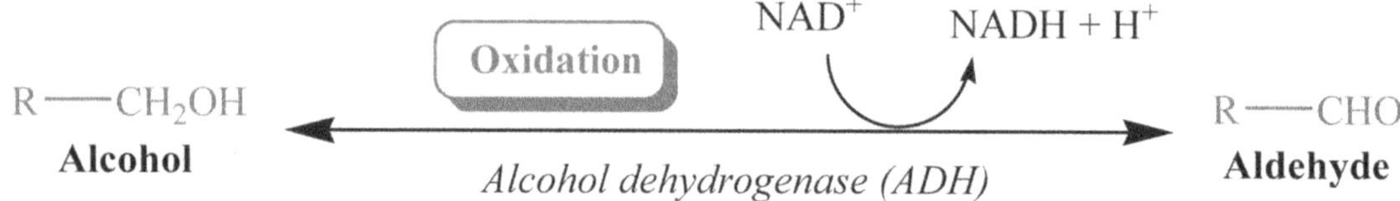

It is otherwise known as *creatine kinase* or *CK*. It catalyzes the interconversion of creatine phosphate or phosphocreatine into creatine.

There are two iso-enzymes available for *alcohol dehydrogenase*. *$\alpha\beta_1$-ADH* is present in white Americans and Europeans and *$\alpha\beta_2$-ADH* is present in Japanese and Chinese (Orientals). The *$\alpha\beta_2$-ADH* iso-enzymes more rapidly converts alcohol into aldehydes. Among oriental accumulation of acetaldehyde is associated with tachycardia and facial flushing. This is not common in whites. The increased sensitivity of Japanese and Chinese to alcohol is due to the presence of *$\alpha\beta_2$-ADH* iso-enzymes.

Applications of Enzymes

The applications of enzymes are broadly classified into five major categories 1) Therapeutic applications, 2) Analytical applications, 3) Applications in genetic manipulation, 4) Industrial applications, 5) Diagnostic applications.

1. **Therapeutic applications:**

   Various enzymes are therapeutically useful for the treatment of various diseases. They are,

   (a) From *streptococcus, streptokinase* was prepared and is used for clearing blood clots. *Streptokinase* is an enzyme which activates the conversion of plasma plasminogen into plasmin. This plasmin activates the conversion of fibrin clot into soluble products.

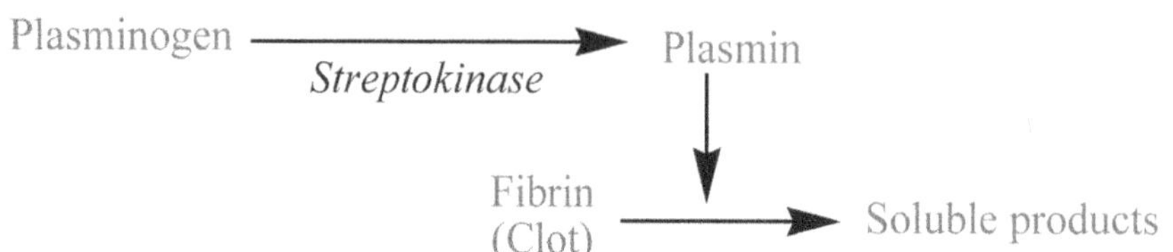

(b) Tumor cells are dependent on asparagine of the host's plasma for their multiplications. *Asparaginase* drastically decreases the host's plasma asparagine which may lead to decreased viability of the tumor cells. Hence, *asparaginase* enzyme is used in the treatment of leukemias.

(c) *Papain* is used as an anti-inflammatory agent.

(d) Enzyme α_1*-antitrypsin* is used for the treatment of emphysema.

(e) Pancreatic enzymes like *lipase* and *trypsin* are used for the digestion in pancreatic diseases.

2. **Analytical applications:**

In the clinical laboratories some of the enzymes are used for the measurements of drugs, substrates and even the activities of other enzymes also. Compared to the conventional chemical methods, enzymatic methods are more accurate and specific for the estimation of various biochemical compounds like glucose, urea, uric acid, cholesterol, etc.

(a) Plasma glucose is estimated by using *glucose oxidase* and *peroxidase* enzymes.

(b) Few of these enzymes are immobilized by binding with insoluble solid matrix. Stability and catalytic activity of enzymes are not affected by this solid matrix. The commonly used solid matrixes are beaded gels and cyanogen bromide activated sepharose. Without losing the activity the bound enzymes can be preserved for long periods. *Glucose oxidase* and *peroxidase*, immobilized and coated on a strip of paper is used clinically for the detection of glucose in urine. Based on the concentration of glucose, the intensity of blue color varies. Hence, strip method is useful for semi-quantitative estimation of glucose in urine.

$$\text{Glucose} \xrightarrow{\textit{Glucose oxidase}} \text{Glucuronic acid} + H_2O_2$$

$$\underset{\textbf{(Colorless)}}{o\text{-Toluidine} + H_2O_2} \xrightarrow{\textit{Peroxidase}} \underset{\textbf{(Blue color)}}{\text{Oxidized toluidine} + H_2O}$$

(c) *Urease* is used for the estimation of urea.

(d) Uric acid is estimated using *uricase* enzymes.

(e) *Lipase* is used for the estimation of triglycerides.

(f) Bacterial contamination of food substances is identified by *luciferase* enzymes.

(g) In the analytical technique ELISA, *horse radish peroxidase* or *alkaline phosphatase* are useful.

3. **Applications in genetic manipulation:**

Some of the enzymes also play a role in the genetic engineering.

(a) *Restriction endonucleases* are useful for gene transfer and DNA finger printing.

(b) *Taq DNA polymerase is* useful for the *polymerase* chain reactions.

4. **Industrial applications:**

In industries, enzymes can be used as catalytic agents.

(a) For preparation of cheese, enzyme *rennin* is used in industries.

(b) In food industries α*-amylase* is used.

(c) High fructose syrups are produced by using *glucose isomerase.*

(d) Washing powders are produced in industries with the help of enzyme *proteases.*

5. **Diagnostic applications:**

Clinically the enzyme activities in biological fluids are more important. There are two classes of enzymes present in the circulation. They are 1) Plasma functional or plasma specific enzymes, 2) Plasma non-functional or non-plasma specific enzymes.

Plasma functional or plasma specific enzymes: In general, the activities of these enzymes are high in plasma than in the tissues. It is mainly synthesized in liver and enters into the circulation to perform specific functions. **Example:** *Lipoprotein lipase, plasmin, thrombin, choline esterase, ceruloplasmin,* etc.

Plasma non-functional or non-plasma specific enzymes: In general concentration of these enzymes are high in tissues compared to plasma either low or absent. **Example:** Digestive enzymes like *amylase, pepsin, trypsin, lipase,* etc. and constitutive enzymes like *lactate dehydrogenase (LDH), transaminase, acid and alkaline phosphatase (ACP or ALP), creatine phosphokinase (CPK),* etc. For the diagnosis or prognosis of many diseases these plasmas non-functional or non-plasma specific enzymes are very useful. The balance between the enzyme synthesis and its release in the normal cell turnover is indicated by the normal serum level of enzymes.

Elevated serum level enzymes in diagnosis: The serum enzyme levels may increase due to cellular damage, proliferation of cells, increased synthesis of enzymes and increased rate of cell turnover. Generally, to detect the cellular damages serum enzymes are used conveniently as markers which help in the diagnosis of diseases. The followings are some important examples of elevated serum level enzymes used for the diagnosis purpose.

(a) Increased serum *amylase* is seen in acute pancreatitis, chronic pancreatitis, acute parotitis (mumps), severe diabetic ketoacidosis and obstruction of pancreatic duct.

(b) Increased serum *lipase* is seen in acute pancreatitis and moderate elevation seen in carcinoma of pancreas.

(c) In acute hepatitis of viral or toxic origin, cirrhosis of liver and jaundice serum *alanine transaminase (ALT)* or *serum glutamate pyruvate transaminase (SGPT)* is elevated. It is more specific for diagnosis of liver diseases because it is a cytosomal enzyme.

(d) Serum *aspartate transaminase (AST)* or *serum glutamate oxaloacetate transaminase (SGOT)* is elevated in liver diseases and myocardial infarction. It is more specific for diagnosis of heart diseases because it is found in both cytostome and mitochondria.

(e) In some liver and bone disease *serum alkaline phosphatase (ALP)* is elevated. Hence it is useful for the diagnosis of rickets, obstructive jaundice, carcinoma of bone and hyperparathyroidism.

(f) *Serum acid phosphatase (ACP)* is elevated in the prostate cancer. Hence, tartrate labile *ACP* is used for the prognosis and diagnosis of prostate cancer.

(g) *Creatine kinase (CK)* is elevated in myocardial infarction and hence, useful for the diagnosis of myocardial infarction.

(h) *Lactate dehydrogenase (LDH)* is useful for the diagnosis of myocardial infarction, infective hepatitis, leukemia and muscular dystrophy.

(i) Serum *aldolase* is elevated in muscular dystrophy.

(j) In hepatitis, serum *5-nucleotidase* level is elevated.

(k) Alcohol sensitively is detected by using *γ-glutamyl transpeptidase (GGT)*. It is also elevated in obstructive jaundice and infective hepatitis.

Decreased serum level enzymes in diagnosis: Sometimes due to congenital deficiency or decreased enzyme synthesis the plasma level of enzymes may decrease than normal. This is also useful for the diagnosis of certain diseases.

(a) In liver diseases *amylase* serum level is decreased.

(b) Serum *pseudocholinesterase (ChE II)* is decreased in cirrhosis of liver, liver cancer, viral hepatitis and malnutrition.

(c) Wilson disease is diagnosed from decreased serum *ceruloplasmin.*

(d) Decreased *glucose-6-phosphate dehydrogenase (G-6-PD)* in RBC is useful for the diagnosis of congenital deficiency with hemolytic anemia.

Estimation of enzymes in other body fluids and tissues: Estimation of enzymes in other body fluids and tissues other than serum or plasma is also used for diagnosis of several diseases.

(a) In acute pancreatitis urinary *amylase* is increased and in renal graft dysfunction urinary *β-N-acetylgalactosidase* is elevated. *B-Glucuronidase* is increased in the urinary bladder cancer and pancreatic cancer.

(b) Meningitis is diagnosed using *lactate dehydrogenase (LDH)* in cerebrospinal fluid (CSF).

(c) Gastric carcinoma is diagnosed from elevated *β-glucuronidase.*
(d) Cystic fibrosis is diagnosed from decreased fetal *trypsin* levels.
(e) Type - I glycogen storage disease is diagnosed from decreased *glucose-6-phosphatase* in liver.
(f) In McArdle's disease muscle *phosphorylase* activity is decreased.
(g) Thiamine deficiencies are diagnosed using decreased *transketolase* activity.
(h) For the diagnosis of in born error cultured fibroblasts and amniotic cells are frequently used. **Example:** In cultured amniotic cells deficiency of *phenylalanine hydroxylase* is observed in phenylketonuria.

Enzyme patterns in important diseases: It is better to estimate few (three or more) enzymes instead of single enzymes for the better diagnosis of a particular disease. The followings are the enzyme patterns in important diseases.

(a) Myocardial infarction is diagnosed from elevated serum levels of *creatine phosphokinase (CPK), aspartate transaminase (AST)* and *lactate dehydrogenase (LDH)*. For the early diagnosis of myocardial infarction, the protein *cardiac troponins* are highly useful. Similarly, the protein *myoglobin* is also an early marker for the diagnosis of myocardial infarction.
(b) The elevated serum level of *alanine transaminase (ALT), aspartate transaminase (AST)* and *lactate dehydrogenase (LDH)* are useful for the diagnosis of liver dysfunction due to jaundice, toxic hepatitis, cirrhosis and hepatic necrosis. Alcoholic liver diseases are diagnosed using serum *γ-glutamyl transpeptidase (GGT). Alkaline phosphatase* and *5-nucleotidase* are elevated markedly in intrahepatic and extrahepatic cholestasis.
(c) Serum levels of *creatine phosphokinase (CPK), aldolase* and *aspartate transaminase (ATA)* are elevated in muscular dystrophies.
(d) Prostate cancer is diagnosed from elevated serum *acid phosphatase (ACP)*. For lung cancer, neuroblastoma, pheochromocytoma, etc. neuron specific *enolase* is serving as a marker.

PROBABLE QUESTIONS

PART – A: Multiple Choice Questions

1. Which one is the functional unit of the enzyme?
   (a) Apo-enzyme (b) Holo-enzyme
   (c) Co-enzyme (d) Iso-enzyme
2. Which of the following is non-protein part of the enzyme?
   (a) Apo-enzyme (b) Co-enzyme
   (c) Holo-enzyme (d) Iso-zyme
3. Which part of enzyme is responsible for specificity of enzyme?
   (a) Co-enzyme (b) Holo-enzyme
   (c) Apo-enzyme (d) Iso-enzyme
4. Which of the following co-enzyme is not involved in hydrogen transfer?
   (a) FMN (b) FAD
   (c) NAD^+ (d) FH_4
5. Which word may be memorized to remember the six classes of enzymes in correct order.
   (a) OLLITH (b) OHLITL
   (c) OLTHIL (d) OTHLIL

6. Which of the following statement is incorrect?
   (a) Enzymes increases the activation energy
   (b) Enzymes decreases the activation energy
   (c) Enzymes are colloidal in nature
   (d) Enzymes are thermo liable in nature
7. What indicates low Km value?
   (a) Strong affinity between enzyme & co-enzyme
   (b) Weak affinity between enzyme & co-enzyme
   (c) Strong affinity between enzyme & substrate
   (d) Weak affinity between enzyme & substrate
8. Disulfiram is a very good example for which type of enzyme inhibition?
   (a) Irreversible
   (b) Reversible
   (c) Competitive
   (d) Non-competitive
9. Which enzyme is useful for the diagnosis of obstructive jaundice?
   (a) *Acid phosphatase*
   (b) *Alkaline phosphatase*
   (c) *SGOT*
   (d) *SGPT*
10. Which of the following is true about Michaelis-Menten kinetics?
    (a) K_m, the Michaelis constant, is defined as that concentration of substrate at which enzyme is working at maximum velocity
    (b) It describes single substrate enzymes
    (c) K_m, the Michaelis constant is defined as the dissociation constant of the enzyme-substrate complex
    (d) It assumes covalent binding occurs between enzyme and substrate
11. When the velocity of enzyme activity is plotted against substrate concentration, which of the following is obtained?
    (a) Hyperbolic curve
    (b) Parabola
    (c) Straight line with positive slope
    (d) Straight line with negative slope
12. The rate determining step of Michaelis-Menten kinetics is __________
    (a) The complex dissociation step to produce products
    (b) The complex formation step
    (c) The product formation step
    (d) None of the mentioned
13. The molecule which acts directly on an enzyme to lower its catalytic rate is __________
    (a) Repressor
    (b) Inhibitor
    (c) Modulator
    (d) Regulator
14. Which of the following is an example for irreversible inhibitor?
    (a) Disulfiram
    (b) Oseltamivir
    (c) Protease inhibitors
    (d) DIPF
15. Which of the following is an example of reversible inhibitor?
    (a) DIPF
    (b) Penicillin
    (c) Iodoacetamide
    (d) Protease inhibitors
16. Where does inhibitor binds on enzyme in mixed inhibition?
    (a) At active site
    (b) Allosteric site
    (c) Does not bind on enzyme
    (d) Binds on substrate

17. The catalytic efficiency of two distinct enzymes can be compared based on which of the following factor?
    (a) K_m
    (b) Product formation
    (c) Size of the enzymes
    (d) pH of optimum value
18. What is the general mechanism of an enzyme?
    (a) It acts by reducing the activation energy
    (b) It acts by increasing the activation energy
    (c) It acts by decreasing the pH
    (d) It acts by increasing the pH
19. The allosteric inhibitor of an enzyme ___________
    (a) Causes the enzyme to work faster
    (b) Binds to the active site
    (c) Participates in feedback regulation
    (d) Denatures the enzyme
20. Which of the following is false about allosteric feedback inhibition?
    (a) Bacterial enzyme system is the first known example
    (b) Conversion of L-leucine to L-isoleucine
    (c) *Threonine dehydratase* is inhibited by isoleucine
    (d) If the isoleucine concentration decreases, the rate of threonine dehydration increases
21. Fischer's "lock and key" model of the enzyme action implies that
    (a) The active site is complementary in shape to that of substance only after interaction
    (b) The active site is complementary in shape to that of substance
    (c) Substrates change conformation prior to active site interaction
    (d) The active site is flexible and adjusts to substrate
22. A sigmoidal plot of substrate concentration ([S]) verses reaction velocity (V) may indicate
    (a) Michaelis-Menten kinetics
    (b) Co-operative binding
    (c) Competitive inhibition
    (d) Non-competitive inhibition
23. An inducer is absent in the type of enzyme
    (a) Allosteric enzyme
    (b) Constitutive enzyme
    (c) Co-operative enzyme
    (d) Isoenzymic enzyme
24. In reversible non-competitive enzyme activity inhibition
    (a) V_{max} is increased
    (b) K_m is increased
    (c) K_m is decreased
    (d) Concentration of active enzyme is reduced
25. Co-enzymes are
    (a) Heat stable, dialyzable, non-protein organic molecules
    (b) Soluble, colloidal, protein molecules
    (c) Structural analogue of enzymes
    (d) Different forms of enzymes
26. An example of hydrogen transferring co-enzyme is
    (a) CoA
    (b) NAD^+
    (c) Biotin
    (d) TPP
27. An example of group transferring co-enzyme is
    (a) NAD^+
    (b) $NADP^+$
    (c) FAD
    (d) CoA
28. *Co-carboxylase* is
    (a) Thiamine pyrophosphate
    (b) Pyridoxal phosphate
    (c) Biotin
    (d) CoA

29. A co-enzyme containing non aromatic hetero ring is
   (a) ATP (b) NAD
   (c) FMN (d) Biotin
30. A co-enzyme containing aromatic hetero ring is
   (a) TPP (b) Lipoic acid
   (c) Co-enzyme Q (d) Biotin
31. Iso-enzymes are
   (a) Chemically, immunologically and electrophoretically different forms of an enzyme
   (b) Different forms of an enzyme similar in all properties
   (c) Catalyzing different reactions
   (d) Having the same quaternary structures like the enzymes
32. Iso-enzymes can be characterized by
   (a) Proteins lacking enzymatic activity that are necessary for the activation of enzymes
   (b) Proteolytic enzymes activated by hydrolysis
   (c) Enzymes with identical primary structure
   (d) Similar enzymes that catalyze different reaction
33. The iso-enzymes LDH_5 is elevated in
   (a) Myocardial infarction (b) Peptic ulcer
   (c) Liver disease (d) Infectious disease
34. Lineweaver - Burk double reciprocal plot is related to
   (a) Substrate concentration (b) Enzyme activity
   (c) Temperature (d) Both (a) and (b)
35. The co-enzyme not involved in the formation of acetyl-CoA from pyruvate is
   (a) TPP (b) Biotin
   (c) NAD^+ (d) FAD
36. Characteristic features of active site are
   (a) Flexible in nature (b) Site of binding
   (c) Acidic (d) Both (a) and (b)
37. Which of the following is an example of enzyme inhibition?
   (a) Reversible inhibition (b) Irreversible inhibition
   (c) Allosteric inhibition (d) All of these
38. Which of the following co-enzyme takes part in hydrogen transfer reactions?
   (a) Tetrahydrofolate (b) Co-enzyme A
   (c) Co-enzyme Q (d) Biotin
39. Which of the following co-enzyme takes part in oxidation-reduction reactions?
   (a) Pyridoxal phosphate (b) Lipoic acid
   (c) Thiamin diphosphate (d) None of these
40. A co-enzyme required in transamination reactions is
   (a) Co-enzyme A (b) Co-enzyme Q
   (c) Biotin (d) Pyridoxal phosphate

41. Co-enzyme A contains a vitamin which is
    (a) Thiamin (b) Ascorbic acid
    (c) Pantothenic acid (d) Niacinamide

Key for Multiple Choice Questions

1. (b)	2. (b)	3. (c)	4. (d)	5. (d)
6. (b)	7. (c)	8. (a)	9. (b)	10. (b)
11. (a)	12. (a)	13. (b)	14. (d)	15. (d)
16. (b)	17. (a)	18. (a)	19. (c)	20. (b)
21. (b)	22. (b)	23. (b)	24. (d)	25. (a)
26. (b)	27. (d)	28. (c)	29. (d)	30. (a)
31. (a)	32. (b)	33. (c)	34. (d)	35. (b)
36. (d)	37. (d)	38. (c)	39. (b)	40. (d)
41. (c)				

PART – B: Short Answers

1. What is intra-cellular enzyme & extra-cellular enzyme?
2. What is monomeric & oligomeric enzyme?
3. Explain multi enzyme complex with suitable examples.
4. Explain the term "enzyme kinetics".
5. What are co-enzymes? Write the biochemical role of nicotinamide co-enzymes.
6. Define Michaelis-Menten constant and write its significance.
7. Note on Lineweaver–Burk double reciprocal plot.
8. What is competitive enzyme inhibition?
9. Write a note on suicide inhibition.
10. Explain allosteric enzyme inhibition.
11. Define constitutive enzyme and adaptive enzyme.
12. Define enzyme induction and repression.
13. What is iso-enzyme? Write clinical applications of iso-enzymes.
14. Write a short note on non-vitamin co-enzyme.
15. With suitable example explain about co-enzymes and co-factors.
16. How many classes of enzymes are there according to the IUB?
17. Give a brief account of co-enzymes and iso-enzymes.
18. Explain enzyme inhibition.
19. List out various therapeutic applications of enzymes.

PART – C: Long Answers

1. Explain the characteristics of reversible enzyme inhibition with their kinetics.
2. Explain the nomenclature and classification of enzymes.
3. Describe different types of enzyme inhibitors. How do you distinguish a competitive inhibitor from non-competitive inhibitor?
4. Explain about diagnostic & therapeutic applications of enzymes & iso-enzymes.

5. Define & classify enzymes.
6. Write the clinical applications of enzymes.
7. Define & explain the following: a) Enzymes, b) Iso-enzymes, c) Co-enzymes.
8. Explain kinetics, mechanism of action & inhibition of enzymes.
9. What are enzymes? Classify enzymes with examples. Explain the mechanism of enzyme action.
10. Write briefly on activators & deactivators of enzymes.
11. Explain the clinical significance of enzymes, iso-enzymes & co-enzymes.
12. What are co-enzymes? Give the example & explain their significance.
13. What is regression, induction & control of enzyme synthesis.
14. Sketch the clinical applications of enzymes & iso-enzymes.
15. Discuss briefly on the mechanism of enzyme repression & induction.
16. Explain the various properties of enzymes.
17. Write a detailed note on nomenclature of enzymes.
18. How are enzymes regulated in biological systems?

www.ingramcontent.com/pod-product-compliance
Lightning Source LLC
LaVergne TN
LVHW080851240726
843527LV00052B/302

* 9 7 8 9 3 9 5 0 3 9 3 6 9 *